D1541631

HEALTH CARE ETHICS

A Guide for Decision Makers

Contributors

Fredrick R. Abrams

Terrence F. Ackerman

Gary R. Anderson

Michael D. Bromberg

E. Richard Brown

Michael R. Callahan

Susan N. Chernoff

Leah L. Curtin

Carol Estwing Ferrans

Ruth L. Garvey

Valerie A. Glesnes-Anderson

Thomas G. Goodwin

Luke Gregory

Marc D. Hiller

George A. Kanoti

Andrew Moss Kaunitz

Karen Rose Koppel Kaunitz

Barbara Sue Koppel

Joseph W. Kukura

Walter J. McNerney

Mark D. Nelson

J. Phillip O'Brien

Kevin D. O'Rourke

David A. Ogden

Susan R. Peterson

William H. Roach, Jr.

Jamie A. Savaiano

Robert L. Schwartz

K. Bruce Stickler

Jennifer A. Stiller

Janicemarie K. Vinicky

Sylvia Ridlen Wenston

HEALTH CARE ETHICS

A Guide for Decision Makers

Edited by

Gary R. Anderson, PhD
Hunter College
School of Social Work
City University of New York

Valerie A. Glesnes-Anderson, MHSA
West Essex General Hospital
Livingston, New Jersey

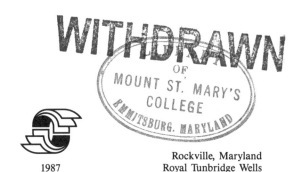

AN ASPEN PUBLICATION®
Aspen Publishers, Inc.

1987

Rockville, Maryland
Royal Tunbridge Wells

Library of Congress Cataloging-in-Publication Data

Health care ethics.

"An Aspen publication."
Includes bibliographies and index.
1. Medical ethics. 2. Medicine—Decision making.
I. Anderson, Gary R., 1952-   . II. Glesnes-Anderson,
Valerie A. [DNLM: 1. Decision Making, Organizational.
2. Delivery of Health Care. 3. Ethics, Medical.
W 84.1 H4355]
R724.H336   1987   174'2   87-1011
ISBN: 0-87189-630-3

Editorial Services: Marsha Davies

Library of Congress Catalog Card Number: 87-1011
ISBN: 0-87189-630-3

Printed in the United States of America

1   2   3   4   5

Table of Contents

Preface

Today's headlines are filled with significant medical advancements and consequent ethical concerns. Health care issues are as diverse and critical as deciding to terminate treatment for the very old, choosing not to treat developmentally disabled newborns, refusing medical treatment, and adopting health care delivery policies that may constrict patient options. These decisions, involving medicine, health care institutions, and morality, invoke intense emotions affecting thousands of patients and their families. Consequently, life-and-death decisions confront health care providers in an often disturbing manner. Hospital administrators, managers, physicians, nurses, and the full complement of allied professionals who serve patients need to understand the complex issues and choices that are increasingly part of the American health care experience.

Today's health care professional cannot afford to be ignorant of complex ethical dilemmas. Current concern has resulted in an emphasis on ethics committees. While extremely positive, the establishment of committees does not necessarily result in an understanding of issues or provide a context for thinking for noncommittee members. Consequently, in addition to clear information that leads to a better understanding of issues, there is a need for practical guidance concerning not only difficult decisions but also the process of making those decisions. The discussion of ethics at a purely theoretical or philosophical level might not provide the understandable guidance needed by professionals who must make decisions despite dilemmas.

The purpose of this book is to assist health care professionals in understanding some of the complex contemporary issues that they confront and to provide guidance in making decisions. These issues are described and analyzed in the context of philosophical principles and methods in language that is understandable to the professional who is unfamiliar with the study of philosophy and ethics.

The first chapters provide a framework for thinking—discussing issues and principles that cut across a number of contemporary ethical dilemmas. The context for later issue analysis is set by addressing the emerging place of ethics in health care. Key principles from the law and from philosophy offer guidelines for administrative decision making and introduce recurrent themes in the book. Administrators' values and the role of values in decision making are also highlighted.

The next chapters discuss and illustrate the contemporary and controversial issue of access to health care. Fueled by changes in reimbursement and political priorities, these issues shape the environment in which health care is delivered and, consequently, need to be understood. These issues of access are outside the typical discussion of biomedical ethics but are increasingly central to ethical issues in American health care. Of crucial importance to administrators, policy makers, and planners, decisions about access made at management and legislative levels will have a significant impact on the work and choices of health care clinicians. The access section of this book begins with a detailed overview of issues, including the role of prevention services and the physician's role as patient advocate. The section also considers the issue of reimbursement, analyzing the impact of prospective payment on health care and considering the evolving issue of rationing.

Access issues are illustrated further by the treatment of dialysis patients. The implications of funding for patient access to medical services is presented with a consideration of "quality of life" as a criterion in making decisions and allocating scarce resources. A related presentation places contemporary headlines about organ procurement and transplantation in historical perspective to inform readers about the current transplantation controversies.

Few issues evoke such discomfort and strong reactions by the public and by health care professionals as those addressing life and death. The third section of this book explores (1) a patient's refusal of treatment and how administrators can respond; (2) withholding or withdrawing treatment from incompetent patients; and (3) various definitions of death. It also reviews the controversies and the difficulties in decision making, suggests guidelines, and provides information such as a survey of state laws on definitions of death.

Chapters on informed consent and confidentiality address other patient care issues. These issues and others can fit under the broad umbrella of paternalism, which raises questions of patient autonomy and competency in decision making. A specific chapter on paternalism lays out some philosophical issues leading to the next chapters that specify the interplay between law and policy to minimize paternalism in health care settings.

A section on professional management issues covers a range of concerns. Two chapters devoted to opposing views present the key controversies in the development of profit motives and for-profit ownership in health care.

Other chapters address issues more specific to hospital functioning: conflict of interest; discharge planning, concerns about harm to patients, and appropriate considerations for such planning; and whistle-blowing, a controversial subject rarely discussed in the literature. Like access issues, these topics raise areas of ethical inquiry for health care managers beyond the often presented areas of biomedical ethics. This broader approach acknowledges the importance of ethical concerns for health care professionals and underscores our contention that while the physician/patient aspect of ethical issues is important, health care professionals cannot abdicate their ethical responsibilities to physicians.

This guidebook's concluding section is designed to go beyond detailing controversies to suggesting possible courses of action. Each chapter provides guidance and specific plans. These action plans include (1) practical guidance on institutional ethics committees; (2) the issues to consider with regard to hiring or retaining a professionally trained ethicist; (3) the role of codes of ethics in guiding professional behavior; and (4) models for decision making by administrators, building on the foundation principles in the first chapters. These chapters, combined with earlier guidelines and suggestions, avoid simplistic solutions—such as relegating ethical concerns to ethics committees—while presenting viewpoints with merit and practicality.

Any book of this nature will necessarily limit the length of what could be exhaustive discussions. The goal of this book is to provide information on important contemporary ethical concerns in health care, offer an understanding of key principles for resolving dilemmas, and give guidance for responding to some of the troubling situations increasingly confronting health care professionals.

The book is not intended to replace consultation with appropriate advisors when facing specific dilemmas, and guidelines for seeking consultation are addressed in a number of chapters. We intend to provide a direct, informative guide that will assist health care executives and challenge professionals to increase their knowledge for informed decision making and action in response to ethical issues in health care delivery.

Acknowledgments

Editing a book requires the cooperation of many talented and busy professionals. We thank the contributors for their enthusiastic response to their topics and their patience with demands made upon them. A special note of thanks is due to Walter McNerney, who served as critic, mentor, and friend through the conceptualization of this volume.

We would like to thank the staff at West Essex General Hospital for their valuable assistance, Dr. Charles Steiner for his stimulatingly clear thinking, and Doree Kline for consistent and timely support. The early stages of creating this book were facilitated by the gracious assistance of Shirley Hicks, Maria Valdes, and Laura Ferreira at St. James Hospital. Research, guidance, and literature monitoring throughout the construction of this volume were simplified by the depth, knowledge, and insight of a talented librarian, Betty Garrison.

A special note of appreciation is due to: Dean Harold Lewis of the Hunter College School of Social Work, New York City, whose leadership and support were instrumental in addressing ethical thinking and dilemmas; the leadership of the Health Corporation of the Archdiocese of Newark; the administrative staff at Catholic Guardian Society (Brooklyn/Queens), specifically Dr. Catherine White, William Guarinello, Phillip Georgini, and Ellen Murphy-Hackett; our parents; Marilyn Hines and Lauren Marie Anderson.

Part I
Framework for Thinking

Chapter 1

Ethics in Health Care

Walter J. McNerney, MHA

Ethical issues often involve conflicting right and wrong imperatives that cannot be resolved simultaneously. The ethical issues that arise in the health field are especially complex. It is not easy to distinguish the relative rights of the patient, family, institution, and community, nor to establish at what level public or private decisions should be made.

This chapter focuses on two major propositions regarding ethical issues in the context of health administration:

1. Health care administrators are obligated, professionally and by institutional imperative, to become involved in and provide leadership in ethical issues. Currently, too few administrators involve themselves or lead sufficiently.
2. Long-standing concerns with the rights of patients and physicians have overshadowed the critical importance of the institutional management process in dealing with ethical issues. A balance is necessary to ensure sound management while protecting the rights of those who depend on the hospital.

Health administrators and allied professionals face a difficult dilemma in deciding what constitutes ethical issues.[1] Attempting to resolve questions of ethics when they are too broadly construed can turn an institution upside down. Yet an institution that limits its self-scrutiny can lose its social perspective, and a responsible, enabling middle ground is hard to achieve.

However ethical issues are defined, we must bear in mind that over time the public will hold institutions—including health care institutions—accountable for just conduct. Even in today's climate of cost containment, the public will ultimately castigate those that fail to be responsive even more aggressively than if their costs were out of line.

ETHICAL CHOICES IN PERSPECTIVE

Ethical questions have been discussed in the medical and lay literature for centuries. One of the constant ideals held forth to physicians since classical times

3

is "to help, or at least do no harm." A fifteenth century moral theologian, Saint Antoninus of Florence, advises that "succor must be given, following the rules of charity, to those who are in danger, however stubborn they may be."[2]

A more generic principle, central to the mission of health care, has been fairness. This principle supports equity in and access to health care. Fairness guides physicians' commitment to being available to patients and to providing quality care to the best of their ability.

These principles have been on the health care agenda from the beginning. They have afforded rational guideposts for action over time, although conflicts among them may generate thorny ethical issues. While most such dilemmas have rested largely with physicians and other clinical providers, changes in the environment—including societal values, advances in medical technology, and increasing economic and financial pressures—have contributed to requiring administrative decision making for their resolution.[3]

The degree to which certain practices are considered right or wrong has changed over time. Today all-out efforts are often made to prolong the lives of infants, no matter how frail they are, and often despite the fact that the family may fear severe handicap more than death itself. But infanticide was practiced widely until the Middle Ages and selectively until the mid-1800s in England, reflecting "society's continued ambivalence toward the inherent sanctity of life and realistic judgement on the quality of life."[4] In more recent years, many decisions involving the life or death of the young and old, decisions now highly visible and contentious, were made quietly by families and physicians in a less litigious environment.

Until the 1980s, health care ethics generally centered on the physician, the patient, and on a few communitywide considerations such as health as a right. Only in the last few years has the span of ethical issues grown to embrace questions of institutional ethics, and only recently have administrators been substantively involved. These changes in how ethics is viewed reflect several influences:

1. Burgeoning technology has made it possible to extend life beyond old limits and has, in the process, increased the range and complexity of options for prolonging life.
2. A more competitive health field places greater emphasis on price and priorities. Competition is being driven at an increasing pace by scarce resources such as federal government and state government deficits and by employer concerns over escalating fringe benefit costs. Providers are forced to make choices.
3. More sophisticated buyers, both public and private, are more demanding, better informed, and less in awe of doctors and hospitals. They are making assertive choices among the options produced by competition, and they are more aware of the limitations of medicine.

4. A greater supply of than demand for physicians and hospital beds makes providers more interested in, and less resistant to, innovative schemes.

5. Public policy in the United States favors competition and thus heightens interest in considerations of cost versus benefit.

Growing concern with ethical issues reflects a growing anxiety and uncertainty among health institutions and physicians in general, fostered by rapid change. As the power base shifts from practitioner to institution, it is not always clear who is responsible for what.

Further, a better educated public is less willing to allow professionals complete freedom in deciding key issues. Concern over consumer rights and individual rights is widespread. There is growing tension among income, age, sex, and ethnic groups. Specific issues have gained high visibility, such as the right to guns versus the right to know who has them, and the right to know versus the right to privacy. We are coming to realize that there are severe limits to self-aggrandizement and that the institutions that endure are those that come to grips with existential questions of obligation and justice.

Most fields of endeavor entail ethical concerns comparable with those found in the health field. A growing number of businesses seek out the regular counsel of ministers, philosophers, and other "right thinkers." Increasingly, corporations reverberate with serious talk about the integrity of the corporate culture. This trend started with revelations of such inappropriate political behavior as the Watergate scandal, combined with a mounting number of environmental problems. Chief executive officers discovered that an image of integrity no longer sufficed. Companies had to be honest in their dealings or face stiff public reprisals. Codes or good intentions were insufficient; the whole staff had to be imbued with a sense of propriety and honor.

Business, law, and engineering schools, as well as medical schools, discuss ethics. In some major universities, undergraduates are required to take courses that address "the overwhelming questions." Recently, the National Council on the Humanities convened philosophers to discuss ethical issues. At least one major executive of American enterprise, James Burke, chairman and chief executive officer of Johnson and Johnson, believes that a corporate credo "geared to service to society"—a credo in which people can believe—not only minimizes alien objectives but leads to a better service or product; that is, it is better business. Johnson and Johnson's credo spells out responsibilities to customers, employees, communities, and stockholders, in that order. Polaroid holds regular conferences to address moral questions raised by new technology.

Such issues as the following become part of the practice of management: Is the individual dehumanized by the corporation, as the corporation tries to meet its purposes? What is the proper balance of the needs of individuals and the requirements of the organization? How does one minimize paternalism and accord dignity to the individual? What processes promote fairness?[5] In essence, a company acting in good conscience stands a better chance of succeeding if it has a long history of community concern.

ETHICAL ISSUES OF CONCERN TO HEALTH PROVIDERS

The list of ethical issues confronting health care professionals in recent years is extensive. With considerable overlap, the issues tend to fall under three headings: individual, institutional, and community. A few examples under each heading should suffice to show the dimensions and textures involved.

Questions of ethics focusing on the individual address such issues as: What are the limits of the patient's right to privacy? Under what circumstances can a patient refuse treatment? Who is competent to refuse treatment on a patient's behalf? Should life be extended by artificial means when that life holds little or no promise of normal function or the treatment causes acute suffering? What is the proper balance between survival and the quality of life?

Institutional issues include: Given limited resources, who should be admitted? Who should not? Is ability to pay the critical factor? How does the administrator deal with inappropriate use of scarce goods and services when, in effect, use for one purpose makes it impossible to serve another? As a hospital administrator, how does one cope with the proper balance between health promotion and cure when one gets paid for one and not the other? How does one balance provider versus patient rights in deciding whether to provide home care services to residents of dangerous neighborhoods? Under what circumstances does the administrator "blow the whistle" when physicians charge excessive fees? What about excessive hospital fees? In advertising, to what degree is the truth rationalized? In investor-owned institutions, what are the relative rights of the patient and the stockholder? Does the physician as well as the chief executive officer and board member have a conflict of interest? What does the administrator do when medical staff needs are inconsistent with community needs?

Ethical issues under the "community" heading include: How do communities deal with matters of distributive justice? If all persons seeking all the health services they want outstrip community resources to provide these services, do one and all get smaller-but-equal shares, or is a minimum standard of service offered, with variation above it based on ability to pay? How does the community balance demand and need? How does one balance provider rights versus patient rights, in the community interest, when both are legitimate? What is the community's obligation under areawide planning: Simply to promulgate the plan? To screen applications for buildings and services? Or, further, to accept responsibility when there are gaps, such as in nursing home services or home care services that are not being filled, or when the underprivileged lack access to care because of institutional flight to the suburbs? Who are the community's agents; is the administrator of a nonprofit hospital a community agent? When organs or given procedures are in short supply, who gets the implant or service?

These represent only a fraction of the ethical issues providers face. Some questions are narrowly focused. Others lead to the larger questions that plague all countries, such as how to balance social justice and efficiency. All raise the difficult question of the level at which decisions should be made.

LEVELS FOR DECISION MAKING

Ideally, the level at which decisions should be made will vary with the issues involved. Some decisions should more clearly involve the courts than others. Some are more clearly in the domain of the individual and family. Many, however, fall in gray zones, and the process of sorting them out is difficult.

In these gray zones, we must decide to what degree we can entrust issues to national, state, and local governments through use of minimum standards, regulations, laws, and the courts; to nonprofit governing boards, professional societies, and associations, or other voluntary initiatives, such as the Oregon statewide network of concerned persons associated with health planning that addresses ethical issues; to local, less formal processes, involving doctor, nurse, and patient; or to the market, reflecting consumer demand and stockholder rights.

We have a way to go. For example, as George Annas reports, "intermediate appeals courts in California and New Jersey have reached dramatically conflicting conclusions on the legality of withdrawing nutrition from incompetent patients."[6] On their own, hospitals and physicians pursue different paths when facing the same issue, particularly where the issue is complex, as when the patient's capacity to make critical judgments is in question.

While most judges are dedicated to detached and rigorous investigation in sorting out responsibilities, they differ in the degree to which they will entrust this process to others, including hospitals or physicians. Some feel strongly that, in the last analysis, the courts must represent the "morality and conscience of our society."[7]

On the other hand, the recent President's Commission for the Study of Ethical Problems in Medicine and Biomedical and Behavioral Research[8] recommended that there be limits to legal action in general in ensuring that seriously ill infants receive correct care. For example, "although criminal penalties should be available to punish serious errors, the ability of the criminal law to ensure good decision making in individual cases is limited."[9] Also,

> governmental agencies that reimburse for health care may insist that institutions have policies and procedures regarding decision making, but using financial sanctions against institutions to punish an "incorrect" decision in a particular case is likely to be ineffective and to lead to excessively detailed regulations that would involve government reimbursement officials in bedside decision making. Furthermore, such

sanctions could actually penalize other patients and providers in an unjust way.[10]

Thus, the trustee and health care administrator get only relative guidance from the government per se and must confront a host of institutional and community issues that to date have not been subjected to "detached and rigorous investigation."

The lack of guidance gives the health institution flexibility in dealing with ethical issues, but it also provides a license to steal and engage in questionable practices. For those without moral commitment, it represents an opportunity to do little or nothing.

IMPLICATIONS FOR HEALTH ADMINISTRATORS

Health administrators react to ethical issues in a variety of ways. Some meet issues head-on, others turn a deaf ear to them. Health administrators should be obligated to assume leadership in the increasingly important area of ethical issues. Leadership includes:

- knowing what is going on
- identifying ethical issues and groups of issues and helping to put them in perspective
- establishing procedures and processes to deal with the issues, including determining who should make decisions in particular situations
- demonstrating how to deal with conflicts (persistent investigation and negotiation versus order and command) and how to prevent specialized interests from getting in the way
- educating participants and giving them support
- monitoring progress on a continuing basis
- including ethical issues on the board and medical staff agendas

Furthermore, because each ethical instance differs from all others, the administrator should work toward relatively specific guidelines. For example, it is not enough to say that there should be an ethics committee in the hospital. Guidelines are needed in regard to its authority, organization, staffing, and methods of operation and documentation. If a committee is not appropriate in particular circumstances, who should make decisions, using what procedures, needs to be made explicitly clear.

Such administrative initiatives require the administrator to have a great deal of sensitivity. Some families feel differently about death than others. Persons dying alone usually receive less treatment.[11] Alternate physicians and consultants are more likely to order active treatment than those who have had continuing contact with the patient.[12] Boards of trustees and individual board members differ in their perceptions of ethical issues, reflecting various backgrounds; the administrator must take the differences into account in educating them. To some physicians, negotiation of complex issues is an unfamiliar process; to some, it is a sign of weakness.

The necessity for a strong administrative role in matters of ethics arises from at least two "givens" of institutional operation. First, if the ethical structure and climate of the health institution are not sound, ethical issues will get out of hand and absorb excessive time, a situation inimical to the mission of the institution and ultimately detrimental to the community. Second, not only do misdirected, low-morale institutions fail to recognize or deal adequately with ethical problems, they create them. Just as ethical problems tend to occur when physician/patient relations are poor, so it is when institutional initiatives and tone are inadequate.

Thus, coping with ethical issues requires far more than an ethics committee, confined largely to matters of patient care. It requires:

- well-informed governance with understood roles
- strong management involving, for example, strategic planning, a strong human resource program, and a strong data base
- a strong sense of mutual destiny between the institution and the medical staff
- a health administrator evaluation process conducted by the board or owner that holds the administrator explicitly accountable for ethical issues
- a reasonably democratic process throughout the institution that respects the maturity of the individual employee and medical staff as well as the patient, minimizes the stultifying effect of bureaucracy, and fosters an ability to listen and empathize as well as counsel
- a pervasive attitude of open and respectful communication—essential to resolution of tough issues

The health administrator cannot deal with every ethical issue that arises. But if the institution is well managed, the administrator can contribute, in a major way, toward the likelihood that sound decisions will be made and that other decisions will be rendered unnecessary. Furthermore, given the limited roles of the judicial system and the market, it is quite likely that if the health administrator does not act, no one will. Failure to act is, of course, often an ethical consideration itself.

The management of health institutions involves far more than cost containment and efficiency. Yet, while the demands of cost containment on management have been extensively discussed, the demands of morality and justice have not. It is time to put the various dimensions in proper perspective.

CONCLUSION

For the past few years, United States health institutions have been on a heady, market-oriented ride. They have become accustomed to a new language involving vertical integration, restructuring, and diversification. They are learning to market their services.

A discussion of ethics is not only healthy in its own right; it serves to remind us that, as important as our new enthusiasm for change is, there is more to health management than crisp efficiency. In the health field, perhaps more than any other, management involves moral values and ethical choices. It involves deep commitment and personal courage. It involves a resolve to be just and right, not only a resolve to win.

As the resolution of ethical issues becomes secular and moves from private domains toward the public realm of courts, commissions, and legislatures, it would be a tragic mistake for health executives and other health professionals to undervalue the importance of personal ethical commitment—commitment rooted firmly in the concepts of human dignity and the common good.[13]

NOTES

1. This chapter is adapted from "Managing Ethical Dilemmas" from *Journal of Health Administration Education*, Vol. 3, no. 3, pp. 331–340, with permission of Association of University Programs in Health Administration, © Summer 1985.

2. D.W. Amundsen, "The Physician's Obligation to Prolong Life: A Medical Duty Without Classical Roots," *The Hastings Center Report* 8, no. 4 (1978):28.

3. Marc Hiller, "Ethics and Health Care Administration: Issues in Education and Practice," *Journal of Health Administration Education* 2, no. 2 (1984):147, 148.

4. W.A. Silverman, "Mismatched Attitudes About Neonatal Death," *The Hastings Center Report* 11, no. 6 (1981):13.

5. J.W. Hennessey, Jr., "Moral Dilemmas in Modern Management" (Typescript of speech delivered at the University of New Hampshire, February 21, 1980).

6. George L. Annas, "Nonfeeding: Lawful Killing in California, Homicide in New Jersey," *The Hastings Center Report* 13, no. 6 (1983):19.

7. *Superintendent of Belchertown State School v. Joseph Saikewicz*, 1977 Mass. Adv. Sh. 2461, 370 N.E.2d 417 (1977).

8. President's Commission for the Study of Ethical Problems in Medicine and Biomedical and Behavioral Research, *Deciding to Forego Life-Sustaining Treatment: Ethical, Medical and Legal Issues in Treatment Decisions* (Washington D.C.: Government Printing Office, March 1983).

9. Ibid.

10. Ibid.

11. N. Brown and D. Thompson, "Nontreatment of Fever in Extended Care Facilities," *New England Journal of Medicine* 300, no. 22 (1979):1249.

12. Ibid.

13. R. Fox and D. Willis, "Personhood, Medicine, and American Society," *Milbank Memorial Fund Quarterly* 61, no. 1 (1983):137, 138.

Chapter 2

A Practical Guide to Legal Considerations in Ethical Issues

Jennifer A. Stiller, JD

Because the moral and ethical issues raised by advances in medical technology are complex and make most of us uncomfortable, we tend to turn to lawyers in search of absolute answers. The law, however, rarely provides such answers.

Despite this, there are two reasons why the law must be considered in decisions regarding consent to treatment, withholding of treatment, or termination of treatment. First, and of most day-to-day concern, it is generally desirable to avoid being sued. A basic understanding of the legal principles underlying the law of torts (private wrongs) will enable those actually engaged in treatment decisions to know when a lawyer should be consulted. Second, one must keep in mind the strictures of the criminal law—fortunately it is of more concern in theory than in practice, but it could conceivably be invoked in situations involving termination of treatment or late-term abortion.

The purpose of this chapter is to provide an overview to enable the lay person to better understand what ''the law'' is and how it works, so that necessary legal considerations can be integrated into the ethical decision-making process.

SOURCES OF THE LAW

Nonlawyers often envision the law as a vast library containing books of rules. They want concrete answers to practical questions: Is such-and-such legal? Will someone sue me if I do thus-and-so? Lawyers have earned an unwarranted reputation for evasiveness because they generally answer, ''It depends'' or ''Maybe.''

The reason that lawyers so rarely give definite answers may be found in the nature of the law itself. There is no book of rules; or rather, to the extent that there are such books, they are only the beginning of a lawyer's analysis, not the end. An understanding of what the law is and how it develops is necessary to evaluate meaningfully the significance of key judicial decisions discussed in Parts II and III of this book.

Judge-Made Law

It makes sense to begin where our law itself began: with the common law. This is the name given to an immense and variegated body of law developed over centuries by English, and later American, judges. Cases arose, as they do today, out of disputes between people and, in deciding those cases, the judges would look to earlier cases involving similar disputes and attempt to glean from them general principles that could be applied to the case at hand. At the time the United States became an independent nation, the vast bulk of English—and hence American—law was case law, the recorded decisions of the judges. Tort law, the law concerning suits among private individuals seeking compensation for negligent or intentional wrongful acts committed by one person against another, was then and is today largely judge-made law.

Because tort law is of common law origin, the answer to a particular question ("Is such-and-such legal?") will at best be a lawyer's educated guess based on knowledge of the relevant case law. To find "the law," the attorney researches the case law of the applicable jurisdiction (usually the local state), sometimes extending that research to include significant cases in other states as well. Having read the case law, the lawyer then tries to assess how a judge would be likely to apply those precedents if the problem the lawyer is concerned with ever went to court.

When judges write opinions in areas where there is little if any prior case law, they do so knowing that their opinions will provide guidelines for future behavior by people who are not parties to the case they are deciding. This is particularly true in medicolegal jurisprudence, where a carefully reasoned opinion by a judge in a legally influential state such as California, New York, New Jersey, Massachusetts, or Illinois may have far-reaching implications for the development of the law in other jurisdictions.

One further aspect of tort law is worthy of mention. Although this branch of law antedated the creation of the modern insurance industry by several centuries and developed as a means of providing compensation for people who were injured through another person's acts of omission or commission, judges have increasingly recognized that tort law can also play a major role in influencing people's behavior. For example, if a manufacturer can be successfully sued by a customer who is injured because, not being aware of the danger and of steps that could be taken to mitigate it, he uses a dangerous product in an unsafe manner, the manufacturer is more likely to place warning labels and instructions for safe use on the product's container.

In health care, this behavior-influencing aspect of tort law can be seen every time a patient signs a written consent form or a doctor practices "defensive medicine" by ordering a diagnostic test of small potential value just to demonstrate that every possibility has been explored.

Statute Law

In addition to the common law, modern American law contains a substantial body of statutory law. Statutes—laws enacted by a legislative body such as Congress—may fill in areas not covered by the traditional common law, or they may amend or abolish common law principles. Thus, when a newspaper article refers to a bill that would abolish or modify the principle of "joint or several liability," it is describing a proposed statutory change to a common law principle. In addition to the laws enacted by the legislative branch, statutory law also includes regulations, which come into being when a statute authorizes an executive official (such as the secretary of the U.S. Department of Health and Human Services) or an administrative agency (such as the Food and Drug Administration) to adopt them. Regulations have the force of law, unless a court finds that they are inconsistent with the authorizing statute or were adopted without compliance with established rulemaking procedures.

Because the United States has a federal system of government, every American is governed by at least two levels of statutory law: federal laws passed by Congress, and state laws enacted by the local state legislature. (In addition, there may be local government statutes, which are called ordinances. These are generally not relevant to medical treatment decisions.)

In the United States, all criminal law is statutory. Thus, no one may be imprisoned unless he or she has violated a state or federal criminal statute.

"Hybrid" Law

Much of modern American law is a kind of hybrid between statutory law and common law. That is because, after the legislature passes a statute, litigation will inevitably arise under it, and the courts will have to interpret what the legislature meant when it enacted the law. Sometimes the legislature will have passed two statutes that seem to be somewhat inconsistent, and the courts will have to interpret the two provisions, either (as is preferred) by figuring out a way that both statutes can apply, or by ruling that the later law impliedly repealed the former.

To see how all this applies in practice, let us consider the case of a 17-year-old Pennsylvania girl who is pregnant and wants an abortion. Can she consent to this procedure herself, or is she a minor whose parents must give the consent for her? In 1973, immediately following the Supreme Court's landmark decision in *Roe v. Wade*,[1] the only law on the books in Pennsylvania that was relevant to this question was a 1970 statute that provided:

> Any minor who is eighteen years of age or older, or has graduated
> from high school, or has married, or has been pregnant, may give

effective consent to medical, dental and health services for himself or herself, and the consent of no other person shall be necessary.[2]

Assuming that the minor in question is still in high school and has never married, is a young woman who is currently pregnant covered by the words "has been pregnant?" A lawyer trying to answer this question in late 1973 and reading this statute would have found no case law interpreting it. Accordingly, he or she would have consulted the general law concerning minors' consent to medical treatment, that is, the case law as it existed in Pennsylvania at the time. Because then, as now, the general common law rule was that a dependent minor is not legally capable of giving consent to medical treatment, the careful lawyer would have advised the physician to obtain consent from at least one of the girl's parents before performing the procedure.

In September 1974 the Pennsylvania General Assembly passed the Abortion Control Act of 1974.[3] With regard to pregnant minors, that statute provided:

> (a) No abortion shall be performed upon any person in the absence of the written consent of . . . (ii) one parent or person in loco parentis of such person if such person is under eighteen years of age and unmarried, unless the abortion is certified by a licensed physician as necessary in order to preserve the life of the mother.
>
> . . .
>
> (e) Whoever performs an abortion without consent as required in subsection (a) of this section shall be guilty of a misdemeanor of the first degree. . . .[4]

This would seem to be fairly clear; not only may the 17-year-old not consent to the abortion, but the doctor may be thrown in jail if he or she performs the abortion without obtaining the specified consent.

As might be expected, however, the passage of the Abortion Control Act did not end the development of the law in this area. Shortly after the statute was passed, the enforcement of this provision was enjoined by the U.S. District Court for the Eastern District of Pennsylvania, which ruled that the statute conflicted with the United States Constitution, as articulated in *Roe v. Wade*, and hence was invalid.[5] In so deciding, the court interpreted the general minors' consent law quoted above to rule that the words "has been pregnant" include a person who *is currently* pregnant, and therefore, a minor could consent to an abortion. Thus, the law of Pennsylvania became that articulated by the federal court, and a pregnant minor could authorize her own abortion without parental consent.

This situation prevailed until late 1982, when the 1974 act was repealed and a new Abortion Control Act went into effect.[6] The new statute contained a lengthy section providing that an abortion could not be performed (except in a medical emergency) if the pregnant woman was less than 18 years of age and "not emancipated," unless the consent of both the pregnant woman and one of her parents were obtained. The statute further provided a mechanism whereby the pregnant minor could obtain court consent in lieu of parental consent if both of her parents or guardians refused consent or if she elected not to seek their consent.[7] In addition, the new abortion control law contained the following "penalty" provision:

> Any person who performs an abortion upon a woman who is an une-mancipated minor . . . to whom this section applies either with knowl-edge that she is a minor . . . , or with reckless disregard or negligence as to whether she is a minor . . . , and who intentionally, knowingly or recklessly fails to conform to any requirement of this section is guilty of "unprofessional conduct" and his license for the practice of medicine and surgery shall be suspended . . . for a period of at least three months. Failure to comply with the requirements of this section is prima facie evidence of failure to obtain informed consent and of interference with family relations in appropriate civil actions. The law of this Commonwealth shall not be construed to preclude the award of exemplary damages or damages for emotional distress even if un-accompanied by physical complications in any appropriate civil action relevant to violations of this section. Nothing in this section shall be construed to limit the common law rights of parents.[8]

This statutory provision provides an excellent example of "hybrid" law. First, the General Assembly has overruled a court's interpretation of a previous statute, by reinstituting the requirement for parental consent. In doing so, the legislature has incorporated by reference a common law concept—emancipation of minors. (State law on whether and when a minor becomes "emancipated," that is, treated by the law as an adult even though he or she is younger than the age of majority, is generally set forth not in statutes but in case law. In general, courts will infer emancipation from such indicia of adult status as economic independence, living apart from one's parents, and marriage.)

What does this mean in practical terms? Normally, providing treatment to a person who is not legally empowered to consent to that treatment may be con-sidered the tort of "battery"—an unauthorized touching. Thus, the inhibiting effect of a possible civil lawsuit will cause the physician's lawyer to advise him or her to "be on the safe side" and obtain consents from as many potential plaintiffs as possible. In the case of abortion, however, the Pennsylvania General Assembly has provided more stringent penalties. First, it imposes a statutory penalty: the physician's license may be suspended. Second, the legislature has made clear that it wishes all the available common law inhibitions to physician action to remain valid, even though the statute provides this special penalty. In fact, the legislature has gone even further, by stating that failure to comply with the statutory requirements will constitute "prima facie evidence" of tortious behavior. This means that if the person who is suing the doctor can prove that the doctor did not comply with the statute, no further additional proof would be necessary. (The physician would, however, be allowed to put forth evidence to rebut such a finding.) Thus, the legislature has used the inherent inhibiting effect of tort law to enforce its desire that physicians obtain parental consent before performing an abortion on an unemancipated minor.

BASIC PRINCIPLES OF TORT LAW RELEVANT TO MEDICAL TREATMENT

Much of the law applicable to complex medical treatment decisions is judge-made law, although there may be state statutes (such as the Pennsylvania Abortion Control Act provision discussed above) that are also relevant. The law of each state will thus turn heavily on that state's particular case law precedents. However, some general principles of tort law are commonly applicable.

The law starts from the premise that the patient has a right to determine what medical treatment he or she should receive. Thus, as long ago as 1914, Justice Benjamin Cardozo wrote:

> Every human being of adult years and sound mind has a right to determine what shall be done with his own body, and a surgeon who performs an operation without his patient's consent commits an assault and battery for which he is liable in damages.[9]

Inherent in the individual's right to consent to medical treatment is the right to refuse treatment, even if the inevitable result of that refusal is death.[10] There are, however, some instances where courts will intervene and order life-saving or life-prolonging treatment for a competent individual, if the court finds a compelling state interest outweighs the individual's rights to privacy and self-determination. For example, courts have frequently intervened, in the interest of the patient's unborn child or dependent minor children, to order a necessary blood transfusion for a Jehovah's Witness who has refused such treatment on religious grounds.[11]

To the law, the touching of a person's body that is incident to medical treatment is, if not authorized by the patient, no different from the unauthorized touching that might occur when a person is assaulted by a mugger or hit by a negligently operated car. Any of these "touchings" would be considered the tort of battery. The "touching" incident to medical care is rendered permissible under the law by the patient's informed consent to treatment. However, if the patient, because of some mental incapacity, is unable to understand the nature of consent and whatever is consented to, the "consent" is meaningless.

In general, the law presumes that an adult is competent for any purpose unless he has been adjudicated otherwise by a court. However, in many states, a person who has been adjudicated incompetent to handle his financial affairs may nonetheless be competent to consent—or withhold consent—to medical treatment.[12]

Minors—people under the age of majority as defined by state statute—are unable by virtue of their age to give effective consent to medical treatment and must rely on their parents or guardians to grant consent for them. However, as noted above, many states have enacted special statutes that allow minors to grant consent for treatment in certain specified circumstances. It is not uncommon for such statutes to authorize medical personnel to treat even very young children without obtaining consent if a life-threatening emergency exists.

To obtain an informed consent, the physician generally should have discussed with the patient the diagnosis, proposed treatment, risks, and treatment alternatives. The patient should have understood the discussion and agreed to the plan of treatment. It is the physician's responsibility to obtain informed consent, even though hospital nurses frequently undertake the task of securing signatures to consent forms. Such forms are, however, only evidence of informed consent; if a patient signs a form without being aware of its contents, there may be no valid consent despite the signature.

A PRACTICAL APPROACH TO LEGAL ISSUES

A facility involved in treating patients with chronic disease or terminal illness faces different ethical and legal considerations than a pediatric tertiary care hospital. To ensure proper consideration of the legal implications of treatment decisions, a three-step approach is often helpful:

1. Ascertain current policies and practices.
2. Learn the law.
3. Develop policies and procedures for dealing with problems as they arise.

Such an approach will enable the institution to tailor its decision-making process to the particular legal requirements applicable to it.

Ascertaining Current Policies and Practices

The institution's review of the legal soundness of its policies necessarily starts with a review of both those policies and the degree to which they are being followed in practice. Unless a unified effort has been made at some point in the past to develop institutionwide standards, practices for obtaining proxy consents for incompetent individuals, determining incompetence, assessing degree of informed consent, and documenting a patient's refusal of recommended treatment may vary from department to department or even from physician to physician. Even where the institution has standardized consent forms, review may turn up some deviations from standard practice. Thus, periodic review of what is actually happening on the treatment units can be a useful exercise.

Although it is not strictly necessary to undertake this step before the facility's attorney begins his or her review of the law, it will be helpful to the attorney to know, before reading the cases, what is actually going on in the institution. This will help to focus the lawyer's attention on whether or not particular practices really need to be revised, or whether they are legally acceptable.

Learning the Law

It is important that key decision makers within the institution have a good understanding of what laws apply to the treatment decisions made within it. This is best accomplished by asking the institution's attorney to review the law and provide a synopsis of applicable points to appropriate hospital personnel. Once a comprehensive review of this kind has been conducted, the attorney need only stay abreast of current developments and advise appropriate personnel as they occur.

An individualized legal review is necessary because both the institution's activities and the state in which it is located can affect what the law is. For example, a comprehensive summary of legal principles prepared for a hospital without an obstetric service need not consider the case law, statutes, or regulations relating to withholding of treatment from severely defective newborns. The attorney's review should include:

- review of home state statutes and regulations (if any)
- review of home state case law
- review of key case law from other jurisdictions on any relevant issue for which home state case law is not dispositive
- review of applicable federal statutes and regulations

State statutes are often a good starting point for this analysis, if only because many attorneys frequently overlook them. Review of state statutes should include subjects such as:

- informed consent
- physician licensure statute
- statutory definition of "death"
- abortion
- sterilization
- incompetency

- commitment procedures for the mentally ill
- peer review
- Good Samaritan law
- "living will" statute
- newborn infant protection act
- child abuse laws
- emergency medical services

In addition, there may be regulations promulgated by the state public health department, perhaps under the hospital licensure statute, that relate to patient consents for treatment or refusal of treatment.

It is often useful to conduct this review of state statutes prior to researching the case law, because a recent statute may overturn or modify case law precedents. Review of state case law should include:

- informed consent
- patient's right to refuse consent
- proxy or substitute consent for an incompetent
- what constitutes incompetence for medical consent purposes
- minors' ability to consent to medical treatment
- standards for emancipation of minors
- parental refusal of consent for minor child
- obligations of physicians and health care facility in connection with obtaining informed consent
- termination or withholding of extraordinary means to preserve life
- what procedures are considered extraordinary means to preserve life

Depending on the nature of the institution, some of these issues will be of more concern than others. Where a state does not have either statutory or case law on an important point (such as, for example, whether a relative can authorize removal of a respirator from a comatose patient), the lawyer must also review key precedents from other states in conjunction with whatever local case law there is, in an effort to reach an informed judgment as to what the state's courts are likely to do in a given situation.

Finally, federal statutes and regulations may affect the following:

- clinical drug trials
- withholding treatment from defective newborns
- sterilization procedures performed on Medical Assistance recipients
- duty to provide treatment in emergency room
- human experimentation

Developing Policies and Procedures

The purpose of the legal review is to enable the institution's decision makers to know, to the extent possible, what legal standards are likely to apply before the situation arises in which those standards need to be applied. The development of institutional policies and procedures in effect creates a legal triage system, enabling treatment personnel to handle all but the most legally complex decisions without the need for further involvement by a lawyer.

Institutional policies and procedures will usually involve the development of standard procedures for obtaining consents and requirements for retaining consent documents in the patient's medical record. In addition, it is usually helpful for an institution to have standard consent and release of liability forms, which may include the following:

- consent to hospital admission
- consent to surgery
- consents to specific procedures
- release of liability for refusal of treatment
- release of liability for discharge against medical advice
- release from liability for refusal to permit blood transfusion
- authorization for medical care for minor

From a purely practical point of view, there is less likely to be a lawsuit if there is no potential plaintiff, and there is less likely to be a potential plaintiff if any party who has an interest in the outcome of the treatment decision participates actively in the decision-making process and agrees with it. Subordinate members of the treatment team should not be ignored or, even worse, coerced into participating in a course of action that they find morally repugnant. An institution with an atmosphere that encourages lower-level personnel to air their deep concerns is less likely to find that such personnel have filed a "Baby Doe"–type complaint with state or federal authorities or urged a politically ambitious local prosecutor to file a murder charge against a physician who terminates treatment to a brain-dead patient.

In general, when the decision is one of giving consent to treatment, there is no need to obtain additional consent from the patient's next of kin unless there is some reason to doubt the patient's mental competency. In such a case, it is often helpful to obtain the consent of the patient's close relatives—the spouse, parent(s), or one or (preferably) more of the patient's adult children. The kin should indicate by their signatures that they agree both with the patient's decision and with the informed nature of the patient's consent (which includes an affirmation of the patient's apparent competency).

The institution should also have policies concerning what to do if a patient refuses to consent to treatment. In general (unless state law provides otherwise), such a refusal should be honored. However, policies will need to specify the procedures to be followed if the patient refuses treatment but both the treating physicians and the patient's family believe that treatment is necessary. Institutional policy should also specify what is to be done in an emergency, where delay would result in a seriously adverse effect on the patient or on the therapeutic process, to the material detriment of the patient's health. Finally, there should be policies for dealing with situations where the patient is, or appears to be, incompetent to give informed consent to treatment.

CONCLUSION

Understanding the applicable law and developing policies and procedures consistent with it will enable the health care institution to keep most difficult decisions regarding consent to treatment, withholding of treatment, or termination of treatment out of the hands of lawyers and under the control of the people who are most affected—patients, their families, and their physicians. By knowing general legal principles applicable to their state and their institution, hospital decision makers will be better equipped to know which situations can be handled on the institutional level and which ones are so legally problematic that they require a lawyer's assistance.

NOTES

1. Roe v. Wade, 410 U.S. 113 (1973).

2. 35 PA. STAT. ANN. §10101 (Purdon 1977).

3. 35 PA. STAT. ANN. §§6601–6608 (Purdon 1977).

4. 35 PA. STAT. ANN. §6603(a)(ii), (e) (Purdon 1977).

5. Planned Parenthood Ass'n v. Fitzpatrick, 401 F.Supp. 554 (E.D. Pa. 1975), *aff'd* 428 U.S. 901.

6. 18 PA. CONS. STAT. ANN. §§3201–3220 (Supp. 1986).

7. 18 PA. CONS. STAT. ANN. §3206 (Supp. 1986).

8. 18 PA. CONS. STAT. ANN. §3206(i) (Supp. 1986).

9. Schloendorff v. The Society of New York Hospital, 211 N.Y. 125, 129, 105 N.E. 92, 93, 133 N.Y.S. 1143, 1145 (1914).

10. *See* Satz v. Perlmutter, 362 So. 2d 160 (Fla. App. 1978).

11. *See, e.g.,* Raleigh Fitkin-Paul Morgan Memorial Hospital v. Anderson, 42 N.J. 421, 201 A.2d 537 (1963), *cert. denied* 377 U.S. 985 (1964); Application of the President and Directors of Georgetown College, 331 F.2d 1000 (D.C. Cir. 1964), *cert. denied* 337 U.S. 978 (1964).

12. *See* In Re Yetter, 62 Pa. D & C. 2d 619 (1973); Lane v. Cantura, 376 N.W. 2d 1232 (Mass. 1978); In Re Quackenbush, 156 N.J. Super. 282, 383 A.2d 785 (1978).

BIBLIOGRAPHY

American Bar Association Forum Committee on Health Law, *Critical Care Decision Making in Hospitals* (Chicago, 1986).

Chapter 3

Applying Philosophy to Ethical Dilemmas

Sylvia Ridlen Wenston, PhD

INTRODUCTION

Health care professionals often face situations where they are unsure about how to proceed. In some cases, uncertainty is the result of inadequate knowledge, lack of factual clarity, or lack of relevant information. In other cases, however, additional information is not enough: the professional faces an ethical dilemma and must decide among competing moral claims or obligations.

While situations involving ethical problems are extremely complex, two conceptual tools are helpful in clarifying, analyzing, and deciding ethical questions. First, ethical principles provide a standard by which to evaluate the ethical implications of alternatives. Second, methods of ethical analysis provide systematic ways to think about ethical questions and possible solutions. In combination, these two conceptual tools can enhance clear thinking and principled decision making, thus guiding and justifying a health care professional's action.

This chapter considers the nature and sources of ethical problems and responsibility, the ethical principles applied in biomedical ethics, and two of the primary methods of philosophical ethical analysis.

MORALITY, ETHICS, AND SPECIALIZED ROLES

"Morals" and "ethics" are familiar terms, but differences between them may be less clear. Morality refers to one's personal or private system of values, or convictions about how one "ought" to behave in relation to others. For instance, most people think they should tell the truth, should not cheat or steal, and should keep promises. (Of course, there may be specific situations when one thinks one ought to make exceptions to these general guides to behavior—but they are exceptions.) Failure to act in accordance with one's morals leads to feelings of guilt or pangs of conscience.

Morals are intrapersonal; that is, their force comes from internal feelings that arise when a person has or hasn't acted in accordance with them. When a person lies or breaks a promise, even if nobody else finds out and no harm results to others, it is common to feel at least a little guilty or uneasy about having lied or broken that promise.

Morals are not based on specialized roles or responsibilities but are acquired by being a person in a society that has established and accepted norms for behavior. Thus, there is a general set of norms or mores from which every able member of society derives and internalizes a sense of right and wrong. For instance, most parents teach their children that lying is wrong. They may punish or otherwise correct their children for lying. Later, as adults, those grown children generally tell the truth—and when they don't they feel guilty or anxious. They also try to keep it a secret when they do lie, knowing that such behavior is not socially or morally approved.

Such norms and their internalization have social utility: if everyone lied without compunction, social regulations would be much more complex and dysfunctional. Internalization is also essential, since it is impossible to have external policing of most behavior.

Ethics, on the other hand, is a system of values that guides behavior in relationships among people, in accordance with certain social roles. Ethics is relative to particular roles: different roles call for different ethical standards. For instance, a manager who learns sensitive information about an employee in the context of the work relationship is bound, in sharing that information, by role expectations and rules of confidentiality. The manager's nonprofessional spouse, learning the same information from a mutual acquaintance, is not constrained in the same way.

Professional Ethics

By definition, professionals are bound by ethical standards. One attribute of a profession is its ethical code.[1] Most professional codes are articulated by major organizations to which many or most of the professionals belong. For example, an association of doctors, the American Medical Association, has articulated the code governing physicians' ethical behavior. For nurses, the American Nurses' Association has performed the same function. By articulating standards in a code of ethics, professions establish expectations for every member of the profession and provide a basis for the evaluation of professional behavior.

Organizational Ethics

Social organizations and institutions also have ethical obligations.[2] Organizational ethics are based on the selection and pursuit of organizational purposes and functions, in consideration of the many people and groups the organization affects.[3] Organizational ethics are put into practice by employees, who are bound by these moral and ethical obligations in their roles as employees.

Hospitals, for instance, are ethically obligated to maximize patients' health. They also have obligations to their employees, communities, and, if they are teaching institutions, to their students. These ethical obligations are separate from, but may be reinforced by, legal, political, business, or other considerations.

Hospital administrators, because of their role in the hospital, are expected to further the organization's purposes and to assist other employees in doing the same. Administrators are also expected to work toward fulfilling the hospital's obligations to patients, doctors, employees, students, governing bodies, the community, and others with significant interests in the hospital. Administrators have special obligations to exercise their power—derived from their position, responsibility, and relationships—responsibly and ethically.[4]

ETHICAL DILEMMAS AND RELATED PROBLEMS DEFINED

It is not always easy to know when one faces problems with ethical or moral elements. Difficult problems, whether of ethics or of practice, raise feelings of anxiety and uncertainty. There are two sorts of problems that have ethical or moral implications and clearly lend themselves to ethical analysis. Situations where two parties have conflicting and irreconcilable interests pose the clearest sort of ethical dilemma. The interests of a pregnant woman, for whom bearing a child jeopardizes her health or the quality of her life in profound ways, may be irreconcilable with the interests of the fetus she carries. In this type of case, no matter what course of action is selected, the interests of one party must yield to the interests of the other. These are true ethical dilemmas.

More commonly encountered are situations where practice must be conducted, or decisions made, in uncertainty, and the consequences of a decision may have a significant impact on others. The information that would make clear the best course of action to take may be unavailable, inadequate, or nonexistent. Despite this, however, decisions must be made. Ethical dimensions are present in such problems when the effects of action may put others at risk, harm others, lead to a violation of rights, or have other ethical implications. In such instances, the goal may be positive, but the probability of achieving good rather than harm may be unclear.

GUIDES TO MORAL AND ETHICAL BEHAVIOR

When faced with ethical dilemmas, what should the health care professional do? To make a carefully reasoned and principled decision, ethical principles should be considered.

Ethical Principles for Professionals and Organizations

One's personal feelings, in the form of one's own moral system, are likely to provide the first ideas about what should be done. Private morality is necessary but not sufficient for professionals to act responsibly. A set of ethical principles, shared by the profession as a group and consistent with the profession's mandate, is needed if members of that profession are to behave ethically.

In addition to moral standards that guide hospital administrators as individuals, ethical principles are needed to guide behavior when ethical conflicts arise within professional or organizational contexts. These principles should help one decide how best to meet the organizational and professional ethical mandates. To be useful, such principles must have certain qualities:

1. They must reflect shared and highly valued purposes overriding most other considerations.[5]
2. They should be universalizable.[6] In other words, to be moral or ethical in nature, a guide to behavior must require that all situations that are similar in relevant ways be treated alike. Morality and ethics are not idiosyncratic and arbitrary, but generalizable and durable.
3. They should refer directly to the welfare of others.[7] The focus of concern is on others rather than on the self.

Beauchamp and Childress have articulated a system of four principles relevant to biomedical ethical questions: (1) autonomy, (2) beneficence, (3) nonmaleficence, and (4) justice.[8] These principles reflect strong values, are universalizable, and are framed in terms of the welfare of others. They are readily usable by a variety of health care professionals involved in decision making in hospital settings.

Autonomy

Many philosophers have written about the important ethical concept of autonomy. Autonomous people are self-governing; they exercise control over their actions and circumstances. As an ethical principle, autonomy guides us to respect others as autonomous[9] and to enhance, support, or restore autonomy insofar as possible.

The American Hospital Association's Patient's Bill of Rights lists a number of rights that hospitals should support.[10] These rights are clearly aimed at protecting and supporting patients' personal autonomy in the belief that patients' health and recovery will be enhanced as a result. Many of these pertain to information to which patients are entitled, including explanation of bills, hospital rules and regulations, and several others.

Informed consent is also listed as a patient's right.[11] Ethically, informed consent is based on the principle of autonomy. Autonomous decisions to give consent for risky procedures require disclosure of adequate and relevant information that must be comprehended by the patient.[12] Furthermore, to be autonomous, such decisions must be made voluntarily, without coercion or undue influence. In legal terms, informed consent can be given only by someone who is mentally competent to make such a decision.[13]

Confidentiality—another patient right[14]—is also grounded in the principle of autonomy; individuals have a right to control the dissemination of personal or sensitive information about them.[15]

Professionals must also have some degree of autonomy if they are to fulfill their own ethical mandates. Each profession has its own code of ethics, to which its members are bound. The hospital's obligation to its professional employees includes granting needed professional autonomy.

Limits to Autonomy

Although important, autonomy is not an absolute ethical principle. It is a "prima facie" principle: it should be followed unless there are other, overriding considerations or principles in a specific situation.

Being guided by the principle of autonomy may be inappropriate when doing so would threaten the autonomy or well-being of others. A person who sets out to steal a car can be stopped from doing so with moral (and legal) justification. So, too, a person who drives with flagrant disregard for the safety of others can justifiably be prevented from such autonomous action. Recently, a company that arbitrarily decided to stop its retirees' benefits because of financial problems was ordered by the courts to reinstate them. As these examples suggest, many situations pertaining to the bounds of autonomy have legal implications that reinforce moral considerations.

Organizational autonomy is not absolute either. While organizations like hospitals are free to define their own goals, ethical constraints on this autonomy exist. Organizational goals should be selected with consideration for community needs and existing resources. Goals should obviously reflect social rather than antisocial purposes.[16] The autonomy of other organizations should also be respected.

A potential problem for clinicians concerned about patient autonomy may be a failure to recognize situations when conditions for autonomy are not met. For example, it seems inappropriate to use the principle of individual autonomy as a guide when a person is mentally incompetent or unable to make decisions voluntarily or rationally. Similarly, an organization in severe financial crisis may not realistically be capable of making autonomous decisions. Autonomy isn't always possible, either for individuals or organizations. When autonomy is not possible, a second important ethical principle, beneficence, might often be more helpful.

Beneficence

Beneficence directs the actor to try to do good, to further the welfare or well-being of others. This may be accomplished by making positive contributions or by acting to remove or prevent harm.[17] A stranger who sees a child about to be hit by a truck and rushes to save him is acting in accordance with beneficence. So is a person who stops at the scene of an accident to offer assistance. Beneficence is the principle that underlies the goals of many social and health care organizations.

In medical settings, beneficence is very often expressed in the form of paternalism. Paternalism is, very simply put, doing what one believes is for someone else's good, without necessarily having obtained the other person's knowledge or consent.[18] A commonly cited example is when a doctor decides not to tell a patient the truth about his or her condition in the honest belief that this paternalistic action will protect the patient from distress or other negative reactions.

To be justifiable, paternalistic behavior must prevent significantly more harm to the other than it causes, and one must also be prepared to allow it in all such similar cases.[19] Paternalism is not justifiable when the action primarily serves the interests of the person being paternalistic.

Limits to Beneficence

Although not all philosophers agree to what degree beneficence is required, it is clearly accepted as a moral ideal. However, like autonomy, beneficence is not an absolute moral duty. There are times when other considerations override beneficence. Some philosophers have made a good argument that, at the minimum, beneficence can be said to be morally required when one can act so as to prevent significant harm but without taking significant risk oneself.[20]

One's role affects one's obligations to act beneficently: historically, doctors have had a moral and ethical duty of beneficence toward their patients. A physician treating a patient with a highly dangerous and contagious disease is ethically obliged to risk some personal harm;[21] the patient's friends, on the other hand, may have no such ethical obligation to put themselves at personal risk to help their friend.

Nonmaleficence

Another fundamental ethical principle, so obvious that it is often overlooked or taken for granted, is nonmaleficence.[22] This principle guides individuals and organizations to not harm others. It is different from beneficence in that it is not concerned with improving others' well-being but only with avoiding the infliction of harm.[23] It seems a basic assumption that underlies all helping professions and social organizations, though it is rarely made explicit.

Limits to Nonmaleficence

At times, of course, a situation may arise where one is justified in inflicting harm for long-term benefit (e.g., surgery) or to protect others from harm. For these reasons, nonmaleficence is, like the other principles, a "prima facie" principle, a guide to action that should be followed unless there are overriding reasons to act differently.

Justice

Justice is Beauchamp and Childress's fourth major ethical principle.[24] Justice has to do with how people are treated when their interests compete and are compared with the interests of others. Most often, justice is equated with fairness or merit. Aristotle said justice consists of treating equals equally, and unequals unequally but in proportion to their relevant differences.[25]

There is considerable disagreement among philosophers, politicians, and others as to how to determine proportionality or what constitutes relevant differences. Some have suggested that just treatment should be determined according to need, contribution, effort, merit, or by other systems.[26] Whatever the system of distribution or allocation, to be just, individuals must be treated impartially and fairly, not in an arbitrary or capricious manner. Justice toward individuals, or comparative justice, is the concern of much of our judicial system.[27] One murderer should not be treated differently from another murderer, if the two crimes were essentially similar in all important ways.

Distributive Justice

Similar to the previous three principles, comparative justice guides behavior in relation to other individuals. For example, an administrator might be concerned to treat all employees fairly or to develop an evaluation system such that merit raises are given only to those who deserve them.

However, there is another important element of the principle of justice. It has to do with the bigger picture of individuals in relation to group and society. Distributive justice refers to how benefits and burdens are distributed among all members of the social order, not simply individuals. It follows that, when resources are scarce, how one individual is treated must be fair compared with how others are treated. No one person should get a disproportional share of society's resources or benefits.[28]

For the hospital administrator, the principle of distributive justice is particularly and increasingly relevant. As allocation of health care dollars and other resources becomes ever more important, the hospital administrator's role requires a consideration of individual versus organizational or societal needs. For example, the cost of patients' medical care under diagnosis-related groups (DRGs) may put some patient needs and related physician goals for patients into conflict with the hospital's financial needs and interests.

Since clinicians' roles require them to advocate for individual patients,[29] it falls most logically on hospital administrators to work toward a balance between individual patient needs and the hospital's survival needs—which are, in the long-term and general sense, patients' and doctors' needs as well. At the same time, assuring access to needed services remains an ethical obligation of the hospital. The ethical principle of justice may be helpful when faced with hard ethical decisions about how to respond to competing needs when allocating resources for patient services and care.

Prioritizing Principles

Very often, ethical problems entail conflicts between principles. Should one further individual autonomy or social justice? Autonomy or beneficence? Such choices among highly valued principles are hard, because there are usually compelling reasons to support each of them. Scholars have used several different approaches to prioritizing moral and ethical principles.

John Rawls developed an influential theory of social justice, which he identified as a basic societal structure. A system of justice directs the distribution of rights, duties, and the advantages deriving from social cooperation.[30] Indeed, in a just society as Rawls conceived it, individual rights to equal treatment for all citizens are an unquestioned goal.[31] There are few potential conflicts in Rawls's just society with the other ethical principles discussed here. Justice is the structure for achieving those things that rational beings want.

Lewis observed that trust is fundamental both to ethical practice by helping professions and to a functional, just society.[32] He offered several principles for professional practice designed to further trust and social justice. To illustrate his approach, he argued that clients can't trust professionals unless the professionals provide full information about resources that might be of help to the client. All Lewis's principles are similarly designed to guide practice in very practical ways, so as to further trust and social justice.[33]

After considering the nature of ethical problems faced by social workers, Reamer proposed partial guidelines for prioritizing conflicting values.[34] While Reamer did not use Beauchamp and Childress's principles, his guidelines can be interpreted in the same terms nonetheless. Reamer indicated that protection of individual autonomy, and the capacities necessary for it, should take precedence over individual well-being (beneficence). Indeed, Reamer's wording suggests that he may see individual autonomy as the single most important ethical guideline for social workers to follow. However, he made no specific reference to the principles of justice or nonmaleficence.

Having reviewed other scholars' thinking, I would like to offer my own general guide for prioritizing ethical principles for helping professionals, in the following order:

1. Nonmaleficence seems to be the most fundamental ethical principle for those in helping professions and organizations, as the only ethical justification for harming those who seek help is when short-term harm results in long-term benefit.
2. The second most important principle is comparative justice. Without justice, the possibilities for social living are greatly reduced. And without social living, personal autonomy is also reduced. Justice is a necessary means to the end of individual rights. In fact, failure to act justly toward individuals may be couched in terms of violation of autonomy and rights. It is hard to think of compelling reasons for helping professionals to violate the principle of comparative justice.
3. The principle of individual autonomy is very highly valued: we all want to be self-determining in our daily lives and resist efforts to detract from our self-governance. The principle of individual autonomy should be violated only under extreme circumstances.
4. Beneficence is an important guide to professional and organizational action, especially when the conditions for autonomous action are lacking. Beneficence seems an essential ideal and function of professional relationships, at least to the degree that the professional does not risk significant personal harm. In general, however, beneficence should not supersede nonmaleficence, justice, or truly autonomous action. The professional role requires that these ethical principles be furthered, using beneficence to accomplish this if necessary.

The principle of distributive justice must be considered separately because it includes societal as well as individual dimensions. Distributive justice may require prioritization according to roles.[35] Distributive justice may be particularly important for those in roles with an organizational focus. Clinicians, whose primary concern is with treating patients, may be less concerned with the principle of distributive justice.

The conflicts most likely to arise—and most problematic to resolve—are between distributive justice and individual autonomy. Individuals' and society's needs and rights are so interdependent that it is hard to choose—or justify choosing—one over the other. Perhaps there are no satisfactory answers, but separating the responsibilities by clinical and organizational roles may make for a clearer debate.

MODELS OF ETHICAL THINKING

Ethical principles serve as a standard by which the merits of alternative courses of action can be judged. However, a systematic approach to thinking about ethical questions is also necessary to prevent arbitrary, self-serving, or poorly analyzed conclusions.

Consequentialism or Teleology

There are two common ways to think through ethical questions. The first, teleology or consequentialism, is used in many (not only ethical) situations. According to consequentialism, morally right action is whatever action leads to the maximum balance of good over evil.[36] "Good" and "evil" are not restricted to the moral senses of the words but refer to whatever is humanly desirable or undesirable.[37]

The most common form of consequentialism is utilitarianism, a type of cost-benefit analysis. When deciding, using a utilitarian analysis, one weighs ethical and other costs against the benefits of all feasible alternatives.[38] Questions like the following guide a utilitarian analysis: What will be the effects of each course of action? Will they be positive or negative? For whom? Will one course of action result in more good than any other? What will do the least harm?

Critique

Clearly, utilitarian analyses depend on being able to measure and balance good and bad consequences. This means that utilitarianism, and consequentialism more generally, are hard to use, because it is not always easy to weigh the relative merits of one course of action against those of an alternative.

Being able to quantify consequences is implicit in this form of analysis, and quantification is not really meaningful or possible in many ethical dilemmas. Because of the lack of formal quantitative mechanisms and the complexity of real situations, utilitarians sometimes end up using (deontological) rules of thumb.[39]

Moreover, utilitarianism relies on an attitude of "generalized benevolence," the assumption that decision makers consider their own happiness or good neither more nor less than that of others. This may be neither logical nor realistic.[40] If such an attitude does not exist among decision makers, those who are deemed less valuable in society—like the poor, mentally ill, or disabled—might often lose when their well-being must compete with that of more valued people. Decisions couched in ethical terms may actually be a self-serving rationalization when the generalized benevolence attitude is absent.

Deontology

The other major approach to ethical analysis, deontology, is ethical analysis according to a moral code or rules. By such a procedure, one would ask: What rules (legal, moral or ethical, religious) are relevant to this situation? What do these rules tell me to do? Is there any reason these rules are not fully applicable? If so, are there other rules that apply?

The consequences of actions are not important in a deontological analysis. For instance, lying or killing might always be wrong—no matter what the consequences. The Golden Rule (do unto others as you would have them do unto you) is a good example of a deontological moral rule. It is flexible, yet general, and does not concern itself with consequences.

Critique

Deontology is at times too rigid, and its lack of concern with the consequences of action at times may be unsatisfactory. There is also some danger that, in adhering too closely to rules, the purposes for which the rules were promulgated will be defeated. In addition, ethical rules or codes may not give guidance for handling cases of conflict among them.[41]

Both deontology and consequentialism are flawed and can be subject to misuse. Imperfect as they are, however, these are the two predominant models of analysis available for thinking through ethical problems. There are others, and even combinations of these two, but the most useful and important ideas needed for clear ethical thinking can be found in deontology and teleology.

CONCLUSION

Using the models of analysis in conjunction with ethical principles can result in clearer understanding of the ethical implications of a decision or course of action. At times such an analysis can help identify either the most or the least ethical alternative. It can help keep ethical goals clearly in focus in complex situations. It is not realistic, though, to expect that ethical analysis will lead to the only "right" decision or that such analysis will bring an end to all dissent.

Systematic analysis leads to clearer thinking and increased confidence in the justifiability and limitations of decisions. These seem to be significant advantages for those who want and need to act ethically.

NOTES

1. Ernest Greenwood, "Attributes of a Profession," *Social Work* 2 (July 1957):45–55.

2. Charles S. Levy, *Guide to Ethical Decisions and Actions for Social Service Administrators: A Handbook for Managerial Personnel* (New York: Haworth Press, 1982).

3. Ibid.

4. Ibid.

5. Tom L. Beauchamp and James F. Childress, *Principles of Biomedical Ethics*, 2nd ed. (New York: Oxford University Press, 1983).

6. Ibid.

7. Ibid.

8. Ibid.

9. Ibid.

10. American Hospital Association, *A Patient's Bill of Rights* (Chicago, Ill., 1973).

11. Ibid.

12. Beauchamp and Childress, *Principles*.

13. Ibid.

14. American Hospital Association, *Bill of Rights.*

15. Beauchamp and Childress, *Principles.*

16. Levy, *Guide.*

17. Beauchamp and Childress, *Principles.*

18. Ibid.

19. Bernard Gert and Charles M. Culver, "The Justification of Paternalism," *Ethics*, 1979, 199–210.

20. Beauchamp and Childress, *Principles.*

21. Laurence B. McCulloch, "History of Medical Ethics: Britain and the United States in the Eighteenth Century," in *Encyclopedia of Bioethics*, ed. Warren T. Reich (New York: Macmillan Publishing Co., Inc. and The Free Press, 1978) 957–963.

22. Beauchamp and Childress, *Principles.*

23. Ibid.

24. Ibid.

25. Stanley I. Benn, "Justice," in *The Encyclopedia of Philosophy*, Vol. 4. (New York: Macmillan Publishing Co., Inc. and The Free Press, 1972) 298–302.

26. Beauchamp and Childress, *Principles.*

27. Benn, "Justice."

28. John Rawls, *A Theory of Justice* (Cambridge: Harvard University Press, 1971) lays out what is probably the most influential contemporary explanation of distributive justice.

29. Robert M. Veatch, "DRGs and the Ethical Reallocation of Resources," *The Hastings Center Report* 16 (1986):32–40.

30. Rawls, *Theory.*

31. Ibid.

32. Harold Lewis, "Morality and the Politics of Practice," *Social Casework*, July 1972, 404–417.

33. Ibid.

34. Frederic Reamer, "Ethical Dilemmas in Social Work Practice," *Social Work* 28, no. 1 (Jan–Feb. 1983):31–35.

35. Veatch, "DRGs."

36. William K. Frankena, *Ethics*, 2nd ed. (Englewood Cliffs: Prentice-Hall Inc., 1973).

37. J.J.C. Smart, "Utilitarianism," in *The Encyclopedia of Philosophy*, Vol. 8 (New York: Macmillan Publishing Co., Inc. and The Free Press, 1972) 206–212.

38. Ibid.

39. Ibid.

40. Ibid.

41. Robert G. Olson, "Deontological Ethics," in *The Encyclopedia of Philosophy*, Vol. 2 (New York: Macmillan Publishing Co., Inc. and The Free Press, 1972) 343.

BIBLIOGRAPHY

Bok, Sissela. *Lying: Moral Choice in Public and Private Life.* New York: Random House Inc., 1978.

Rokeach, Milton. *The Nature of Human Values.* New York: The Free Press, 1973.

Taylor, Paul W. *Principles of Ethics: An Introduction.* Belmont, CA: Wadsworth Publishing Company, 1975.

Chapter 4

Health Care Managers' Values and Decision Making

Luke Gregory, MBA, MHA

Each of us makes decisions daily. We purchase houses, cars, and televisions, select vacation sites, and elect club presidents and city officials. We discuss these choices with family or friends, make evaluations, compare alternatives, and ultimately satisfy our desires either by achieving our goals or accepting compromises. Undoubtedly, some of these decisions are wrong, but equally many are right or appear right.

Often the accuracy of this decision-making process is difficult to predict. We either fail to fully explore the information available or we do not anticipate or measure the consequences of our action. As one reflects upon past decisions this does not appear so disturbing, since most decisions are relatively insignificant. But when decisions truly affect people and their lives, all sources of information and every possible consequence must be examined. This obsession occurs because we recognize that lives are not routine and that the typical decision-making model is not adequate. Our process must be expanded to include an ethical dimension. We are not concerned with the relative worth or "rightness" of a decision, but we desire to know the ultimate truth. This truth is the good or the benchmark necessary to validate our decisions.

Ancient Greek philosophy is the foundation for our modern understanding of ethics. Aristotle (ironically, the son of a physician) first described the process for discovering this good.

> Every act and every inquiry, and similarly every action and pursuit, is thought to aim at some good; and for this reason the good has rightly been declared to be that at which all things aim.[1]

Paul Lehmann, a twentieth century philosopher, echoes Aristotle's notion that all things define the good. He describes ethics as the process that makes "human life human."[2] It is not a code or a set of rules; it is a process. It is the task of asking difficult human questions and seeking answers, while recognizing that seldom are comprehensive solutions available. As more opportunities for human interactions occur, a greater number of difficult decisions are demanded.

34

In health care there is an inexhaustible list of dilemmas to confront. Managers who face these hard decisions must recognize that ethics cannot be abdicated to a committee or a courtroom. Ultimately, all decisions can be made only by individuals. In the changing environment of health care the task of making a right decision is difficult, the challenge of making a good decision is overwhelming. But as long as professionals are willing to try, decisions that are right and good will occur.

MANAGING CHANGE

Managing change appears to be health care's current theme. Though change is not new to medicine, it is rather new to the management of health care. No longer are the health care industry and its professionals exempt from the planning and the problems familiar to other mature businesses. Simply operating the facility is no longer adequate for hospital administrators. Success and even survival often depend upon an acceptance of innovation and consequently the management of change.

But as health care leaders accept this new ultimatum they also reflect upon those unique challenges that change has failed to resolve. Health care has always been host to a variety of human dilemmas. Reshaping the system of delivering health care or packaging its services in new boxes will not eliminate these concerns. Issues such as quality of life, care for the poor, and the consequences of technological and medical innovations are not disappearing. These ethical concerns have historically defined our profession and today they are confronting concerns that ultimately will determine our future.

Ironically, this confrontation may encourage managers to include an ethical dimension in their decision-making process. Often, health care managers have excused themselves from many of these traditional concerns by suggesting that only the medical community can adequately evaluate ethical concerns.

Naively, management has ignored the fact that many nonmedical decisions have major ethical implications. Within any hospital, administrative decisions on admission policies, allocations of resources, and developing new services require ethical evaluation. These issues continuously test the strength of an organization's values.

Furthermore, as the health care industry makes its awkward transition from a loosely knit structure of parochial providers to a well-defined structure of multisystems, new ethical concerns will be introduced. Leaders who once concentrated solely on delivering a single product, medical care, must now deliver many products. These products may have many prices and may be sold to many different customers.

Some individuals fear that health care providers may ignore their foundations and abandon their missions because of the demands of the transition. Robert

Cunningham discusses this predicament in his book *The Healing Mission and The Business Ethics*. He concludes that today's hospital trustees and administrators "will need all the business brains they can command, but the salvation of their institutions is the moral estate they have inherited."[3] Cunningham's prophecy is challenging. It requires leaders to reflect as they react to a changing environment. It demands that CEOs have confidence in their decision-making skills and a willingness to expose their judgment to ethical scrutiny. To unite an institution's heritage with its present demands requires sharing personal and institutional values throughout the organization. As these fundamental values permeate all levels of the organization, decision-making skills are enriched. Managers understand that values can influence decisions without distorting logic.

For some critics, it is not appropriate to allow values to intrude into corporate decision making. For them, the nature of business and industry has released managers from moral strictures. Paradoxically, formal organizations appear to be privileged to benefit from the contributions of their employees without being ethically responsible for their decisions. Milton Friedman perceives an organization as essentially amoral. Though Friedman does recognize that there may be value conflicts between the goals of the organization and those of the employee, he does not acknowledge corporate responsibility. For example, he suggests that "if a chemist feels it is immoral to make napalm, he can solve his problem by getting a job where he doesn't have to."[4] To evade the situation as Friedman suggests does not resolve the ethical dilemma.

An organization is exposed to and becomes an actor in an ethical system. If this system is internalized by an organization then it affirms certain values and provides a corridor for interaction. The hospital is the setting of the most crucial dialogue between institutions and individuals. Here it is essential that values penetrate the environment. Hospital managers are not exempt from the confusion, temptations, or trauma that surround their decision making, but they must confront the challenges, not avoid them. Good decisions require endurance as well as aim.

Joe McCue, a former president of Hospital Financial Management Association, suggests that hospitals and other providers must internally examine themselves in order to discover ethical options to guide the organization. McCue recommends a "social audit" or an accounting of an organization's contributions to its community.[5] This audit is an effort to renew institutional values. It encourages managers to develop ethical systems. Unfortunately, the social audit does not provide a model for evaluating actual ethical dilemmas. It is reflective and passive; it reports the actions of the organization after they have occurred. Obviously, there is no single model that unaltered can resolve the predicaments health care managers confront. Yet ethical dilemmas do not vanish as Friedman implies; they must be challenged. Ethically sensitive managers can discover solutions within the parameters of their organization. But such solutions occur only when managers are courageous in their efforts to recognize their own values.

DECISION MAKING AND VALUE SYSTEM

The traditional decision-making process has neglected to recognize the impact of value systems. Even the most unscrupulous professional cannot evade certain expressed values or social customs. Typically, such customs are considered prerequisite for "doing business." For example, a personnel manager will not overtly discriminate in hiring staff. The law prohibits such a practice, but society's condemnation of prejudice initiated this law. All decisions are at least minimally influenced by values.

Decision making is a logical and progressive analysis. But at certain stages the process is exposed to value domination. A typical decision-making model is illustrated in Figure 4-1. In this model, values are generated by several sources: professional rules, social mandates, and institutional philosophy. Each source provides some valuable guidelines for defining ethics in the health care setting.

A value system is not stagnant; it is constantly renewed by the decision maker's environment. Obviously not every decision maker will be influenced equally by values. The point to understand is that there does exist a minimal level of values and these directly influence decision making.

As the model indicates, the decision maker's value system is constructed from a variety of variables. Each variable penetrates the decision maker's evaluation

---

Figure 4-1 Decision-Making Process

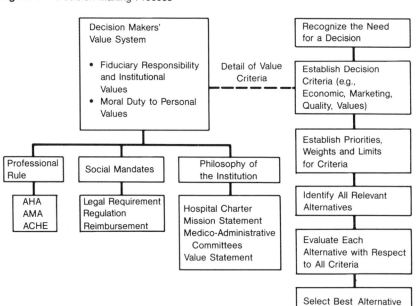

and becomes a determinant of that individual's actions. This conclusion is not astonishing, but neither has it been much explored. In 1982, I surveyed hospital chief executive officers to gain additional insight.[6] The goal was to evaluate administrators' perceptions of the impact of values on managerial decisions. These CEOs were asked to compare their professional ethics with those of other disciplines. Four conclusions were most interesting.

1. Clearly, the respondents perceive ethical dilemmas in the hospital workplace. No CEO denied that ethical implications surround decisions.
2. As CEOs compared themselves with thirteen other professions, they perceived their ethical stature to be outstanding. Collectively, they ranked only the clergy higher than themselves in ethical sensitivity. Tables 4-1 and 4-2 summarize these perceptions.

Table 4-1 Rating Grid of Perceived Professional Ethics, %

	Extremely Unethical	Very Unethical	Moderately Unethical	Half & Half	Moderately Ethical	Very Ethical	Extremely Ethical
Hospital Administrators	0	0	0	0	32	68	0
Physicians	0	0	0	4	52	40	4
Engineers	0	0	0	8	52	40	0
Lawyers	0	0	12	36	40	12	0
Politicians	0	4	36	36	24	0	0
Clergymen	0	0	0	4	4	68	24
Newspaper Reporters	0	12	36	24	24	4	4
TV Reporters	0	12	36	24	26	4	0
Pharmaceutical Salesmen	0	0	4	40	52	4	0
Purchasing Agents*	0	0	0	21	33	46	0
Government Regulating Agents*	0	4	0	38	38	21	0
Corporate Managers	0	0	0	16	60	24	0
Personnel Managers	0	0	0	0	60	40	0
Production Managers	0	0	0	16	68	16	0

*n = 24, all others, n = 25

Table 4-2 Ranking of Professional Groups by Perceived Ethical Stature

Ranking Order	Score
Clergymen	512
Hospital Administrators	468
Physicians	444
Personnel Managers	440
Engineers	432
Purchasing Agents	415
Production Managers	400
Government Regulating Agents	370
Pharmaceutical Salesmen	356
Lawyers	352
Newspaper Reporters	284
Politicians	280
TV Reporters	274

Source: Reprinted with permission from *Hospital and Health Services Administration* (1984:102–119), Copyright © 1984, American College of Healthcare Executives.

3. As CEOs make decisions they have a strong allegiance to the values of their organizations and critically recognize their fiduciary responsibilities. They ''often place secondary interest on personal values in order to support the operation and success of the hospital.''[7] CEOs were asked to respond to a set of eight scenarios, each describing an ethical dilemma and requiring an administrative decision. The structure of the scenario forced the respondent to evaluate institutional and personal values. Examples 1–4 illustrate the CEOs' positions as they confronted difficult predicaments.*

Example 1: A Sweet Deal

Ralph Adams is the administrator at Crossville Hospital. Prior to his work in administration, Adams was a product manager for SGA, a computer company. Presently, Adams is reviewing computers for Crossville's laboratories. McKinsey, a SGA salesman and old friend, visits Adams' office. He offers Adams a computer discounted below actual cost. In exchange for this offer Crossville Hospital is to endorse the equipment, and Adams is to encourage colleagues to review SGA's computers. Adams:

1. is within his rights to make the best business deal
   for the hospital.   11%
2. is vulnerable to criticism by solely making this decision.   27%
3. is attempting to serve two masters.   4%
4. should seek other opinions if he feels uncomfortable
   with the situation.   27%
5. (alternative) _____ 31%

Comment: All respondents were sensitive to the issue of conflict of interest. The

---

*Examples 1–4 are reprinted with permission from *Hospital and Health Services Administration* (1984:102–119), Copyright © 1984, American College of Healthcare Executives.

choices selected and the comments added reveal a concern by the administrators/respondents for their personal job security even though a financial gain for the hospital was possible. One respondent straddled the fence by suggesting a compromise, "Should reveal conflict of interest then recommend best deal for the hospital."

Example 2:   A Conflict of Conscience
Paula Brown, hospital administrator at Mercy Hospital, fundamentally questions the Catholic position on abortion. The policy at Mercy is to refuse any abortion patient. Based upon *Bellin, Allen vs. Sisters of St. Joseph*, Mercy is within its legal rights to have such a policy. Yet, Mercy's physicians often will disguise medical records and falsify documentation in order to perform therapeutic abortions. Brown is aware of these procedures. Should Brown:

1. challenge the physicians despite her present personal
   ambivalence?   38%
2. delay any confrontation until she resolves her own confusion?   0%
3. encourage Board members to resolve the predicament?   35%
4. resign her position because of the present irreconcilable
   dilemma?   8%
5. (alternative) _____   19%

Comment: Though the respondents were divided on the appropriate solution, more than 73% of them believed that this problem should be confronted. It is interesting to note that 38% sought to resolve the dilemma without guidance from the Board of Trustees. Alternative solutions offered varied from "Do nothing" to "It seems to me that the administrator must remain true to her employers as well as to herself." About 8% felt the situation was irreconcilable and the administrator should resign.

Example 3:   Prejudices and Problems
Richard Hunt is the administrator for a small hospital in a southern rural area. Recently, a coalition of foreign nurses offered to help Hunt resolve his nursing shortage. Though this is a solution to a staffing problem, Hunt fears reprisals which the community might present if such an agreement is made. Though Hunt considers himself an affirmative action employer, he is hesitant to challenge community norms. Hunt decides not to pursue the coalition's offer and to continue to struggle with the shortage. His rationale is "Why trade one problem for a bigger problem?" Hunt is:

1. only rationalizing, not confronting his present problem.   30%
2. allowing his perceptions to prejudice his attitude.   12%
3. honest with himself and is correctly approaching the problem.   19%
4. correct in allowing his perceptions of community reprisals to
   affect his attitude.   31%
5. (alternative) _____   8%

Comment: This scenario produced a normal distribution of choices. Apparently, respondents could easily identify with the frustration present in the scenario. The absence of an appropriate professional ethical code is most apparent in these results. Though choices #1 and #4 are opposite in orientation, respondents were divided between the two. The individual ethical perspective was vividly displayed by one comment, "It seems to me that at issue are the health needs of his community which are not resolved by temporizing. Perhaps a frank community-wide discussion of this problem would bring the issue to a successful conclusion."

Example 4: I'll Lose My Job

Smith Hospital has a reputation for outstanding operating room service. Jack Wright, CEO at Smith, has documentation that Dr. Jones, chief anesthesiologist, is personally abusing drugs. Jones' abuse is interfering with his duties. Wright has repeatedly discussed this matter with the Medical Review Committee, but they refused to confront Jones. Therefore, Wright presents the problem to the Board. Without the Committee's evaluation, the Board refuses to initiate any action against Jones. Wright knows that if he pursues the situation any more, it may mean he will lose his job. Wright should:

1. voluntarily leave his position.   0%
2. aggressively continue to pursue the problem.   31%
3. secretly enlist the aid of the medical staff.   19%
4. at this time confront Jones.   27%
5. (alternative) _____ 23%

Comment: The object of this scenario is to measure the appropriateness of utilizing colleagues in problem solving. The respondents were divided as to the correct approach. The comments suggested hesitancy and caution. Two examples are illustrative: "Take no further action at this time" and "Continue to work at enlisting support from medical staff to be able to approach Board. Again legal liability." These statements strongly reveal that our professional code is silent when addressing the administrator/physician interactions.

4.   Professional codes of ethics are not perceived as adequate assistance in making decisions. CEOs made no reference to an institutional policy, charter, mission statement, or professional code for guidelines in reaching a conclusion. This observation has since been verified. Kurt Darr's survey of hospital administrators revealed that 41 percent of the respondents have never used the ACHE Code of Ethics.[8] All of the respondents were either Members or Fellows in the College.

This 1982 survey shows that CEOs perceive themselves as ethical and desire to make good decisions. But it is also obvious that CEOs lack formal guidelines to assist them in their decision-making process. Whether effective guidelines will ever be available is uncertain. It is quite evident that CEOs must implement some structure to define ethical criteria for their organizations. If they encounter difficulty in resolving value conflicts we can assume that their staff members experience this same frustration. A decision model is not adequate to manage an organization. It is critical that employees comprehend the impact of their leaders' actions. They cannot support decisions if they are not aware of the values that influenced the choices. When an organization achieves this realization then the validity of including values in the decision-making process becomes very clear.

IDENTIFYING AND USING ORGANIZATION VALUES

Buried in the archives of every hospital is a mission statement. This document describes the philosophy of the organization and succinctly reveals its traditions.

The nature of the statement allows it to be the ideal vehicle for introducing values in the setting of the organization. Though it is not a list of values, it serves as the foundation for all of the actions and inquiries within the organization. If examined and followed it can aim the organization at the good. The strength of the statement is its uniqueness for each particular organization.

A mission statement will not provide solutions to ethical dilemmas. It can only introduce guidelines. CEOs can use their statements to create an environment receptive to ethical decision making. A list of the ten or twelve fundamental values that truly influence decisions can be constructed. An example of such a value statement is displayed in Exhibit 4-1.

This example is from Northeast Georgia Medical Center, located north of metropolitan Atlanta. Over a period of three years management introduced and now continues to nurture a very strong value-oriented culture management program. Its values demonstrate a recognition of the needs of a variety of constituents: patients, families, physicians, employees, and community. Equally, the statement describes the requirements and commitments necessary for a growing corporation. It clearly provides concrete guidelines for blending intrinsic values into decisions. A value statement is useless if it only reiterates the mission statement. It is critical for the value statement to extract those vital factors that both tradition and reality demand. In turn these factors must be communicated throughout the organization. If a value statement is only a tableau and is not incorporated into the organization's management systems it is incomplete. De-

Exhibit 4-1 Value Statement

WE VALUE . . .

. . . the philosophy that all humans have equal worth.

. . . warm, caring comfort to all patients and their families.

. . . wholistic care of body, mind and spirit.

. . . the philosophy that each person is responsible for his behavior and determines his own degree of success.

. . . open and effective communication.

. . . effective leadership at all organizational levels.

. . . the physical and emotional well-being of employees, demonstrated through competitive salaries and benefits, and a mechanism for personal growth, self-help and wellness.

. . . an attractive, clean, safe hospital with modern technology.

. . . providing a range of services sufficient to meet the health and wellness needs of area citizens.

. . . financial responsibility and cost-effectiveness in meeting the needs of those we serve.

NORTHEAST GEORGIA MEDICAL CENTER

Source: Courtesy of Northeast Georgia Medical Center, Gainesville, GA.

cision models must include values that can be applied. As a value statement is developed it is essential to use and replace those values which no longer serve the organization. This maintenance process should not be a casual effort. It requires management and staff to review the guidance provided by the statement. I strongly recommend that all organizations develop value statements. It is an opportunity to communicate what typically has been described as the intangibles of the organization. The benefits include consistency and completeness in decision making.

IMPLICATIONS

Our health care legacies have provided managers with an intuitive sense for the need to include values in decision making. Our new responsibility is not only to preserve this heritage but to expand its applications.

Having described and illustrated the role of ethics in health care management, I want to explore several implications.

* measurement of values in the decision-making process
* identification of ethical behavior
* development of new methods to introduce ethics into the management setting
* actions for unethical management decision
* influence of administrative decisions or biomedical ethics

Measurement of Values

As shown in Figure 4-1, each decision criterion can be prioritized and weighted. This is a prospective task necessary to provide objectivity to the process. But to verify the total process it is necessary to measure the influence of each criterion retrospectively. No single system can adequately accomplish this analysis of values. In some way managers must begin to describe values and their role in a quantitative manner. Already, many organizations have highly developed financial and planning decision models. It is management's responsibility to use these same skills to design a model that recognizes human values.

Identification of Ethical Behavior

If managers are oriented only toward measuring decisions in terms of right and wrong, it becomes difficult to identify good decisions. This chapter's introduction attempted to define a good decision. This is a continual task. Just as managers must constantly search for the good decision, they must also continue to define their changing role.

For values to be implemented in any organization, managers must develop greater talent in two skills: communications and trust. Ethics is a human process. Managers must learn to listen to their employees, employers, and clients as well as to talk with them. As managers become more dependent upon automated systems to satisfy all of their information needs, they can lose meaningful dialogue on values. Second, as managers we develop relationships based on a high level of trust in order to implement values. If decision makers cannot be confident that their choices will be supported, they will be more hesitant to commit to a value-oriented environment. Management leaders can accomplish their responsibility by stepping into the workplace and demonstrating that good decisions make an organization successful.

New Methods To Introduce Ethics

Managers must move beyond their dependence upon traditional sources, such as attorneys, clergy, and educators, for ethical input. These sources have reminded managers of their ethical responsibilities. However, the penetration of values depends upon managers throughout the work environment rather than exclusive reliance upon experts foreign to the workplace to lead discussions and recommend actions.

Managers must be hearty leaders who can collectively establish a value statement and apply it. Ethics cannot exist on the periphery of an organization. It must be articulated by managers who have the talent and the authority to develop new tools for implementing values.

This implementation will not be adequate unless an organization has a financial commitment to its achievement. Placing new tools into a decision model requires time and creativity. Organizations favoring a decision-making process that includes a recognition of values have made substantial financial investments in developing the process. Equally, the benefits appear to be financially attractive. The decision to construct and implement a new model should be based on its financial feasibility.

For some organizations such a model can be accomplished only in phases. Executing a program in this manner may extend the total implementation, but visibility demonstrates that management is aware of the benefits of an enhanced model.

Actions for Unethical Decision

As ambitious as management may be in identifying and applying values in the workplace, unethical decisions will continue to occur. The response to these actions is part of the entire process of utilizing values. Management must be prepared to address unethical actions for reasons in addition to legal considerations. The strength of a decision model and the vitality of the organization's culture will suffer greatly if appropriate responses do not occur.

Obviously, an organization's personnel policies will guide managers as they uncover ethical improprieties. But two factors are crucial for all organizations. First, the organization should have an overall administrative policy clearly stating the values and the importance of their adherence. Second, management should be flexible in the evaluation of a violation. If we return to our earlier definitions we recall that ethics is a process and that values evolve. Obviously, some improprieties are so very severe that they may destroy a deeply held value. In these cases strong actions are required. Other violations may be less destructive. For this discussion the critical aspect to recognize is that not all values are of equal importance to the organization. Part of the management process associated with applying values is to prioritize and weight them.

Influence of Administrative Ethics in Biomedical Ethical Dilemmas

Perhaps the most important implication is the interaction of administrative and biomedical ethics. As we have said, managers have been reluctant to participate in biomedical dilemmas. But as the environment changes managers will be driven into these decisions. Ultimately, both fields of ethics will probably collapse into a single decision-making process.

This new effort will require increased discussions among all professions. No longer will dilemmas be delegated to a single group for resolution. This area will require an organization to be highly creative as well as dedicated to conflict resolution. An ethics committee is one example of an attempt to create a multidiscipline team to address ethical dilemmas. In most instances these committees limit their discussions to medical issues, a major shortcoming. If a hospital desires to apply values to all decisions, administrative issues require the same conscientious attention as medical ones. Structuring a vehicle to accomplish this goal is essential.

CONCLUSION

Dilemmas, decisions, and values are words that haunt managers. Behind each term lies an abundance of frustration. It would be emotionally desirable to eliminate these terms and ignore their implications, but such action would be to deny our responsibilities as managers. Furthermore, if we agree with Paul Lehmann we would be violating the process that makes "human life human." It would appear that these issues cannot be avoided. Therefore, if we must confront them we need to develop a structure to assist us. Whether this structure is a new decision model or a value statement, the goal is the same: to recognize that many variables influence all actions. Managing the outcome of these actions is the ultimate goal.

As managers examine the decision-making process, they will recognize that values often complicate decision making and what once appeared to be right decisions may become quite inadequate. As the process is explored, management can and should become obsessed with making good decisions by carefully considering the impact of values.

NOTES

1. W.D. Ross, "Aristotle: Ethic Nicomachea," in *Approaches to Ethics*, W.D. Jones et al. (New York: McGraw-Hill, 1969), p. 54.

2. Paul L. Lehmann, *Ethics in a Christian Context* (New York: Harper and Row, 1963).

3. Robert Cunningham, *The Healing Mission and The Business Ethics* (Chicago: Pluribus Press, 1982), p. 302.

4. James M. Humber, "Milton Friedman and the Corporate Executive's Conscience," *Philosophy in Context* 10 (1980):72.

5. H.T. Lindsey, "Social Auditing," *Hospital Financial Management*, May 1979, p. 32.

6. Charles L. Gregory, "Ethics: A Management Tool? A Profile of the Values of Hospital Administrators," *Hospital and Health Services Administration*, March/April 1984, pp. 102–119.

7. Gregory, "Ethics," p. 107.

8. Kurt Darr, "Administrative Ethics and the Health Services Manager," *Hospital and Health Services Administration*, March/April 1984, pp. 120–136.

Part II
Access to Health Care

Chapter 5

Access to Health Care

Fredrick R. Abrams, MD

Access to health care is like one leg of a three-legged stool. It can be looked at individually, but if it is separated from the other two legs, the cost and the quality of health care, like the stool it will not stand alone. Hence, when we consider access, we must frequently range into cost and quality areas. Speaking of one often implies the consequences to the others. Our social and political system locks them together.

THE SPECIAL NATURE OF HEALTH CARE

Why is health care currently of such special consideration that society concerns itself with broad issues of access? The President's Commission for the Study of Ethical Problems in Medicine and Biomedical and Behavioral Research addressed the issues of securing access to health care in three volumes. The special importance of health care is attributed to its role in relieving suffering, preventing premature death, restoring function, increasing opportunity, providing information about an individual's condition, and giving evidence of mutual empathy and compassion. Because of its special importance, health care must not, the commission concluded, be left to the marketplace, thus becoming virtually the only facet of American life for which such an exception is asked.

THE STANDARD OF HEALTH CARE

In discussing the securing of health care, the President's Commission noted two important traditions, (1) responsibility for oneself and (2) the obligation of the community to the individual. Their recommended standard was phrased as "access for all to an adequate level of care without the imposition of excessive burdens."

The undefined factor in the President's Commission's excellent publication, that is, the "adequate level," remained unspecified. But it was made clear that this remains undefined because it will change, depending on the macroallocation of health care funds in competition with other worthy societal needs, the effectiveness of various treatments in dealing with particular problems, and how society sees health needs.

Clearly, in legislating the translation of the ethical obligation to provide access to health care into a civil right, the access cannot mean all beneficial care. Society would be overwhelmed by the diversion of so many resources to health care. The backlash would create an atmosphere of total abrogation of any ethical imperatives. We are seeing harbingers of this in the evolution of Medicare, begun as an equal distribution of goods (medical care) regardless of ability to pay. Cost-plus reimbursement gave a blank check to providers whose incentives were to test the far reaches of marginally beneficial care, since both patients and providers could only gain.

Then the prospective payment plans changed the incentives, at least for hospitals, by offering a package rate tied to a diagnosis. Any money saved is "profit" for the hospital. The less spent on the patient, the more the hospital benefits. Some hospitals are even offering to "split the difference" with doctors who save money.[1] This is a small example of the governmental backlash to runaway spending and the resulting ingenuity of providers, by adopting a business rather than a medical ethic, to modify behavior accordingly.

MACROALLOCATION—SOCIETAL AMBIGUITY

There is sharp disagreement between those who feel there is an ethical basis for ranking health care first in societal allocations, and those who feel that cross-cultural comparisons indicate little consensus for a universal ethical imperative ranking health care so high. Clearly, members of our own society vary greatly in ranking health when one considers the spectrum of health-risky behavior in which they participate. Shelp[2] discusses the subterfuges involved in politically determined macroallocation when values are in conflict. He points out that pluralistic societies selecting from two conflicting values try to preserve the appearance that neither fundamental value has been abandoned. Society uses a two-step technique. First, it determines how much will be produced (either because of true scarcity or because of preference in priority); then it decides who gets it. Society pretends that the rationing is unavoidable and no longer a choice. Thus, we have been told that the fraction of the Gross National Product devoted to health care has reached its limit.

When a society doesn't address the issue of allocation, economics fills in the vacuum. This has been the trend since the halcyon days of Medicaid and Medicare. Is that the best basis for distributing such a basic need? If we require copayments, or decrease services, or make Medicaid qualifications more stringent, are we truly containing costs or simply shifting them? Does depriving the indigent of care cost more in future work hours lost to society, long-term incapacity at greater expense, or permanent members of welfare rolls? Might not many of us end up as medically indigent if a catastrophic illness occurs? All of us hope to be among the elderly. Should we not protect the elderly now, and ourselves in the future? If we were truly to contain costs, shouldn't the limitations apply to all citizens? We would certainly learn quickly whether 10.5 percent of the Gross National Product is too much to spend if we cut back on the portion that affected the wealthy and the insured, rather than the often politically weak poor of our society, from whichever ethnic or age group they come.

There are at least two sorts of economic concerns that appear to be primary in discussing macroallocative health care expenditures. One is the economic consequences, regardless of who is paying the bill, of using progressively more resources for medical care. For example, it is said that our automotive industry has such a large commitment to health care that our production costs cannot compete with the Japanese production costs, less burdened by health care for their factory workers. The second consideration is our society's perceived obligation to assure that care is available from public funds to all of its members. That means higher taxes or the sacrifice of other national needs that such a commitment necessitates. The cost of good medical care will continue to be high despite efficiencies.

Few have as rigorously questioned the marginal benefit of chrome trim on automobiles, or the unusable and unsafe horsepower available at premium prices. Money for health care recirculates in the economy in the same way as that from the automotive industry. No one appears to want to limit those who want to purchase more than a basic decent minimum of transportation. The difference clearly is that we *do* feel health care is so basic a human need that we feel a moral obligation to provide it to our citizens. It comes out of taxpayers' pockets, unlike automobiles, and it is expensive. Jellinek takes "yet another look at medical cost inflation" and explores the idea that medical markets have incorrectly been assumed to be inefficient because they have not been correctable by either regulation or competition.[3] He proposes that this inefficiency is preferred and perpetuated because the medical care serves a need other than producing health. He speculates that it is a "societal concession" in exchange for the rise in depersonalization and alienation imposed on the individual by post–World War II industrial and economic development. This seeming willingness to value individual human life highly, even by spending inefficiently, becomes an important form of adjustment of the social contract.

MACROALLOCATIONS WITHIN THE HEALTH CARE BUDGET

Within the health care budget, allocations are made to two types of health-seeking interventions. They are (1) prevention and (2) care. Childress points out that the lion's share, about 90 percent, of the federal health budget has gone to the health *care* system, and the remainder was divided among *preventive* allocations to human biology, life-style, and environment. This apparently illogical allocation occurs, he explains, because the reinforcement of fundamental values under many circumstances appears to be more appealing to our society than the achievement of goals, a similar interpretation to that of Jellinek.[4]

Why society prefers sometimes to ignore utility and efficiency is influenced by four factors in resource allocation:

1. Symbolism comes from our penchant for valuing identified versus statistical lives.[5] Using the mining industry, Childress points out that more money will be spent in rescue work after a disaster than would have been needed to avoid one. The myth is that society will not sacrifice lives for mere money. This is less threatened by a failure to allocate for prevention when the inevitable victims are unknown, than if society stinted in rescue efforts for identified people in peril.
2. Fairness arises when, because of inherent dangers in certain jobs assigned by society, we try to balance the hazard by overcompensating allocations when health damage results, even when the expenditures are clearly not efficient.
3. Equal access is exemplified by the fact that treating known hypertensives would be more cost-effective to prevent cardiovascular morbidity and mortality than screening for new cases of hypertension. This would inevitably be disadvantageous to the poor population that, because of limited access, would remain undiagnosed. Thus, perhaps more expensive but preferably more just allocation methods must be found.
4. Liberty is often treasured more than health and, when respected, puts strains on the efficient utilization of resources. (1) Important goals, (2) strong evidence that restrictions on liberty will have the desired result, and (3) using the least coercion are the minimal requisites for overriding the presumption permitting voluntary risk taking. Thus, this valued principle works against efficient utilization of funds if only the goal of good health is considered.

ALLOCATIONS FOR PREVENTION

By now it is conventional wisdom that neither a population's nor a person's health increases proportionately with the dollars invested in health care; that broad and general preventive measures against pathogenic environments and microorganisms yield a much higher return of good health than one-on-one physician-patient intercession; and that health is unquestionably affected by life-style and health-risky behavior and habits. Acknowledging the significant role of prevention, we should try to effect significant changes in personal life-styles by education. We should convince the body politic to change what the President's Commission considers an ethical obligation into a civil right by financing changes to correct the social conditions apparently underlying much of the ill health among the poor.

I am not going to address these important issues at length because, were this all accomplished tomorrow, there would still remain work for the medical professionals. Microorganisms seem to mutate and become insensitive to our magic bullets. And if social conditions were improved so that black youths, whose leading cause of death is homicide, were upgraded to the status of white youths who die in automobile accidents, there would still be a need for physicians and surgeons to treat individuals subject to the trauma of living in our high tech aggressive society.

ALLOCATIONS FOR CARE

I'm going to take the narrow view of access to health care by addressing only that portion of health care defined as crisis or rescue intervention. As it becomes increasingly clear that our society resists increases in the macroallocation to health care, it must face the issues it skirted earlier in this evolution. How shall limited funds be allocated within health care? End-stage renal disease (ESRD) illustrates the dilemma well. Unable to face the ethical and political ramifications of rationing life-saving technology in the 1960s, Congress chose to fund dialysis for all who desired and needed it. Now fewer than 2.5 percent of patients covered by Medicare Part B consume over 9 percent of the expenditures. Despite this disproportionate use of funds, consideration for discontinuing the program has been diverted instead to developing techniques within the allocation for ESRD to improve cost effectiveness. In this way, more patients can be treated within the old limits. There is a shift to home care, which is cheaper, and increasing pressure to acquire kidney donors. Not only is the quality of life after a transplant improved, it also turns out to be much cheaper in the long run. These developments are commendable, and the practice of determining cost effectiveness has been too long delayed by the hypnotic effect of high tech in the belief that it is per se the solution. Cost effectiveness is valuable information for comparing two techniques to treat the same condition, for example, dialysis versus transplant. It can also be used to compare two health care innovations equally desirable to different populations, such as heart transplant versus kidney transplant. When cost-benefit analysis is considered, everything is translated into money as the lowest common denominator, sometimes omitting the quality of life factors and intrinsically bearing an age bias.[6]

A few years ago the federal government appeared unlikely to do more ESRD-type problem solving. A brief flirtation by then HEW Secretary Pat Harris with financing heart transplants ended within months when a little study uncovered the rest of the iceberg, namely the social and economic implications of financing a new and increasingly useful technique. With the advent of a new secretary of HHS, Otis Bowen, a change in policy was announced. By declaring heart transplants nonexperimental, the way was cleared for Medicare and insurance funding. Not unlike the beginnings of the ESRD program, a modest $5 million was envisioned for 65 transplants the first year, anticipated to grow within five years to 143 transplants per year at a cost of $25 million. Age rationing was set forth as a limitation, based on the scientific reason that the prognosis is better in younger patients. Patients over 55 will rarely be chosen, we have been told.

This answers the argument that Medicare rejection of heart transplants as a standard procedure has discriminated against the poor who could not afford a $100,000 operation. But if the total Medicare pie is not increased, what programs must be eliminated to accommodate this new demand? Although it is now limited by the number of hearts available (already the demand has exceeded the supply), social policy will change that. There were 103 transplants in 1982, 730 in 1985, and 300 in the first quarter of 1986. Norman Shumway, M.D., who heads the program at Stanford, estimates that 3,000 persons per year could benefit from this procedure. Recall that the modest ESRD program cost $250 million when initiated and now approaches $2 billion annually. What program will be eliminated to accommodate 3,000 heart transplants annually, if no additional funds will be appropriated?

TECHNOLOGY

Technology has been hailed as the boon and damned as the bane of cost containment. Much technology is devoted to chronic disease to aid in increasing function. These procedures do not cure. To some degree they make the "big picture" worse, since they allow the fatally ill to become chronically ill (for example, treatment of meningomyelocele, shunts for hydrocephalus, renal dialysis). In other cases they increase productivity (for example, the use of artificial joints in an otherwise incapacitated patient).

Inefficient evaluations of technology also contribute to the expense, since without planned programs technology is tried willy-nilly, and much money is spent until techniques are proven useless. Gastric freezing for ulcerative disease of the stomach was used for several years before it was proven to have no lasting benefits, and complications on occasion were more serious than the illness for which it was being employed.

Having a total hip replacement is clearly more expensive than limping and taking pain killers. In a young person, it would be economically sound to make him or her productive. In an older retired person, the mathematics would weigh against it.

An examination of this simple comparison and your own intuition tells you that strict economics does not apply to these health decisions. The intrinsic age bias has been discussed perceptively in an article by Avorn,[7] the title of which,

"Benefit and Cost Analysis in Geriatric Care: Turning Age Discrimination into Health Policy," sums up its message succinctly.

It is critical in the interests of good medicine even prior to good economics to continue to evaluate medical care on a scientific basis. Consensus conferences, controlled evaluation of new instrumentation and techniques, comparisons of alternative treatments for cost effectiveness without losing sight of safety and efficacy, and other data-gathering and disseminating techniques will continue to draw medicine away from its earlier character of an anecdotally-based cottage industry.

Using information primarily drawn from a report by Ruby et al.,[8] I believe that discussion can be extrapolated to technology across the entire spectrum of health care. The Office of Technology Assessment estimated that prior to the acceptance of heart transplantation in 1986, 30 percent of all Medicare inflation was due to new technology, and 50 percent of hospital cost inflation. The pressures for increasing use of technology include (1) the large investments made by industry, (2) the ability of industry to promote products, (3) the exciting and glamorous accomplishments of high tech, (4) the real improvement in health that can occur, (5) the fact that those entrusted to perform high tech procedures can command higher fees, and (6) the fact that hospitals also can obtain higher fees. Even the DRGs initially gave and continue to give more coverage for high tech procedures than for cognitive functions. There are strong political pressures for more coverage of the high tech, high visibility procedures. These incentives have put the pressures on for inappropriate uses, with excess surgical procedures, excessive use of laboratory procedures, and prolonged hospital stays.

Third party coverage of various technologies also serves to promote their use. For example, dialysis quintupled from 1972 to 1980, after Medicare approved payment, and similarly transplants tripled. The standards for approval of technology include (1) that they are effective and safe and (2) that they are not experimental. By and large, in Medicare, these are under the supervision of Health Care Finance Administration (HCFA). The third and fourth requisites are supervised by the contractors for HCFA. They are (3) that the procedure is medically necessary in the individual case and (4) that it is applied by accepted standards in an appropriate setting. No cost criteria are included in these coverage decisions.

An example of the other side of the coin was illustrated by Garraway et al.[9] They demonstrated that new technology reduced the cost of diagnosing subdural hematoma. While health costs in the United States rose 87 percent in general, the CT (CAT scan) resulted in a 15 percent decrease in costs.

In a very comprehensive article, Evans noted that the assessment of any emerging technology must include:

(1) the potential need for the procedure, device, instrument or drug,

(2) the relevant constraints on the availability of the technology (e.g.,

absence of donor organs for transplantation, location of treatment facilities, shortage of trained personnel), (3) the cost-effectiveness, cost-
benefit of the technology assessed in terms of both economic and social
costs, including lives saved, (4) the legal issues pertaining to the adoption and availability of the technology, including risks associated with
its use (e.g., "Where will the technology be made available?; Who is
eligible to receive the technology?; What risks does the recipient incur
in the use of the technology?), and (5) the ethical issues concerning
the selection of recipients of the technology, the allocation of resources
to health care programs, and individual patient rights to health care
regardless of costs and availability. Failure to consider these issues
will make it extraordinarily difficult to anticipate the long-term implications of any emerging or existing technology.[10]

Himmelstein and Woolhandler made a very thought-provoking analysis regarding assessment of technology. They pointed out the results of the Rand
Study, which demonstrated that free health care led to only a slight decrease in
early death for a few people at high risk, and therefore significant cost containment could be achieved by increasing copayments. Coupled with this was the
report of the research testing of cholestyramine, widely hailed as a breakthrough
in coronary disease prevention. The authors speculated that the reception of both
studies was highly colored by the public clamor for cost containment and, in
the second case, for control of heart disease. The former supported inequality
of access due to inability to pay, by implying that little difference in outcome
resulted from copayment requirements. The latter was profitable for the pharmaceutical industry and conformed to a familiar medical model. They then
demonstrated by careful analysis that the cost effectiveness of free care in preventing premature death was actually 3 to 100 times more effective than cholestyramine. Pointing out that the cholestyramine trial was not subject to cost
comparisons, but that free care was compared with highly cost-effective blood
pressure screens, they discussed the implicit value judgments, saying

> Alternative policies would have different health and cost consequences
> that should be analyzed, made explicit, and publicly debated. Perhaps
> the American people and their physicians would choose to condemn
> 30 people to early deaths for lack of free care so that three well-insured
> patients could take cholestyramine and live or a hospital might max-
> imize its DRG income. We doubt it. In facing painful decisions about
> containment of health care costs, the facets of the health care system
> excluded from rigorous evaluation and comparison may be as important
> as the results of the evaluations that are carried out.[11]

This raises issues very much like those in the newly approved heart transplant
program. Who will be denied access to basic care, so that a small number of

patients will have heart transplants? Of course, no one need be denied if no ceiling is placed on health care macroallocation.

This concern was raised by William Knaus: "As more and more of our national wealth is being allocated to sophisticated medical services like intensive care, it becomes more likely that the extraordinary demands of a few desperately ill individuals or the indiscriminate application of a new expensive treatment will threaten the availability of basic medical services."[12] This raises certain issues of distributive justice. Certainly, any technology developed with taxpayers' dollars ought to be available to all citizens. Having put $200 million into the artificial heart, now captured by corporate medicine at Humana, it would be unfair to deny citizens access to the perfected end product. Perhaps now is the time for broad reevaluation. Perhaps now we should decide what technology ought to be government-funded, and therefore justly shared with all citizens. If the government is unwilling to guarantee its citizens the benefits of certain research, perhaps it would be better not to fund it and to concentrate common monies on equal access to the care that is currently available.

THE IMPACT OF AN AGING SOCIETY

The demographics of our aging population are creating a problem, the sheer magnitude of which suggests that previous solutions will not suffice. Without speculating widely on reasons beyond generalities of better nutrition, housing, public health measures such as the decline in smoking, and good treatment and prevention for infectious disease, the fact remains that life expectancy has increased in the United States so that a child born in 1983 could expect to live 74.6 years. The extremes are represented by the white female whose life expectancy would be 78.7 years and the black male whose life expectancy would be 65.4 years. In fact, races other than the white have had more years added proportionately, but they began and continue at a lower expectancy, making a strong correlation with socioeconomic status. Whereas 8 percent of the population was over 65 in 1950, 12 percent will be by the year 2000, and the old old (over 75) increase disproportionately. This group, not unexpectedly, consumes considerable resources over an extended period of time. In our general population one out of ten persons is limited in performing major life activities. In those over 65, nearly two out of five have such a major limitation. This limitation is defined as being unable to carry on a major life activity in working, or managing a household, or attending school. A significant evolution also is apparent in the allocation of health resources, formerly largely devoted to acute diseases. Now over 80 percent of health resources are devoted to care and treatment of chronic disease.

THE HARVARD MEDICARE PROJECT

For this reason, studies such as the Harvard Medicare Project are extremely valuable for improving access to medical care.[13] The premise of the study is: "That government must continue to play an important part in insuring that elderly people have adequate access to health care services and adequate protection against the costs of illness." The authors' three goals are (1) cost control, (2) fairness in allocation, and (3) simplicity in administration of the program.

Addressing the issues of copayments and premiums, they point out that co-payments have increased tenfold, burdening the sickest the most. Copayments have no relation to income, so the burden on the poor is disproportionate. They serve as a deterrent to care in the lowest income brackets, and those with chronic illnesses, knowing they will outspend the deductible, find them no deterrent to using care, which was one of the initial purposes. Although premiums have increased from $3 to $15 a month, they have not risen proportionately to co-payments. The authors recommend that premiums be increased, since they are predictable, not disproportionately weighing on the sicker patients, and they can be related to income. Regarding long-term care, they point out that 25 percent of health care costs for the elderly were for the long term. Medicare pays only small amounts for home care and almost none of the non-M.D. outpatient care. Medicaid payments vary from state to state, but many times a patient must be impoverished to qualify.

Blumenthal et al. point out that private insurance fails by being too costly by the time a person purchases it in consideration of later years; that, fearing overuse, companies don't offer a full range of services; and that retirees generally are purchasing individual, rather than group, insurance, and this adds additional costs. They suggest that increased access would be made possible by two major reforms. (1) Extended nursing home insurance could be a mandatory insurance coverage, and those who are living in such facilities would pay 80 percent of their Social Security to the facility. Various copayments and admission screening boards could avoid inappropriate use. (2) The 10 to 20 percent of nursing home inhabitants who are there because there is no outpatient service could be served by long-term outpatient care coverage.

They further suggest an annual physical exam with specified components demonstrated to be effective screening techniques. They recommend reforms in physician payments first by encouraging patients to enroll in a prepaid plan, then by setting a relative value scale with a total federal target budget adopted yearly to recover any excess spending from the previous year, and finally, by instituting mandatory assignment. Reforms in hospital payments would result from a better-designed prospective payment system, with more state participation under federal regulation, including state and federal systems for the uninsured. Finally, HMOs would be encouraged to take Medicare patients, but they would be regulated to prevent discriminatory selection by avoiding costly patients, and peer review organizations would continue to evaluate quality.

THE POLITICAL PROCESS AND ACCESS

Clearly, the "trickle down" philosophy of economics has had a good deal of impact in a different sense in the provision of medical care. The emphasis on cost containment in health care, whatever the consequence, seems to have spread from Washington throughout the country. John Iglehart said,

> The Federal Government's open-ended commitment to finance medical care for the nation's elderly population and eligible poor people has been reduced by wholesale reductions in spending . . . these changes in health policy reflect three important trends: The government's preference for cutting spending by reducing payments for care rather than paring benefits, a stronger congressional commitment to health programs targeted for the poor than administration policies would afford, and overall, a demonstration that health care as a political issue has lost some of its allure as costs have spiraled . . . on the whole . . . the important change is that Congress has abandoned its established practice of protecting health care programs from the budgetary knife.[14]

Has there been real cost containment, or have economic pressures simply resulted in decreased access? And has this decreased access had health consequences?

In 1982 California eliminated 270,000 medically indigent adults from Medicaid and transferred responsibility to the counties, accompanied with block grants equal to 70 percent of the estimated funds that would have been allotted to Medicaid. A group of researchers from UCLA followed 186 adults who were discontinued from Medicaid eligibility and compared them with 109 adults who were able to continue at the UCLA clinic because they had funding other than Medicaid.[15] After six months, the general health of the indigents had worsened, and the study concluded that such cutbacks have serious medical implications.

A 1982 article on Medicaid says that it has been far more valuable than commonly realized. This article also points out that policymakers can choose two general strategies for cutting costs:

> To reduce substantially the numbers of poor and nearly-poor people who are covered by public sector health programs and to reduce the comprehensiveness of the health benefits currently provided to these recipients. . . . The second strategy is to make highly-selective, professionally-determined cuts where they will do the least harm, and to change some of our current arrangements for providing health care to

change some of our current arrangements for providing health care to the poor.[16]

Eli Ginzberg pointed out that former Medicaid eligibles' costs had not been contained; they were simply shifted to the indigents themselves, to philanthropy, to doctors and hospitals. When none of these are operative, there is simply no access.[17] Techniques such as the certificate of need for new technology, for example CAT scans, give little thought to the danger and cost of patient transport and the value of eliminating invasive procedures such as pneumoencephalograms. I have already referred to work such as that by Garraway et al.[18] demonstrating that impeding the use of such technology can in fact interfere with true cost containment.

The difficulty of obtaining real political consensus was demonstrated in the special report "Public Attitudes About Health Care Costs: A Lesson in National Schizophrenia,"[19] in which the authors drew from 15 national public opinion polls conducted between 1981 and 1984 by a number of different national pollsters. They stated that

> most Americans are not troubled by the growing share of the nation's economy that is devoted to health care. In fact, most believe that our society currently spends too little rather than too much for these services. . . . The public is quite enthusiastic (66 percent) about requiring low-income people to use less-costly clinics or HMOs. . . . Only 21 percent of Americans are in favor of rationing costly new technological approaches. In fact, 90 percent of Americans favor the continued development of highly expensive heart, kidney, and other organ transplantations. . . . Though polls show public support for the Medicaid program, in practice, eligibility for Medicaid is closely linked to the nation's welfare programs, and in striking contrast to medical care, welfare is an area in which most Americans (71 percent) want no additional spending.

One of the conclusions from these surveys was that "Americans want the problem of rising health care costs addressed. However, they are unwilling to support the adoption of any solution that would produce a dramatic change in their own medical care arrangements."

The dangers of applying certain economic concepts to medical care are pointed out by several authors. Sabatini warns against devices that obscure the abandonment of basic values.[20] He notes that mathematical equations express ratios without any risk factors. Economic efficiency is justified by limited resources. When placed in a formula with medical values, one or the other value dominates. For example, individuals might benefit significantly from treatment that was economically unsound for a group, but the formula would obscure this.

THE IMPACT OF ECONOMICS ON ACCESS TO HOSPITALS

With the DRG system and tightened requirements for private insurance eligibility and amounts of coverage, hospitals became unable to shift costs, leading to another limitation of access that has gone under the name of "dumping." Journals have published articles with distressing titles like "Economic Considerations in Emergency Care: What Are Hospitals For?"[21] "No Insurance, No Admission,"[22] "Economic and Legal Considerations in Emergency Care,"[23] and "Patient Transfers: Medical Practice as Social Triage."[24] Schiff et al. discuss a dramatic increase in the patients transferred to Cook County Hospital, coincident with state and federal funding reductions that began in 1980.[25] They prospectively followed 467 patients, 89 percent of whom were black or Hispanic, 81 percent unemployed, and 87 percent without adequate insurance. Only 6 percent had written consent to transfer, 22 percent needed intensive care, and 24 percent were unstable at arrival. The average age of the patients was 36, and 78 percent of them were male. The reasons given for transfer: 87 percent had no insurance, 4 percent were transferred for tertiary care. Only 13 percent were insured, compared with 70 percent of regular admissions and 92 percent of patients in short-term general hospitals.

The Schiff study points out that these transfers resulted in an average treatment delay of 5.1 hours, with a range of 1 to 18 hours. Although these patients were accepted in a fine medical facility, clearly some of them suffered by the lack of access at the facility they entered first. Note that the Joint Commission on Accreditation of Hospitals from the American Medical Association states: "Individuals shall be accorded impartial access to treatment or accommodations that are available or medically indicated regardless of race, creed, sex, or national origin, or sources of payment for care."[26] Although we are addressing this primarily from the point of view of access, note that nonreimbursable costs to the hospital were estimated at $24 million, or 12 percent of the total annual budget, demonstrating a shift of costs from private to public hospitals. This, of course, reflects on access later in the fiscal year when budget overruns limit admissions. Relman congratulates the state of Texas, which passed a law in April 1986 insisting on a valid consent and valid medical reasons for transferring patients. He points out that two-thirds of indigent care used to be in private voluntary hospitals but that these institutions, unable to shift costs, have joined the trend to transfer uninsured patients to public institutions.[27] Naturally, these patients had never been welcome at investor-owned hospitals.

The economic crunch has changed access in other ways—witness the report of Hein.[28] Thirty-seven percent of the births in Iowa are in small community hospitals that offer accessible and affordable obstetric service to rural Iowans. Regional systems afford backup for complications, but the statistics of the rural hospitals were favorable regarding neonatal mortality, incidence of low birth weight children, survival of low birth weight children, and neonatal deaths.

However, these services are expensive, since all obstetric programs must have certain essentials that individuals couldn't afford. They include electronic fetal monitoring, life support systems, anesthesia, blood products, promptly available operative services for cesarean section, and standby personnel for unpredictable hours and varying occupancy. There must be a nursery nurse available for even one baby.[29] With new restraints that prevent cost shifting from prospective payment programs such as the DRGs, Hein and Klein feel that, unless the community is willing to subsidize these programs some other way, accessibility will be severely limited for a significant percentage of rural Iowans. If there is a shift to home delivery as a consequence, the quality of care may suffer measurably.[30]

THE IMPACT ON THE PRACTICING PHYSICIAN AND THE ISSUES OF MEDICAL ETHICS, COST CONTAINMENT, AND ACCESS

A letter to the *New England Journal of Medicine*[31] points out that, over three decades, articles dealing with insurance reimbursement, economic policy, and cost have quadrupled in the correspondence file, quintupled in the articles published, and more than doubled in the editorial columns, showing an increasing concern throughout the profession with these issues.

The narrow line between medical decisions and economic decisions is evident in Curran's discussion of a Supreme Court decision in which patients brought suit protesting their transfer from skilled nursing homes to a facility with lower levels of care.[32] The reason, of course, was that programs would not be reimbursed at that lower care level.

The New York Medicaid system has a utilization review program. The patients, however, sought federal constitutional protections of due process. The majority of the Court said that doctors' decisions sending them to lower levels of health care did not represent a state action but rather a medical judgment based on professional standards. The dissenting opinions said that standards of utilization review were developed by state and legislative constructs and were not medical standards. The purpose, they said, was strictly cost containment. Curran, a lawyer, comments: "There is a thin line between activities that can be described as primarily clinical, and others that could reasonably be considered exercises of socio-economic judgment and allocation of public resources." He concludes by asking whether doctors' decisions on behalf of the state ought to be beyond federal due process guarantees. This, of course, raises the question of the physician's role in cost containment. Norman Levinsky points out the increasing pressure on physicians to serve two masters by considering society's needs as well as each patient's needs in deciding limits of medical care. Arguing eloquently that the physicians are required to do everything they believe may benefit each patient within the limits that are selected politically, he takes a position of strong patient advocacy.[33]

Stone points out that, at the very least, the patient has the right to know not only the risks and benefits of alternative treatments but also when cost-benefit analysis is playing a part in the doctor's recommendations. Even then, he feels, "to reveal them may threaten the trust and confidence of patients even in 'caring physicians'" in which case he points out that "caveat emptor" will be more relevant than "primum non nocere" in doctor-patient relationships.[34]

JOINT VENTURES—COST, QUALITY, ACCESS

Economic changes have brought about entirely different aspects of care among the entrepreneurs in the medical profession, the undertaking of "joint ventures." *Physician Financial News* reported on an American Hospital Association survey of 700 hospitals (out of approximately 6,000 hospitals in the United States).[35] Nearly one-third have one or more joint ventures, and 64 percent of the partners in these ventures are physicians. The advantages for the hospitals include increased physician loyalty, expansion of their services, and involvement in primary care. For both doctors and hospitals, joint ventures offer investments and tax shelters. They include such things as private practice organizations; medical buildings; health maintenance organizations; ambulatory care centers, including alcohol rehabilitation, osteoporosis diagnosis and treatment, and weight disorder clinics; individual practice associations; and free-standing surgery, imaging, and emergency clinics. They have grown up most commonly where the competition is greatest.

Their problems are, in economic terms, underutilization and long start-up periods. But there are concerns other than economic concerns related to access because of the business framework and profit motive in which these medical interventions are couched. What will be the physician's first response to an uninsured or indigent patient? Will a physician refer such a patient to a service in which the physician has invested? If he has commitments to business partners, what will be his attitude and what will be his influence regarding the traditional free care offered to the patient unable to pay? In short, will his first consideration be patient or profit?

Relman has pointed out that for-profit health care is now a $35 to $40 billion industry.[36] He notes that physicians must act as discerning purchasing agents for their patients and ensure that no conflict of interest arises. Close attention must be paid to see that the public interest is placed ahead of the stockholders'. Several state legislatures have gone beyond casual admonitions. In California, a physician who owns a five percent or $5,000 interest in an imaging center must inform his patients and mention alternative sites. Michigan bars doctors from referring patients to any imaging center in which the doctor holds a share, and Pennsylvania will not reimburse Medicaid patients if their doctor holds an interest in an MRI center.[37]

MICROALLOCATIONS

By now it is clear that there are layers of macroallocations and layers of microallocations, but at the bottom rung is the allocation under the supervision of the individual physician. This is the first step, and from the patient's point of view, the most important. Here is the gate. Is the physician a guard defending against the enemy, all of those who would enter and consume the wonderful provisions beyond? Or is he or she a host, welcoming reluctant visitors and guiding them through frightening passages and unknown tests until safety and health are attained insofar as possible?

As a group, society would do well to consider themselves as individuals. They ought not enlist the physician to be their collective agent, for placing the physician in that role leaves the isolated patient without help in the struggle to regain health and autonomy. Physicians may properly be called upon to advise society on cost efficiency or to determine which medical omissions impact more upon children or the elderly, urban or rural dwellers, male or female patients, white or black, rich or poor, or a host of other dichotomous groupings that may be considered statistically. But when a single doctor has committed to a single patient, let the loyalty never be divided. No physician in a one-to-one situation should ever have to decide anything more than "Is this treatment appropriate for this patient?" Its availability to that patient may be decided at another level of allocation, but never should a physician be a double agent, serving the state to allocate resources based on the doctor's appraisal of the patient's social value. Victor Fuchs, in referring to such nonphysician decision making, declared: "This shift in the locus of decision-making will inevitably reduce the power of practicing physicians. To the extent that these decisions set the constraints within which individual practitioners function, however, there will be less need for them to ration care to their patients explicitly."[38]

No obfuscation of the source of the decision should be tolerated. If a resource has been interdicted for an age group or a social group, no attempt should be made to disguise a political decision as a medical one.[39] If a corporation employing a physician has made his or her practice subject to time or resource restrictions, and access is thus limited, the patient must have full knowledge of restrictions not made in the patient's interest.[40] If there are incentives, financial or otherwise, for physicians to limit access for reasons conflicting with their patients' best interests, the physicians must never permit their own interests to take precedence.

There will be judgment calls, of course, and a triad of articles and editorials in the *JAMA* considers how bed availability influences decisions to utilize the intensive care unit in a hospital. Ill-considered use by patients with borderline needs is not only an economic drain, but also bad medicine, as the attention of ICU staff is drawn away from properly selected ICU patients deserving full attention to others who clearly could be as well served in less critical hospital environments.[41,42] Knaus points out in his editorial: "Physicians are in the best position to evaluate competing claims for medical care . . . we cannot do it alone . . . American medicine . . . can never provide unlimited services for every one. Choices have to be made among services and between individuals."[43]

Surely this does not mean that the physician uses no judgment in refraining from prescribing clearly marginal diagnostic or treatment techniques. In an article addressing moral conflicts for physicians in cost containment issues (which of course means access to diagnosis or therapy), Morreim points out that when there is true scarcity, some needs will go unmet, but this does not imply moral wrong. If distribution is just, despite sad consequences no one is wrong.[44] Morreim goes on to say, "[the doctor] need not pretend that his own patients' needs preempt the needs of other patients and the requirements of justice, in order to give his own patients a position of very special priority with their relationship." I am not sure I or the patient would understand precisely what he means by that, because "justice" and "needs of other patients" is so abstract when one is not sick. It becomes very concrete when one is competing for a particular resource. But if Morreim has no reservations about his final sentence, I believe it sums it up very nicely: "Though decision-making in Medicine becomes more difficult with the appearance of scarcity and moral conflict, the basic commitment of medicine need not change: to serve one's patients faithfully to the best of one's abilities."

If we were to expand that concept from the individual physician to society at large, addressing the sick among them, we could say something very similar. "Let us treat all the patients among us to the best of our affluent society's ability, fairly and proportionately to the national wealth and other national needs of our society, whose individual citizens place health care high on their own list of resource allocations."

FINAL THOUGHTS

Some time ago a popular beer commercial implied that you had better enjoy their brew while you had the chance, since "you only go around once." I do not want to sound like a beer advertisement. But clearly the advertising agencies know how to connect with the feelings of a significant segment of Americans. And sympathetic vibes occur when we talk about "only going around once." What's more, they are right (with apologies to the growing segment of our population whose religious beliefs include reincarnation). We members of the health care professions had better pay attention to our constituency. With all due respect to our thoughtful and perceptive colleagues who have considered carefully and written extensively on the need for the physician to participate actively in cost containment efforts, our patients don't want us to save money on their care. Abstractly they agree that health care is too expensive, and that money ought to be saved when tax dollars are used to pay for indigent care, but for them no expense, they feel, ought to be spared. It is a matter of odds and stakes. A diagnostic or therapeutic hundred-to-one shot may be inefficient and uneconomical, but "Doc, that's my leg (or stomach, or wife, or child) you're talking about." Cost containment and cost efficiency are wonderful economic terms, but to paraphrase Rashi Fein, we live in a society, not an economy. Because the stakes are high, patients don't care about long odds or expense. A two-tier delivery of health care is inevitable, because politically we cannot prohibit those in the marketplace from buying all the marginally beneficial care they want and can afford. As a nation, however, we will decide, depending on the national conscience, how much of our wealth we will give to make care accessible to those who cannot deal in the marketplace. Here we can talk about efficiencies and odds—but we know when we deny marginal benefits we are denying some people real benefits. Let us make sure, as citizens of a country with representative government, that we enter the political scene to encourage adequate allocations for the politically weak, making at least a "decent minimum" of health care a right for all Americans.

NOTES

1. "Incentive Payment or Kickback," *Medical World News* 26, no. 14 (July 22, 1985):7.

2. Earl E. Shelp, *Justice in Health Care* (Boston: D. Reidel Publishing Co., 1981).

3. B.P.S. Jellinek, "Yet Another Look at Medical Cost Inflation," *New England Journal of Medicine* 307, no. 8 (1982):496–497.

4. J.F. Childress, "Priorities in the Allocation of Health Care Resources," in *Justice and Health Care*, ed. Earl E. Shelp 1981, 131–150.

5. E. Friedman, "Rationing and the Identified Life," *Hospitals*, May 16, 1984, 65–74.

6. J. Avorn, "Benefit and Cost Analysis in Geriatric Care: Turning Age Discrimination into Health Policy," *New England Journal of Medicine* 310, no. 20 (1984):1294–1301.

7. Ibid.

8. G. Ruby, H.D. Banta, and A.K. Burns, "Medicare Coverage, Medicare Costs, and Medical Technology," *Journal of Health Politics, Policy and Law* 10, no. 1 (1985):141–155.

9. M. Garraway et al., "Impact of Computed Tomography on Subdural Hematoma," *Journal of the American Medical Association* 253, no. 16 (1985):2378–2381.

10. R.W. Evans, "Health Care Technology and the Inevitability of Resource Allocation and Rationing Decisions," *Journal of the American Medical Association* 249, no. 15 (1983):2047–2053, and *Journal of the American Medical Association* 249, no. 16 (1983):2208–2219.

11. D.U. Himmelstein, and S. Woolhandler, "Free Care, Cholestyramine, and Health Policy," *New England Journal of Medicine* 311, no. 23 (1983):1511–1514.

12. W.A. Knaus, "Rationing, Justice, and the American Physician," *Journal of the American Medical Association* 255, no. 9 (1986):1176–1177.

13. D. Blumenthal et al., "The Future of Medicare," *New England Journal of Medicine* 314, no. 11 (1986):722–728.

14. John K. Iglehart, "Health Policy Report: Federal Policies and the Poor," *New England Journal of Medicine* 307, no. 13 (1982):836–840.

15. N. Lurie et al., "Termination from Medi-cal—Does it Affect Health?" *New England Journal of Medicine* 311, no. 7 (1984):480–484.

16. D.E. Rogers, R.J. Blendon, and T.W. Maloney, "Who Needs Medicaid?" *New England Journal of Medicine* 307, no. 13 (1982):13–18.

17. Eli Ginzberg, "Cost Containment—Imaginary and Real," *New England Journal of Medicine* 308, no. 20 (1983):1220–1223.

18. M. Garraway, "Impact of CT."

19. R.J. Blendon and D.E. Altman, "Public Attitudes About Health Care Costs: A Lesson in National Schizophrenia," *New England Journal of Medicine* 311, no. 9 (1984):613–616.

20. J. Sabatini, "Ethics and Economic Appraisals in Health Care," *Soc. Sci. Med.* 21, no. 10 (1985):1199–1202.

21. A.S. Relman, "Economic Considerations in Emergency Care: What Are Hospitals For?" *New England Journal of Medicine* 312, no. 6 (1985):372–373.

22. K. Wrenn, "No Insurance, No Admission," *New England Journal of Medicine* 312, no. 6 (1985):373–374.

23. W.J. Curran, "Economic and Legal Considerations in Emergency Care," *New England Journal of Medicine* 312, no. 6 (1985):374–375.

24. D.U. Himmelstein et al., "Patient Transfers: Medical Practice as Social Triage," *American Journal of Public Health* 74 (1984):494–496.

25. R.L. Schiff et al., "Transfers to a Public Hospital," *New England Journal of Medicine* 314, no. 9 (1986):552–557.

26. *Joint Commission on Accreditation of Hospitals Standards* (Chicago: JCAH, 1986), xvi.

27. A. Relman, "Texas Eliminates Dumping," *New England Journal of Medicine* 314, no. 9 (1986):578–579.

28. H.A. Hein, "The Status in Future Small Maternity Services in Iowa," *Journal of the American Medical Association* 255, no. 14 (1986):1899–1903.

29. N.L. Klein, "Small Maternity Services," *Journal of the American Medical Association* 255, no. 14 (1986):1923–1924.

30. Ibid.

31. M.V. Klein and G.W. Small, "Money and Medicine," *New England Journal of Medicine* 311, no. 8 (1984):542.

32. W.J. Curran, "Medical Standards and Medical Ethics in Utilization Review for Nursing Homes," *New England Journal of Medicine* 308, no. 8 (1983):435–436.

33. Norman Levinsky, "The Doctor's Master," *New England Journal of Medicine* 311, no. 24 (1984):1573–1575.

34. A.A. Stone, "Law's Influence on Medicine and Medical Ethics," *New England Journal of Medicine* 312, no. 5 (1985):309–312.

35. *Physician Financial News*, March 15, 1986.

36. A.S. Relman, "The New Medical Industrial Complex," *New England Journal of Medicine* 303, no. 17 (1980):963–970.

37. *Business Week*, July 14, 1986, 70.

38. V.R. Fuchs, "The 'Rationing' of Medical Care," *New England Journal of Medicine* 311, no. 24 (1984):1572–1573.

39. F.R. Abrams, "Patient Advocate or Secret Agent," *Journal of the American Medical Association* (1986) accepted for publication.

40. F.R. Abrams, "Caring for the Sick: An Emerging Industrial Byproduct," *Journal of the American Medical Association* 55, no. 7 (1986):937–938.

41. M.J. Strauss et al., "Rationing of Intensive Care Unit Services: An Everyday Occurrence," *Journal of the American Medical Association* 255, no. 9 (1986):1143–1146.

42. H.T. Engelhardt, Jr. and M.A. Rie, "Intensive Care Units, Scarce Resources, and Conflicting Principles of Justice," *Journal of the American Medical Association* 255, no. 9 (1986):1159–1164.

43. W.A. Knaus, "Rationing."

44. E.H. Morreim, "Cost Containment: Issues of Moral Conflict and Justice for Physicians," in *Theoretical Medicine* No. 6 (Hingham, Mass.: D. Reidel Publishing Co., 1985), 257–259.

Chapter 6

DRGs and the Rationing of Hospital Care

E. Richard Brown, PhD

INTRODUCTION

Do the changes forced on the health care system by Medicare's prospective payment system and other cost containment efforts mean we have entered an era of rationed medical care?

Until the past few years, commercial health insurance companies typically paid hospitals their charges, and Medicare and Blue Cross generously paid hospitals their costs, except some that were disallowed. Under cost-based and charge-based reimbursement methods, hospitals can maximize revenues by doing as much for—and to—patients as possible. This retrospective reimbursement encourages hospitals and doctors to maximize the intensity of hospital care, especially for those portions of the hospital that can be turned into revenue-producing centers. These reimbursement methods are essentially open-ended, generating total program and national expenditures as though providers were drawing on a limitless line of credit. Between 1965 and 1982, total national expenditures for hospital care increased 964 percent, from $12 billion to $135 billion, while the gross national product increased only 444 percent.[1]

Responding to these dramatic increases in hospital costs, which absorbed over 70 percent of Medicare benefits and were thus a major factor in Medicare's growing fiscal crisis, Congress adopted Medicare's present prospective payment system (PPS).[2] In 1983 Medicare began paying hospitals a flat amount for each patient's admission, with the amount dependent mainly on the patient's assignment to one of 468 diagnosis-related groups (DRGs). Each patient's DRG classification is based primarily on his or her principal diagnosis, although some assignments are based in part on surgical procedure, age, sex, and other information that is believed to influence the amount of hospital resources that usually would be used. Once a patient has been assigned a DRG, the hospital's reimbursement amount is substantially determined (unless the patient's costs or length of stay makes his or her case an "outlier").

69

Medicare and other reimbursement systems that pay providers a flat amount per illness episode or per day reverse hospitals' traditional financial incentives. Hospitals are under pressure to weigh more carefully every major purchase and labor expenditure. Every service that was formerly billed separately but is now included in the DRG payment is no longer a source of revenue, only an expense. Under the DRG payment system, hospitals have an incentive to do as little to—and for—a patient as they possibly can. This is clearly rationing.

But is rationing new to health care in the United States? The word "rationing" usually conjures up images of government-imposed allocation systems that result in long waits for scarce resources. We think of long queues for consumer goods in times of war and in many socialist countries even in peacetime. We assume that rationing should be generally unnecessary in a highly industrialized capitalist society. In medicine, many physicians believe, rationing would restrict patients' rights to get the care they need, and it would restrict health professionals' abilities to give the care they deem necessary for their patients.

This view that rationing, especially in medicine, is new or somehow "un-American" doesn't square with reality. Medical care has *always* been rationed in the United States. Rationing is defined in several ways, but it is essentially any method of allocating or distributing resources or goods that are scarcer than the demand for them.

We generally think of rationing as government policies and procedures to control the allocation of scarce goods. Rationing by public policy usually is intended to assure some degree of equity in the distribution of scarce commodities. I will call rationing by deliberate policy "intentional rationing," whether it is based on policy adopted by public agencies (like Congress or the Medicare program) or private ones (like an insurance company or a hospital). But in the absence of deliberate policy, scarce goods are likely to be rationed by market forces, what I will call "nonintentional rationing." Market forces tend to allocate scarce goods or commodities by the ability to pay the prevailing market price, which is called price rationing. In the simplest form of nonintentional rationing, market prices are determined by the demand for the commodity and its supply, but in health care as in other economic sectors, price is also influenced by monopolistic action of producers and sellers and by the availability of subsidies. Health care providers may gain sufficient control of the market for their services to manipulate the supply or price artificially. Alternatively, some public or private "third party" may organize an insurance or subsidy system that protects consumers from the immediate financial impact of purchasing health services.

Thus, the market system in which health care is produced and distributed tends to ration its services and products by the ability to pay for them. These market forces may be modified by public policy, which uses planned rationing methods to achieve publicly determined objectives, or by private action, which manipulates the market through privately planned methods such as insurance programs or monopolistic action. The widespread belief that rationing is imposed by government on medicine is testimony only to how "natural" the market system seems—and how invisible its mechanisms have become. Our initial question should be revised: The issue is not *whether* Medicare's DRG hospital payment system rations care, but rather *how it alters the existing system of rationing.*

FORMS OF RATIONING IN HEALTH CARE

Rationing has several important aspects relevant to health care. First, rationing may be imposed on either of two *subjects*, providers and users. Health care providers may be institutions—like an HMO, hospital, or clinic—or individual practitioners—like a doctor, dentist, or nurse. When rationing is imposed on providers, they must decide whom to treat and whom not to treat and what methods and resources to use. Users, the individual patient and the patient's family, must decide whether to spend money or time obtaining health care instead of spending it some other way, assuming they have the resources to make such a choice in the first place.

Second, rationing may be imposed at different *levels* of society or the health care system. The societal level affects all providers or the whole population within a society or a state; the programmatic level affects only providers and users covered by a particular third party payer, financing program, or service delivery system. These levels are not mutually exclusive, since rationing at any level often requires additional rationing at one or more levels below it.

Third, rationing may employ several *methods*. One involves directly controlling the budget of a national health system, health program, or institution. The budget may be essentially a line item allocation of resources, specifying expenditures from capital construction to laboratory microscopes, from the number of surgeons to the number of ward clerks. Alternatively, only the budget limits may be set, leaving the specific allocation to each level of the system, program, or institution. This approach leaves considerable latitude to each institutional level to decide how best to allocate its available resources, enabling people with more professional or managerial autonomy to make decisions utilizing their technical skills as well as their social values. Capitation payment systems for physicians' services exemplify this more general budgeting method, in which physicians operate within budgetary constraints and merge technical judgments and social values in their daily work. Mechanic calls approaches like this "implicit" rationing because these methods "do not specify what services should be provided or what assessments physicians should make, but achieve their effects by placing greater pressures on doctors to make hard allocation choices."[3]

Nonbudgetary methods are also used to influence the decisions institutions, individual providers, or patients make. One approach involves direct regulation of decision making, such as requiring permits for capital investment and construction (for example, certificate-of-need laws) or regulating the prices of goods and services sold in the health care marketplace (as rate-setting commissions do). Another nonbudgetary approach relies on the market to ration care—financial incentives to influence institutional or individual provider decisions, or the behavior of patients who must weigh the need for health care against other economic and noneconomic needs. For example, in order to restrict the use (and thus total costs) of health services by persons covered by insurance, health insurance plans usually impose exclusions (medical conditions and services not covered), deductibles (out-of-pocket payments required before benefits begin), copayments (a percentage of the costs beyond the deductible for which the patient is responsible), and limitations (upper dollar or service limits for an illness or year beyond which the plan's coverage ends).

It is not enough, however, merely to classify rationing approaches. Imposing rationing on users as opposed to providers, on one level rather than another, and using one method versus another affects who gets care and how much and what kind of care they get. Some important policy questions that we must ask are: Does a particular measure affect the availability of services, that is, the supply and distribution? Does it alter the access to and use of services, that is, the volume of services used by different population groupings? Does it affect the quality of care, for example, the types of care (the mix of particular medical methods or technologies used) or the intensity of care (the amount of given methods or technologies used)? And finally, does it really affect the costs of care? And if it does affect costs, does it affect total system costs, or only one payer's costs? Does it shift costs to other payers, including consumers?

RATIONING IN THE MEDICAL MARKET

In the late 1920s, when virtually no one in the United States was insured for medical expenses, a study by the Committee on the Costs of Medical Care found that persons in upper-income families averaged one and a half times as many hospital admissions each year as members of low- and moderate-income families. Hospital care, as well as other types of medical care, varied directly with income.[4]

The unfettered market system thus rationed hospital care by price to those who could afford it. As a presidential commission on medical ethics concluded half a century later, "When health care is distributed through markets . . . an acceptable distribution is not achieved; indeed, given limitations in the way markets work, this result is practically inevitable."[5] In addition, many working-class and middle-class people who could afford ordinary medical expenses were impoverished by the extraordinary expenses of hospitalization when they simply had to be hospitalized. Simple price rationing also created severe financial instability for hospitals, particularly during frequent downward business cycles. As the Great Depression deepened, many hospitals tottered on the edge of insolvency and some closed their doors. These conditions together created a market for a partial solution—insurance for hospital care.

Private Health Insurance

From their origins in 1929, Blue Cross plans, and later commercial insurance company health plans, grew rapidly. Private insurance socialized the costs of hospital care—that is, it spread each person's financial risks and costs among many thousands of persons—effectively subsidizing individuals' purchase of care from the pooled resources. Insurance thus reduced the effects of price rationing, enabling many more people to use hospital services. It also created a stable financial base for hospitals, enabling them to operate and expand, knowing that their services would be paid for. As the percentage of the population with private hospitalization insurance increased, hospital facilities and use also expanded. Between 1950 and 1965, the number of nonfederal short-term general hospitals increased 14 percent, the number of hospital beds per 1,000 population increased 15 percent, and the rate of admissions rose 24 percent.

But private insurance had its limitations. It reduced but did not eliminate price rationing for those who were relatively well insured. It rationed care by several cost-sharing methods, requiring the insured to weigh the out-of-pocket costs of care against the felt urgency of medical need. And it still left a major portion of the population, especially the elderly and the poor, out of the private health insurance market and therefore left them to the vagaries of price rationing in the market for hospital care.

Government Insurance and Subsidies

In 1965, after years of lobbying by coalitions of labor and the elderly, Congress enacted this country's first broad government health insurance and subsidy programs. Medicare, a federal social insurance program, covers all elderly, disabled, and blind persons. Medicaid, a federal and state welfare program, covers recipients of public assistance under federally subsidized programs for elderly, disabled, and blind persons and families with dependent children, as well as persons in these categories who do not receive welfare cash grants but who are too poor to pay their own medical bills. These programs were intended to increase the economic demand of eligible populations in the medical marketplace, reducing or even eliminating the effects of price rationing.

The combination of private health insurance, Medicare, and Medicaid, as well as expanded public hospital and community health center services, has reduced inequities in the use of health services. Recent national surveys have found that poor adults now make more doctor visits and poor persons of all ages average more hospitalization than the nonpoor. These programs, which were supposed to bring the elderly and the poor into "mainstream" medicine, reduced but did not eliminate the financial barriers by which medical care was rationed.

Cost Containment

From its inception, Medicare adopted rationing methods that prevailed in private health insurance. It included a deductible, copayments, and exclusions of certain services. Within a year of their implementation, Medicare and Medicaid emerged as major expenditures in federal and state budgets. "Cost containment" quickly replaced "equity of access" as the buzz words of the Medicaid program, which was especially vulnerable because it lacked a politically powerful constituency and because it depended on the states for about half its funding. New legislation gave the states more options and power to control and reduce Medicaid costs. This included rationing devices imposed on patients, such as restricting eligibility by reducing maximum income levels or dropping optional groups from Medicaid, eliminating optional medical services, and imposing cost-sharing by patients to discourage the use of services and the purchase of prescription drugs.[6]

Thus, the context in which DRGs were introduced already included an array of rationing devices that variously limit people's access to medical care. Private insurance enrolls most of the population, but with deductibles, copayments, exclusions, and limitations that restrict insured persons' options to seek care at will. Medicare adopted these same restrictions from the beginning, increasing the dollar amounts of the deductibles and copayments over its 20-year history. Medicaid has tightened eligibility and imposed a variety of restrictions on beneficiaries, including limitations, exclusions, and copayments. These rationing devices have been directed at beneficiaries and have reduced, but not eliminated, price rationing.

Other rationing measures have been aimed more at providers. Federal legislation permitted the Medicare and Medicaid programs to change their reimbursement methods to counter the expensive "reasonable costs" reimbursement to hospitals and "reasonable fee" payments to doctors. These changes reduced program expenditures but also applied pressure on providers to ration care by discouraging their participation in these programs or by limiting the number of Medicaid and Medicare beneficiaries they serve. Legislation also authorized utilization review of hospitals and nursing homes and regulation of capital investment in health facilities in order to limit their supply, since there was ample evidence that increases in the supply of hospital beds per 1,000 population leads to increases in hospital utilization rates and ultimately increases the costs of medical care.[7]

THE CONSEQUENCES OF RATIONING

Before we proceed to examine how the introduction of DRGs has altered the rationing of hospital care, it would be helpful to assess the consequences of these different levels and methods of rationing—that is, how they actually affected patients, providers, and costs.

Effects of Recent Rationing Methods

Many of these changes have tended to reverse the previous trend away from price rationing of health care toward more equitable distribution, once again fostering the inequities that were so pervasive in the period before private health insurance and Medicare and Medicaid.

Eligibility for Medicaid

Controlling or reducing eligibility for a third party program is an example of programmatic rationing aimed at users. Cutbacks in Medicaid eligibility, a cost containment strategy that began in the 1970s and accelerated during the Reagan administration, have reduced Medicaid's role in offsetting price rationing.[8] As income limits have been ratcheted downward, the percentage of poor and near poor persons who qualify for Medicaid has declined. In any given month in 1982, only 38 percent of persons living at or below the poverty level—a very bare subsistence standard of living—were covered by Medicaid, 13 percent were enrolled in some type of employer-provided health insurance, and 49 percent had no private or public insurance at all.[9]

Cuts in Medicaid eligibility and the severe economic recession of the early 1980s, combined with the lack of state or federal requirements that employers provide their workers with health insurance, have increased the ranks of the uninsured. In 1984, an estimated 35.1 million Americans under 65 years of age were without health insurance, an increase of more than 22 percent over 1979.[10] Low-income persons with Medicaid see physicians more often than those without any coverage, and loss of Medicaid coverage has been shown to have a measurable and often seriously adverse impact on health status.[11] Thus, cuts in Medicaid eligibility inflict the full brunt of price rationing on low-income people who have no other insurance coverage.

Cost Sharing by Users

Cost sharing is another type of programmatic rationing directed at users, relying on economic incentives to accomplish its purpose. The Rand Health Insurance Experiment demonstrated the effectiveness of cost-sharing methods in reducing use of health services and total costs of care.[12] However, the study also found that such methods had a detrimental impact on the health of low-income people who were in poor health at the beginning of the study.[13] These experimental study findings confirm other evidence from the California Medicaid program (called Medi-Cal), which used copayments for ambulatory services for beneficiaries and substantial deductibles (known as "share of cost") for medically needy recipients. The copayment for ambulatory care was shown to encourage Medi-Cal recipients to postpone needed care and to encourage physicians to hospitalize patients for care that could have been provided on an outpatient basis (because no copayment was charged for inpatient care).[14] Increased shares of costs imposed on Medi-Cal's medically needy patients in 1982 led to widespread observations that such patients were showing up in doctors' offices, clinics, and hospitals less frequently but much sicker than before the increase.[15]

Cost sharing is also significant in the Medicare program. In 1984, Medicare patients who were hospitalized had to pay a deductible of $356, nothing else through the 60th day, $89 a day for 61st through the 90th day, and $178 a day beyond that up to a lifetime total of 60 such "reserve" days. Medicare Part B insurance required a $75 deductible and 20 percent copayment for all *approved* charges. In addition, Medicare beneficiaries pay monthly premiums for Part B, the full cost of services not covered by Medicare, and additional fees that doctors may charge above what Medicare allows.

Cost sharing may decrease costs, at least in some cases and for some payers, but it may also have a detrimental impact on the health of low-income people who forgo needed care. Whereas simple price rationing is a nonintentional method of allocating health care, these public policies intentionally use cost sharing as a controlled, incremental form of price rationing to allocate health care on the basis of ability to pay.

Market Methods Aimed at Providers

Market incentives directed at providers may ration care by limiting its supply to people enrolled in a particular program. Medicaid programs, for example, generally have maintained low reimbursement rates to physicians and other providers. When one payer maintains low reimbursement rates relative to other payers, providers tend to restrict the supply of their services available to that payer's beneficiaries. Low reimbursement rates ration care at the programmatic level, but also at the level of the individual doctor who must decide whether to accept the low rate and care for Medicaid patients, or to allocate his or her time to more lucrative patients. Many physicians have refused to participate in the Medicaid program. In the late 1970s, just 6 percent of all physicians cared for one-third of all Medicaid patients, and 20 percent of all physicians treated no Medicaid patients at all.[16] Thus, maintaining relatively low reimbursement rates for one set of health care users (in this case, Medicaid recipients) tends to dry up the supply of providers willing to treat them, thereby reducing their access to care.

California in 1982 and Illinois in 1984 enacted selective contracting for hospital services to their Medicaid patients. Taking advantage of the low occupancy rates that have increasingly plagued hospitals, they have limited the number of hospitals eligible to treat Medicaid patients by contracting only with those that offered the state a price it found acceptable. Preferred provider organizations (PPOs) are doing the same with their subscribers. Inpatient care is used infrequently, and its use rates are less sensitive to travel distance than ambulatory care. Therefore, although selective contracting may increase the inconvenience of affected hospital users, to the extent that it covers only inpatient care and includes an adequate number and distribution of hospitals, it does not appear to reduce access.[17]

Regulating the Suppliers of Health Care

Nonmarket, regulatory methods have also been used to limit supply and to set rates that hospitals will be reimbursed by all third party payers. They are usually societal in their scope, affecting, for example, all hospitals across all types of programs within a state or country. In recent years, states have required certificates of need (CON) to limit capital investment, which is a major factor in rising hospital costs, and the supply of beds, because more beds result in higher admission rates. CONs have been somewhat effective in slowing the growth in supply of hospital beds, but they have not been effective in limiting other kinds of hospital expense because hospitals are able simply to spend their capital on other cost-generating assets.[18] CONs have thus had little, if any, effect on the rationing of hospital services.

Mandatory setting of reimbursement rates has been far more effective. Across a wide variety of rate-setting programs, states with mandatory programs demonstrated clear reductions in rates of increase in hospital costs per day and per admission.[19] Whether these programs specifically limited hospital use, quality, or profits is unclear.

Budgetary Control

Prospective global budgeting, the exercise of direct budgetary control, has been used infrequently to ration resources to this country's hospitals, but more widely in some other countries. Prospective global budgeting involves an intentional process of allocating annually to hospitals and other provider agencies a basic or complete budget covering capital and operating costs. In the United States, this form of rationing is found mainly in government health systems, such as military, state, and municipal hospitals. Under Canada's national health insurance system, the provincial commissions and departments that administer the insurance program prospectively negotiate global budgets with each hospital.[20]

Comparing the Effects

Each of these rationing methods has a different effect on costs, access, and quality of care. The loss of insurance coverage—whether due to government action that cuts eligibility for Medicaid, unemployment, or employment in a job that does not provide health insurance—has the greatest impact on access to care because it returns those affected (who are mostly very low-income persons) to a price-rationed medical marketplace. It does indeed hold down a single payer's costs and total costs of care, although at a high price in human and social terms.

Cost sharing, which intentionally imposes incremental price rationing on people with third party coverage, may adversely and significantly affect the health of low-income persons, especially those who are already in poorer health. Even for the rest of the population, cost sharing allocates different amounts of care based in part on social class, thus contributing to general inequalities in health care use. However, it does decrease total health care costs for the group subjected to cost sharing—its raison d'être and the source of attractiveness to public and private policy makers.

Rationing by market incentives directed toward providers may also adversely affect the access of particular groups, depending both on whether it is programmatic or societal in scope and on market conditions. Experience in Medicaid programs demonstrates that keeping physician reimbursements low for only one group of patients is likely to reduce that group's access to care in a market in which economic demand exceeds supply. The limited experience to date with selective contracting for hospital care, on the other hand, suggests that such rationing methods will have less detrimental impact when the supply greatly exceeds existing economic demand.

Regulation has proved effective in holding down the costs of hospital care when applied directly to rates paid by third party payers, but it has not been as effective when it focuses on only one aspect of hospitals' own allocation of capital resources (namely, on the number of beds, as many CON laws do). All-payer rate setting, which rations resources per service allocated to hospitals within a given state, is more effective in controlling hospital costs. All-payer methods have the additional advantage of promoting equity because they apply equally to patients with any third party coverage. Those states whose all-payer programs include reimbursement to hospitals for uncompensated care also extend implicit coverage to the uninsured.

Global prospective budgeting is probably the most effective level and form of cost containment, involving political decisions about the share of national resources to be devoted to health care. It thus permits effective control of total costs and relatively great control over the distribution of resources. At the national level, such a system substitutes planning and intentional allocation for market generation of total health expenditures. By itself, systemwide global budgeting does not preclude market organization of health care at subordinate levels. Replacing the market organization of the delivery of health care with a public service model would require a national health service, like the one embodied in the U.S. Health Service bill introduced by Congressman Ronald Dellums (D-Cal.),[21] which would eliminate market autonomy of providers and subject them to a largely democratic planning and policy-making process. These varied cost containment and rationing approaches provided the context within which Medicare introduced its prospective payment system and DRGs.

DRGs AND RATIONING

Medicare's prospective payment system uses financial incentives to control provider behavior. The prospectively set price paid to hospitals for treating all patients with a particular DRG encourages very different behavior than the previous cost-based system because the hospital must bear the financial risks of cost overruns. A hospital whose cost for treating a patient in a particular DRG is below the DRG payment will pocket the difference and reap a profit, but a hospital whose cost is above the DRG payment will lose money on that case. It thus encourages the hospital to monitor closely what it spends caring for each patient.

The introduction of DRGs changed the rationing of hospital care under Medicare as well as the 14 state Medicaid programs and 10 Blue Cross and Blue Shield programs that are implementing or planning similar DRG reimbursement systems.[22] Under the old cost-based reimbursement system, hospitals were paid for all services rendered to Medicare patients while rationing was imposed on Medicare beneficiaries themselves through cost-sharing requirements.[23] The DRG system, on the other hand, provides incentives for hospitals to ration care to Medicare patients. The congressionally sponsored Prospective Payment Assessment Commission (ProPAC), congressional committees, and other analysts and researchers have documented the impact of Medicare's prospective payment system on hospitals, physicians, and patients as well as on Medicare itself.

How Hospitals Have Responded: Cutting Costs

As PPS loomed ahead of them, hospitals began to analyze carefully all the costs of treating patients. Using sophisticated management information systems, hospitals examined the costs of inputs and resources required for each DRG and the impact on the "bottom line" of those costs and the reimbursement for that DRG. In order to gain more control over their costs, many hospitals adopted "product line" management, putting individual managers in charge of coordinating resources across all departments for a particular DRG or group of related DRGs.[24] Hospitals then responded to the new challenges of prospective payment both by cutting their costs and by increasing their revenues. They have cut their expenses in several ways.

First, as expected, PPS accelerated the decline in average length of stay (ALOS) among the elderly. The ALOS for hospital patients 65 years and older fell from 9.9 days in early 1983 to 8.7 days by the third quarter of 1985.[25] ProPAC found that ALOS declined most for preoperative and routine care, 11.9 percent and 7.6 percent respectively, between the period in 1984 before PPS was implemented and the period in 1984 under PPS. Preoperative and routine care are clearly more discretionary and flexible than special and postoperative care, both of which showed virtually no decline over this time period. Regions of the country with above average resource use per DRG had somewhat larger decreases in length of stay.[26] Although these data represent a very incomplete picture of hospital services under DRGs, they do suggest that hospitals first cut those services that are relatively less critical in their efforts to shave their costs.

However, hospitals have cut not only discretionary care. They have achieved their shorter ALOS by pressuring physicians to discharge patients earlier than in the past—often sooner than either physicians or patients believe is good for the patient. Widespread anecdotal reports from hospitals throughout the country suggest, as Senator John Heinz (Rep.-PA) warned, that Medicare patients are being discharged "quicker and sicker," some even prematurely. Senator Heinz's conclusion was based on evidence gathered by the General Accounting Office, including widespread reports and data showing that Medicare patients who were discharged from hospitals to nursing homes after the introduction of PPS had more extensive service needs than Medicare patients before PPS, including more physician visits per case and per week and a greater need for specialized services such as intravenous therapy, catheters, and ventilator care.[27]

ProPAC found similar evidence in newspaper articles, statements from beneficiaries, and interviews with providers, professional review organization representatives, and consumer advocates. They found that many patients felt they were sent home before they felt ready to leave the hospital. Others clearly were discharged without home support or nursing home placement. Some others experienced serious complications that resulted in readmission or death.[28]

Hospitals encouraged these early discharges by pressuring both patients and physicians. In many hospitals, when patients reached the *mean* length of stay for that DRG, they were told that "your DRG is up" and that they must leave or assume the costs of additional days of care. They were not told of their rights to appeal.[29]

Nearly half the internists who responded to an informal survey conducted by the American Society of Internal Medicine (ASIM) during the first year of PPS reported strong pressure by administrators. This included printed forms that appeared in the chart one or two days before the DRG was to "expire," strongly suggesting discharge, and daily notices on how much the hospital was losing as a result of certain patients. Many respondents believed that frail elderly patients and those with Alzheimer's disease were being discharged earlier than medically appropriate. A fourth of the respondents reported that, in their opinions, some early discharges had resulted in increased morbidity and mortality.[30]

Why do physicians succumb to such pressure? At many hospitals, physicians are under heavy peer pressure to reduce length of stay and the use of laboratory tests and drugs. These pressures include using sophisticated severity-of-illness indexes to monitor and compare physician practice patterns; having medical directors and directors of quality assurance and utilization review explain to erring physicians the extent to which their costs exceed the average costs for patients in that DRG; and imposing new rules that require more frequent writing of orders and explanations for ordering costly or repeated tests.[31] There is little evidence that forcing physicians to consider carefully whether a procedure is really needed has harmed any patients. To the extent that such policies have reduced unnecessary and invasive procedures, patients undoubtedly benefit while costs are controlled.

However, many hospitals have made staff privileges conditional on acceptable practice patterns. Physicians who keep their patients in the hospital "too long" or utilize "too many" ancillary services and other hospital resources in treating patients may find themselves without a hospital in which to practice, a policy that so far has been upheld by the courts. "In the past, the criteria for obtaining medical staff privileges here have been based on excellence in practice and teaching," according to William Credé, an internist and director of quality assurance at Yale–New Haven Hospital. "In the future, physicians with records of inappropriate overutilization are going to find it more difficult to get privileges—not just here but at any hospital."[32] Some hospitals have adopted a more insidious policy of sharing the hospital's profits with physicians who keep the costs of treating patients below the amount of DRG reimbursements. While policies providing kickbacks for nontreatment are possibly illegal, the threat of losing hospital privileges is probably unethical. Furthermore, patients may doubt whether to trust the judgment of doctors who are under duress to become society's agents of cost containment.[33]

In addition to reducing length of stay and the use of ancillary services, hospitals also reduced staffing to cut costs. The average increase in total inpatient expenses declined from 13.6 percent per year for the period 1976–1982 to 5.5 percent per year during 1983–1985. This was due mainly to a reduction in costs per admission, since expenses per patient day did not decline significantly during this period, reflecting the concentration of fixed costs across fewer hospital days. One of the main inputs that hospitals targeted were labor costs, changing the composition of their labor forces and reducing full time equivalents (FTEs) an average of 1.3 percent per year during 1983–1985, compared with an average annual increase of 4.3 percent for 1971–1982. FTEs per admission have not matched the decline in total personnel because the number of admissions and patient days fell even faster.[34] Nevertheless, about half the respondents in the ASIM informal survey reported short staffing of nurses and lab technicians in their hospitals.[35]

The trend toward earlier discharges has also meant a rise in discharges to nursing homes and use of home health care. However, the inadequacy of discharge planning in many hospitals, the lack of sufficient nursing home beds and home health services, and Medicare's discouragement of such services have greatly limited their use. In many, if not most, parts of the country, home health services and skilled nursing facility (SNF) beds are in short supply, especially those certified for Medicare reimbursement as providing the required level of skilled care.[36]

But even when beds are available for Medicare patients who are about to be discharged from a hospital, Medicare reimbursement may be denied for a variety of reasons. Medicare coverage is provided only after a hospitalization of three or more days; with pressures for early discharge, many patients who need nursing home care do not meet the hospitalization requirement. In addition, earlier discharges mean that more patients need "heavy care" and are more costly for the receiving nursing home. Nursing homes are reluctant to take such patients. They are also reluctant to take Medicare patients who may not have sufficient private funds and who would therefore become Medicaid patients when their 20 days of fully reimbursed Medicare coverage ends. They are reluctant because Medicaid reimbursement is much lower. Finally, reimbursement for SNF care may be denied by fiscal intermediaries because Medicare now requires them to screen beneficiaries for eligibility based on their potential for rehabilitation, a process that in many states allegedly has left some patients without care despite their inability to care for themselves. "Whether a Medicare patient is considered covered for SNF benefits," claimed Louis Krieger, representing the American Association of Retired Persons, "varies so greatly from case to case and region to region that it has made the benefit an illusion." Requirements imposed on home health services and eligibility for their care reportedly have made their availability to Medicare patients just as uncertain.[37]

Thus, hospitals' efforts to cut their costs in response to PPS have many ramifications that affect Medicare patients and the rationing of health care. In order to shorten length of stay many hospitals are pushing Medicare patients out "quicker and sicker," but appropriate and necessary posthospital care is not adequately available and accessible. Hospitals are also reducing staffing, with uncertain consequences for patient care but definite speed-up pressures for staff. Medicare is squeezing hospitals at one end, while it is squeezing nursing homes and home health agencies at the other end. In the middle, hospitals and nursing homes are in turn squeezing Medicare patients. Hospitals have become the rationing agents of Medicare, and they have coerced and cajoled physicians into joining them in this role.

Professional review organizations (PROs) are responsible for assuring the quality of care under PPS. However, most PROs were the old professional standards review organizations, created to protect Medicare from paying for excessive utilization. That made a lot of sense when the incentives were entirely on the side of overtreatment, but it has not worked well to stem abuses of undertreatment. PROs are still responsible for limiting utilization, and, according to ProPAC, many of them seem to give that objective a higher priority than ensuring that all necessary services are delivered. The orientation of PROs thus compounds the tendencies of DRGs that already encourage less care than patients need. Furthermore, neither PROs nor any other agency has been delegated the responsibility by Medicare to assess the quality of posthospital care by nursing homes and home health care agencies.[38]

How Hospitals Have Responded: Increasing Revenues

In addition to cutting the costs of their inputs, hospitals have adopted several strategies to increase revenues. First, responding to the incentives in the present DRG payment policies, hospitals now generally take care of only one main problem per admission, preferring to readmit the patient later to deal with other medical conditions and collect additional revenues. As one hospital administrator explained, "Since no extra payment is extended for the treatment of needs not related to the principal diagnosis, there is strong impetus for ignoring a recognized, but unrelated need, and readmitting the patient later to correct that problem, thus creating an additional admission, unnecessary expense, and prolonged inconvenience to the patient."[39] In this way, hospitals provide only those services for which they are being reimbursed and generate more revenues.

Second, under PPS hospitals now perform some medical and surgical procedures as outpatient services that were previously done on an inpatient basis. For example, in 1984, outpatient surgery accounted for 25 percent of all surgical procedures, nearly double the proportion in 1980. And contrary to expectations, the number of admissions among people over 65 years of age has declined, reversing the gradual but steady increase up to 1984.[40] Although it is difficult to pinpoint the exact causes of these changes, technological developments have undoubtedly made it safer to perform more procedures on an outpatient basis, while the financial incentives created by DRG payments for inpatient care have provided a strong stimulus for hospitals to do so. Some procedures—such as diagnostic workups, minor surgeries, and preoperative procedures—may be more lucratively performed without admitting a patient to the hospital if the DRG payment has a lower revenue-to-average cost ratio than the outpatient reimbursement, which is still cost-based.

Third, hospitals are using management information systems to monitor carefully the costs of all DRGs in relation to their reimbursements. Assessing the extent to which each DRG "product line" is a loser or a profit-making winner, hospitals may then decide whether to drop, maintain, or add a given service. "Marketplace competition to attract those physicians who specialize in profitable product lines will increase," predict some hospital finance experts, "while the treatment of unprofitable product lines may be curtailed or even discontinued. This 'skimming' and 'dumping' is an acknowledged consequence of a system that encourages hospitals to gravitate toward profitable product lines and abandon loss leaders, regardless of the need for these services."[41] A fifth of the internists in the ASIM informal survey reported that their hospitals had decided not to treat certain types of illness or encouraged physicians to admit patients with certain illnesses to other hospitals.[42] Although this makes perfect business sense under the DRG reimbursement system, it is a far cry from public health planning assessments of whether a health service is needed in a particular community. And it is even a step removed from previous market analyses of the economic demand for a service that provides a reasonable reimbursement. It is the kind of decision analysis that has resulted in investor-owned chain hospitals providing a narrower range of services than not-for-profit or public hospitals.[43]

Finally, hospitals have begun aggressive efforts to increase the use of their profitable services. Hospital advertising budgets in 1985 were one-third greater than in 1984, averaging $64,000 per hospital. Hospitals are also becoming vertically integrated. Their vertical integration includes developing "feeder" services such as free-standing surgicenters and emergicenters, joint ventures with physicians in office buildings and diagnostic centers, physician referral services to steer prospective patients to doctors with admitting privileges in that hospital, and closed- or preferred-service arrangements with health maintenance organizations, preferred provider organizations, and individual practice associations. In addition to increasing the flow at the front end, hospitals have developed "receiver" services such as SNFs and home health service agencies to generate additional revenues as they reduce lengths of stay.[44]

Although hospitals' efforts to generate additional revenues are less problematic than their cost-cutting strategies, even some of these methods affect the rationing of health care. One new form of rationing is to treat only one major medical problem per hospitalization, prolonging suffering and adding to the inconvenience of patients. This problem could be remedied by modifying reimbursement policies to take account of multiple medical conditions.

A second effect is the exaggerated emphasis on increasing profitable product lines and their use and reducing "DRG losers," a pressure that will further distort the kinds of health services available in communities throughout the country. This effect seems inherent in the DRG reimbursement system, and it is very consistent with the market organization of health care. Hospitals are relatively autonomous units within a marketplace that buys and sells health care as commodities. Except for a relatively small amount of public planning and regulation, the system still functions largely through economic incentives rather than a technical process to measure need and an accountable political process to allocate health care resources. In a market system of health care, this seems like a reasonable way of doing business, although it appears irrational from a public health perspective.

DRGs and the Costs of Medicare

What has been the financial impact of PPS? To see the full picture, we must examine its financial impact on Medicare beneficiaries and hospitals as well as on the Medicare program.

Financial Consequences for Beneficiaries

In addition to some patients being discharged before medically appropriate, many Medicare patients and their families must bear greater out-of-pocket financial costs due to PPS. ProPAC found that "a larger portion of health care costs have been shifted to beneficiaries through higher premiums for Medicare supplemental coverage and through larger deductibles, greater use of services with coinsurance, and use of services not covered by Medicare." They pay more for each hospital admission because the decreased length of stay has increased the average cost per day, pushing the "one day of care" deductible up from $400 in 1985 to $492 in 1986, twice the rate of increase in the previous year. Although most Medicare beneficiaries have supplemental private insurance to cover this cost, the premiums for that insurance have risen in response to the increased deductible. The shifting of some procedures and services from an inpatient to an outpatient basis has increased beneficiaries' coinsurance payments under Medicare Part B. And out-of-pocket expenses have grown due to the increased use of health services that are not covered by Medicare, such as long-term SNF and home health services.[45]

Finally, many families find that they have to provide more care to sicker elderly patients who are discharged without adequate nursing home or home health care. This may represent a financial cost to working families if one member must stay at home to care for the elderly patient, or it may mean a physical hardship on an elderly spouse who might also be quite frail or ill.

Financial Consequences for Medicare

The growth in Medicare spending has slowed since PPS was gradually implemented beginning in 1983. Medicare's Hospital Insurance Trust Fund disbursements in fiscal year 1985 were nearly 5 percent lower than the agency had predicted just two years earlier. Between 1983 and 1985, Medicare spending grew at an average rate of 11.8 percent per year, rather than the expected 13.6 percent rate. A continuing increase in Medicare expenditures for nursing home and home health services was apparent in 1984, but it was not greater than average increases during the previous ten years.[46] Although the decline in Medicare spending was undoubtedly strongly influenced by PPS, other changes in health care also helped reduce total costs. Medicare PPS, changes in state Medicaid and private third party reimbursement methods, and growing pressures from employer health care coalitions all influenced hospital-based medical practice. The separate effects of each one are difficult to discern.

Financial Consequences for Hospitals

Through all these changes, most hospitals are doing quite well. Hospitals that provide a disproportionate share of the care to Medicaid and uninsured patients— especially public hospitals—may suffer under the present DRG payments, unless the "disproportionate share hospitals" adjustment recommended by ProPAC and adopted by Congress is implemented by the federal government, which the Reagan administration refused to do through 1986.[47] In addition, there is evidence that recent changes affecting all hospitals have had an adverse impact on rural and small urban hospitals.[48] But most hospitals are not experiencing financial difficulties. In 1984, hospitals reported an average operating margin ratio (operating revenues less operating expenses, divided by operating revenue) of .031, a 35 percent increase over the 1983 ratio and the biggest gain in some years.[49] The Department of Health and Human Services' inspector general analyzed data from more than 2,000 hospitals and reported that the average hospital made a profit of 15 percent on Medicare services in 1984, about three times the average profit margin for all patient services in recent years.[50] Under PPS, Medicare reimburses hospitals for capital-related costs as a "pass through" on top of the DRG payment, encouraging hospitals to make investments and to substitute capital for operating costs whenever possible.[51]

DRG rates in the first year of PPS have been weighted toward hospital- and region-specific average costs, to allow hospitals in higher-cost areas to adjust more gradually to the change. However, beginning in October 1987, Medicare will have completed its transition to national rates, favoring hospitals in lower-cost areas. Thus, hospitals in general have found PPS a profitable change, albeit one that has caused organizational strain. Nevertheless, the financial conditions of individual hospitals may change as the transition to national rates is completed and if additional rate increases are reduced or denied as a result of federal budget cuts, as in fiscal year 1986–87.

CONCLUSION

Prospective payment suggests some of the problems that must be resolved in imposing rationing in a medical system organized along market principles. The medical care market system leaves each unit—each hospital, doctor, drug company—free to produce and distribute its goods or services, without much concern for those who do not have access to care or for any larger social benefit. Price rationing had prevented the elderly, disabled, and poor from getting much of the care they needed. The enactment of Medicare replaced unrestricted price rationing for the elderly and the disabled with an insurance program, but it intentionally imposed incremental price rationing in the form of copayments on beneficiaries as a way to control utilization and costs. Nevertheless, Medicare's cost-based reimbursement, together with supplemental insurance coverage for beneficiaries, encouraged hospitals and physicians to circumvent the utilization and cost controls of copayments, generating a long rapidly rising curve of program costs. PPS seemed like a solution that would protect the government from fiscal disaster without changing the basic market organization of medical care.

PPS fixed Medicare's payments for each episode of hospitalization. In the process, it employed market incentives that changed hospitals' and doctors' behavior, encouraging them to ration health care for elderly and disabled Medicare beneficiaries. Whereas Medicare previously imposed copayments on Medicare patients as a method of rationing care, hospitals and doctors themselves have now been made rationers of care, doing less for patients rather than more. Seeking to reduce their costs in order to make ends meet and pocket a profit, hospitals have pressured physicians and their patients to decrease length of stay and the use of ancillary services. Acting as relatively autonomous market entities without responsibility for the availability of posthospitalization care, hospitals have generated increased medical and financial difficulties for patients and their families. They have also put a strain on nursing homes and home health agencies.

Who will protect the patient's interests in this system? As before, it is assumed that the medical profession's competence and commitment to service, hospitals' competence and government licensing procedures, and the market's "Invisible Hand" will find some satisfactory equilibrium which will provide optimum care to the patient. There is good reason to be skeptical of such premises whether the financial incentives are for less treatment, as under PPS, or for more treatment, as under fee-for-service and cost-based reimbursement. Regulatory quality review and assurance procedures are needed to protect patients from the abuses inherent in a market-oriented hospital financing system such as PPS, but they have been inadequate at best and have had the opposite orientation at worst.

Hospitals, physicians, nurses, and regulatory agencies cannot be expected to be the guarantors of patients' fundamental needs and interests. As we have seen, the relative autonomy granted to the medical profession, hospitals, and other producers of medical services and products enables them to protect their interests no matter how we tinker with the market system. Ultimately, replacing the market system with a more rational national health system can provide opportunities for all relevant interests—community members and patients as well as doctors, nurses, administrators, and other health workers—to be involved in allocating societal and community health resources. But we can begin even now to move in that direction by including in decision making the groups that have been most ignored. Patients and their families, together with their communities, should be involved in every aspect of medical decision making, from life-and-death treatment decisions in the hospital to national policy decisions concerning whether or not to develop major new medical technologies. Organizations of senior citizens and the disabled as well as other groups at local and national levels can monitor the implementation of the present DRG system, develop alternatives to it such as national health insurance or national health service legislation, and organize themselves politically to secure passage. The introduction of prospective payment makes our present rationing system more visible, and that may agitate us sufficiently to work together toward a better solution.

NOTES

1. R.M. Gibson, K.R. Levit, H. Lazenby, and D.R. Waldo, "National Health Expenditures, 1983," *Health Care Financing Review* 6, no. 2 (Winter 1984):1–29.

2. Pub. L. No. 98-21, the Social Security Amendments of 1983, established case-based hospital rate setting for Medicare, known as the prospective payment system. Although Medicare calls the payment method "prospective," it actually is paid retrospectively for a patient whose episode of illness has been treated. It is prospective in the sense that the reimbursement amount for each DRG is set in advance of a patient's admission.

3. D. Mechanic, "Approaches to Controlling the Costs of Medical Care: Short-Range and Long-Range Alternatives," *New England Journal of Medicine* 298 (1978):249–254.

4. I.S. Falk, C.R. Rorem, and M.D. Ring, *The Costs of Medical Care*, Committee on the Costs of Medical Care Publication No. 27 (Chicago: University of Chicago Press, 1933), 599.

5. President's Commission for the Study of Ethical Problems in Medicine and Biomedical and Behavioral Research, *Securing Access to Health Care: A Report on the Ethical Implications of Differences in the Availability of Health Services*, vol. 1 (Washington, D.C.: U.S. Government Printing Office, March 1983), 26.

6. S.F. Loebs "Medicaid—A Survey of Indicators and Issues," in *The Medicaid Experience*, ed. A.D. Spiegel (Rockville, Md.: Aspen Publishers, Inc., 1979), 10–16.

7. M.I. Roemer and M. Shain, *Hospital Utilization Under Insurance* (Chicago: American Hospital Association, 1959), and P.B. Ginsburg and D.M. Koretz, "Bed Availability and Hospital Utilization: Estimates of the 'Roemer Effect'," *Health Care Financing Review* 5, no. 1 (1983):87–92.

8. R.R. Bovberg and J. Holahan, *Medicaid in the Reagan Era: Federal Policy and State Choices* (Washington, D.C.: Urban Institute Press, 1982), pp. 25–32, and J. Cromwell, S. Hurdle, and G. Wedig, *Impacts of Economic and Programmatic Changes on Medicaid Enrollments* (Chestnut Hill, Mass.: Center for Health Economics Research, 1984).

9. T.C.W. Joe, J. Meltzer, and P. Yu, "Arbitrary Access to Care: The Case for Reforming Medicaid," *Health Affairs* 4, no. 1 (1985):59–74.

10. U.S. Bureau of the Census, *1984 Current Population Survey* (Washington, D.C.: U.S. Government Printing Office, 1984).

11. R.J. Blendon et al., "Uncompensated Care by Hospitals or Public Insurance for the Poor: Does It Make a Difference?" *New England Journal of Medicine* 314 (1986):1160–1163; N. Lurie et al., "Termination from Medi-Cal: Does It Affect Health?" *New England Journal of Medicine* 311 (1984):480–484; N. Lurie et al., "Termination of Medi-Cal Benefits: A Follow-up Study One Year Later," *New England Journal of Medicine* 314 (1986):1266–1268.

12. J.P. Newhouse et al., "Some Interim Results from a Controlled Trial of Cost Sharing in Health Insurance," *New England Journal of Medicine* 305 (1981):1501–1507.

13. M.F. Shapiro, J.E. Ware, and C.D. Sherbourne, "Effects of Cost Sharing on Seeking Care for Serious and Minor Symptoms," *Annals of Internal Medicine* 104 (1986):246–251.

14. M.I. Roemer et al., "Copayments for Ambulatory Care: Penny-Wise and Pound-Foolish," *Medical Care* 13 (1975):457–466.

15. C. Bellavita, "California's Health Policy Reform and the Poor," *Public Affairs Report* 24 (1983):1–9, and H. Blum et al., *Medi-Cal Legislation Report* (Berkeley: University of California, Institute for Governmental Studies, May 1983).

16. J. Mitchell and J. Cromwell, "Medicaid Mills: Fact or Fiction?" *Health Care Financing Review* 2, no. 1 (1980):37–49, and J. Hadley, "Physician Participation in Medicaid: Evidence from California," *Health Services Research* 14 (1979):266–280.

17. E.R. Brown, W.T. Price, and M.R. Cousineau, "Medi-Cal Hospital Contracting: Did It Achieve Its Legislative Objectives?" *Western Journal of Medicine* 143 (1985):118–124; and L. Johns, M.D. Anderson, and R.A. Derson, "Selective Contracting in California: Experience in the Second Year," *Inquiry* 22 (1985):335–347.

18. J.J. Aaron and W.B. Schwartz, *The Painful Prescription: Rationing Hospital Care* (Washington, D.C.: The Brookings Institution, 1984), 5.

19. C.L. Eby and D.R. Cohodes, "What Do We Know About Rate-Setting?" *Journal of Health Politics, Policy and Law* 10, no. 2 (1985):299–328, and J. Cromwell and H. Hewes, "Medicare Expenditures and Utilization Under State Hospital Rate Setting," *Health Care Financing Review* 7, no. 1 (1985):97–109.

20. R. Roemer and M.I. Roemer, *Health Manpower Policy Under National Health Insurance— The Canadian Experience* (Washington, D.C.: U.S. Department of Health, Education, and Welfare, 1977); C.B. Mueller, "Some Effects of Health Insurance in Canada—From Private Enterprise Toward Public Accountability," *New England Journal of Medicine* 298 (1978):535–539; G.H. Hatcher, "Canadian Approaches to Health Policy Decisions—National Health Insurance," *American Journal of Public Health* 68 (1978):881–889; and E. Vayda, "The Canadian Health Care System: An Overview," *Journal of Public Health Policy* 7 (1986):205–210.

21. H.R. 2049, 99th Congress.

22. *Medicare Prospective Payment and the American Health Care System—Report to the Congress* (Washington, D.C.: Prospective Payment Assessment Commission, February 1986), 77. (Hereafter called "ProPAC Report.")

23. There were exceptions in the implementation of this policy. Under the old system, Medicare imposed deductibles and copayments on recipients. However, hospitals could choose to waive those deductibles and copayments in order to make their services available to low-income elderly patients who did not have "Medigap" insurance or Medicaid. Some hospitals did adopt this policy following negotiations with certain senior citizen adovcacy groups that made this a campaign.

24. J.P. Sweeney and J.E. D'Itri, "New Success Factors for Management Under Prospective Payment," *Topics in Health Care Financing* 11, no. 3 (1985):10–21; and J.M. McSweeney, M.B. Hebert, and R.B. Holroyd, "Cost Accounting Strategies Under Prospective Payment System," *Topics in Health Care Financing* 11, no. 3 (1985):28–46; and R.G. Goodrich and G.R. Hastings, "St. Luke's Hospital Reaps Benefits by Using Product Line Management," *Modern Healthcare* 15, no. 4 (1985):157–158.

25. J.K. Iglehart, "Early Experience with Prospective Payment of Hospitals," *New England Journal of Medicine* 314, no. 22 (1986):1460–1464.

26. ProPAC Report, 20 and 34–39.

27. Senator Heinz's statement and the GAO report were included in the report of the hearing by the U.S. House of Representatives, Select Committee on Aging, "Sustaining Quality Health Care Under Cost Containment," Joint Hearing, Feb. 26, 1985 (Washington, D.C.: U.S. Government Printing Office, 1985), 101–106.

28. *Technical Appendixes to the Report and Recommendations to the Secretary, U.S. Department of Health and Human Services* (Washington, D.C.: Prospective Payment Assessment Commission, April 1, 1986), pp. 148–149. (Hereafter "Technical Appendixes, 1986.")

29. Ibid., 149–150.

30. "The Impact of DRGs on Patient Care," A Survey of the American Society of Internal Medicine, March 1984–October 1985 (Washington, D.C.: American Society of Internal Medicine, n.d.).

31. J.R. Jay, "Managers and Physicians Work Together to Reduce Healthcare Costs," *Healthcare Financial Management* 39, no. 2 (1985):40–45; D.P. Wilcox, "Financial Criteria, Medical Care, and Your Patient—The Role of Hospital Medical Staffs," *Texas Medicine* 81, no. 1 (1985):49–51;

L.D. Shaw, "Teaming Up With Administrators To Set Prospective Payment Policy," *Pathologist* 38, no. 6 (1984):352–353; M. Nathanson, "More Hospitals Turn to SOIs, but Experts Question Their Usefulness," *Modern Healthcare* 15, no. 4 (1985):63–75; and M.I. Burken, "A DRG-Based Management Information System," *Pathologist* 38, no. 11 (1984):732–733.

32. J. Long, "What Will You Be Worth to Your Hospital Under DRG?" *Medical Economics* 62, no. 1 (1985):141–151.

33. Wilcox, "Financial Criteria," and Long, "What Will You Be Worth." See also A.R. Dyer, "Patients, Not Costs, Come First," and P. Brazil, "Cost Effective Care Is Better Care," *The Hastings Center Report* 16, no. 1 (1986):5–8.

34. ProPAC Report, 22–24.

35. "The Impact of DRGs on Patient Care."

36. ProPAC Report, 61; and "Home Care Bears Brunt of DRG System," *Hospitals* 59, no. 12 (1985):70–73.

37. U.S. House of Representatives, Select Committee on Aging, "Sustaining Quality Health Care Under Cost Containment," Joint Hearing, Feb. 26, 1985, pp. 22 and 105; and U.S. House of Representatives, Select Committee on Aging, "Health Care Cost Containment: Are America's Aged Protected?" Hearing, July 9, 1985 (Washington, D.C.: U.S. Government Printing Office, 1985), pp. 96–105 and 112–113.

38. ProPAC Report, 63–64.

39. Statement of Ben C. White, U.S. House of Representatives, Select Committee on Aging, "Sustaining Quality Health Care Under Cost Containment," Joint Hearing, Feb. 26, 1985, 65.

40. ProPAC Report, 19 and 21.

41. J.P. Sweeney and J.E. D'Itri, "New Success Factors."

42. "The Impact of DRGs on Patient Care."

43. B.H. Gray, ed., *For-Profit Enterprise in Health Care* (Washington, D.C.: National Academy Press, 1986), 108–109.

44. ProPAC Report, p. 26; and J.P. Sweeney and J.E. D'Itri, "New Success Factors."

45. ProPAC Report, 60.

46. ProPAC Report, 11 and 71.

47. Technical Appendixes, 1986, pp. 57–63; *Technical Appendixes to the Report and Recommendations to the Secretary, U.S. Department of Health and Human Services* (Washington, D.C.: Prospective Payment Assessment Commission, April 1, 1985), pp. 59–66; and ProPAC Report, 37.

48. "Report Details Performance of Small and Rurals," *Hospitals* 60, no. 13 (1986):113.

49. ProPAC Report, 90.

50. R. Steinbrook, "Hospital Medicare Profits Told, Disputed," *Los Angeles Times*, June 2, 1986.

51. ProPAC Report, 53–54.

Chapter 7

Organ Procurement and Transplantation

David A. Ogden, MD, FACP

The development of successful human organ transplantation is one of the outstanding medical achievements of this century. It has also challenged modern morality, provoked a reexamination of professional ethics, and highlighted the conflict between public policy and limited financial resources in health care.

The subject of this book is hospital ethics. The words ethics, ethical, moral, and morality are used in everyday conversation and writing, but perhaps without a sound understanding of their meaning. Most physicians are educated in both the arts and sciences, but are most extensively trained in the sciences of medicine. Therefore, it seemed appropriate to turn to the dictionary to determine that moral means in accordance with the principles of right and wrong, and that ethical means conforming to the moral standards of a group or to professional standards of conduct. It then seemed necessary to find some authoritative basis for the principles of right and wrong. The Bible provides a few brief statements concerning the duty of man to man: "thou shalt love thy neighbor as thyself . . ." (Lev. 19:18), and "whatsoever ye would that men should do to you, do you evenso to them . . ." (Matt. 7:12). These standards, the first from the writing of Moses reflecting God's words to Moses, and the second from Jesus' Sermon on the Mount as told by Matthew, remain valid moral principles of our society. Professional practices and public policy must, I believe, reflect accepted societal principles of right and wrong.

The discussion to follow will be limited to aspects of organ procurement and transplantation of whole body organs only. Currently, kidneys, livers, hearts, lungs, and pancreases are successfully transplanted.

The procurement of organs, criteria for the definition of death, selection of those to receive limited numbers of available organs, and financing of organ transplantation continue to intrigue the public and at the same time pose significant questions and problems of societal ethics and public policy. This chapter will provide a framework of information concerning organ procurement and transplantation and will highlight current questions and suggested practices in this field.

HISTORY OF WHOLE ORGAN TRANSPLANTATION

The first successful whole organ transplant was the transfer of a kidney between identical twins at Peter Bent Brigham Hospital in 1954. This procedure documented the surgical feasibility of whole organ transplantation in the absence of any immunologic barrier. More importantly for this discussion, it initiated the concept of the legal and moral right of a person to consent to organ donation in the absence of coercion and with informed consent, a principle since sustained by various court cases.

A few years later, the successful transplant of a kidney between nonidentical twins at the same hospital demonstrated the first successful abrogation of the immunologic barrier between genetically disparate individuals.[1] The ability to cross the immunologic barrier with some degree of success opened the way in the early 1960s for increasing numbers of sibling, parent, and other living donor renal transplants, and to the use of cadaver organs for transplantation. Simultaneous advances in artificial kidney technology, particularly the development of the Scribner shunt for repetitive chronic blood access, permitted survival of patients with chronic renal failure pending identification and evaluation of potential related donors or the availability of a cadaver organ.

Dialysis and transplantation rapidly transcended the experimental phase and were established as successful therapies for chronic renal failure. Federal policy development proceeded apace. In 1963 the U.S. Veterans Administration announced that it would establish dialysis (and subsequently transplant) centers in a number of academically affiliated VA Hospitals, and by 1972 it was operating 44 dialysis centers and about 15 transplant centers. The U.S. Public Health Service established the kidney disease control program (KDCP) in the late 1960s to fund community dialysis demonstration projects and regional organ acquisition and tissue typing programs. In 1966, the Bureau of the Budget established a committee of experts to analyze the implications of the development of hemodialysis and transplantation for the federal government. This committee's report, widely known as the "Gottschalk Report," was released in the fall of 1967 and recommended that a national treatment benefit program be established by amending Title XVIII of the Social Security Act to cover the victims of end-stage renal disease (ESRD).[2]

The growing need for and use of cadaver organs for kidney transplantation set the stage for early attempts, with limited success, at liver and heart transplants in the latter half of the 1960s. It also led to the enactment of the Uniform Anatomical Gift Act of 1968. This act recognized the legal status of donor cards and living wills and the authority of the next of kin to make a donation when the deceased had not indicated any opposition to donation.

In the 1970s, hemodialysis and renal transplantation grew, slowly at first, and then very rapidly following the passage of PL 92-603, Section 2991, on October 30, 1972. This amended the Social Security Act to extend Medicare coverage to individuals under 65 years of age, fully or currently insured, or entitled to monthly disability benefits, and to their spouses and dependent children, if they had permanent kidney failure and required either dialysis or transplantation. As of July 1, 1973, approximately 11,000 patients were receiving benefits under the End-Stage Renal Disease Program of Medicare. The subsequent growth of this program in beneficiaries and cost is detailed in Table 7-1.

During the same period of the 1970s when dialysis and renal transplantation were increasingly applied as successful therapies for ESRD, other whole organ transplantation remained experimental and of limited success. The first transplantation of the human heart on December 3, 1967, generated considerable public press, but also provoked public, political, and scientific concern about the societal, legal, and professional aspects of transplantation. Clips in my file from 1968 newspapers reveal "Transplant Morality Disputed," "Organ Transplants May Produce Legal Tangle," "Judge Foresees Transplant Crisis," "Slain Man's Heart Use is Criticized," "Death Definition Needed," "Limit Asked for Heart Transplants," and "International Medical Group Sets Severe Standards for Heart Grafts." A leading Vatican theologian questioned the morality of transplants in stating, "This way of using the death of another person, this living waiting for someone to die in order that another one may live . . . conveys somehow a sense of fault."[3] Nobel laureate Joshua Lederberg in 1963 foresaw many of the problems of whole organ transplantation in stating, "When surgeons are able to transplant hearts, who will choose which dying patients get the new ones . . . and who will decide the price?"

Table 7-1 Growth of ESRD Program

Calendar Year	Patients on Dialysis	Transplants Performed	Total Number of Beneficiaries	Medicare Costs ($ millions)
1974			19,000	283
1975			27,000	450
1976			35,000	598
1977			41,000	757
1978			47,000	947
1979	45,565		52,000*	
1980	52,364	4697	57,000*	
1981	58,924	4883	64,000*	1,476
1982	65,765	5358	73,000*	1,661
1983	71,987	6112	82,000*	1,889
1984	78,483	6968	92,000*	1,835

Sources: Office of Financial and Actuarial Analysis, Division of Medicare Cost Estimates, Health Care Financing Administration, 1979; ESRD Medical Information System Facility Survey Tables 1983, HCFA Pub. No. 03178, Department of Health and Human Services, August 1984.

*Author's estimates: includes dialysis patients, new transplants, and surviving transplant recipients remaining as Medicare beneficiaries.

In the first half of the 1980s, improved surgical techniques, technical advances in respiratory and artificial kidney support systems, and particularly improvements in immunosuppressive therapy resulted in increased success with liver and cardiac transplantation. Such transplants are still largely limited to a relatively few academic medical centers but are increasingly viewed as accepted therapies. In 1985, between 600 and 700 liver transplants, and about 750 cardiac transplants were performed in the United States.[4] The one-year survival rate for both of these procedures is approximately 75 percent. During the same year, approximately 7,000 kidney transplants were performed, utilizing 5,250 cadaver and 1,750 living donor organs (figures are estimated by extrapolation of 1983 and 1984 reports of the Health Care Financing Administration).

The increasing activity in whole organ transplantation has created an acute shortage of suitable organs for transplantation. The national and local news media are awash with articles reflecting the issues of increasing voluntary organ donation; the criteria by which recipients of the limited numbers of available organs are selected; and society's agony of whether and how to pay for these expensive therapies. These problems are sharply reminiscent of the situation created by the limited artificial kidney therapy of the early 1960s and the University of Washington Admissions and Policies Committee of the Seattle Artificial Kidney Center, which became known as a life-and-death committee and was sometimes referred to as the God committee. This committee, as initially constituted, consisted of an attorney, a minister, a banker, a housewife, a state government official, a labor leader, and a surgeon. They were charged with determining which persons, all previously found to be medically and psychologically suitable for artificial kidney therapy, should be selected to receive this life-saving therapy.[5] Among the criteria they applied were the rehabilitative potential of the candidates, their relative worth to the community and to their families, and their moral worth.

Importantly, the composition of the committee reflected the concept, still debated today, that the allocation of a scarce medical resource is a community responsibility, not the responsibility of government, of the treating institution, or of the treating health care professionals.

SOURCES OF DONOR ORGANS

The potential sources of whole organs for transplantation are listed as follows:

I. Animals (Nonhuman primates)
II. Man
    A. Cadavers
    B. Unrelated Living Donors (kidney only)
    C. Related Living Donors (kidney only)

Animal Donors

Although very early, crude attempts at whole organ transplants involved kidneys from various animals, in the past 25 years only organs from nonhuman primates have been transplanted to man. Baboon and chimpanzee kidneys and a baboon heart have been transplanted, all only experimentally when no other suitable organ could be found, and with extremely limited success.[6] Although a few patients survived for a few months with animal kidney transplants, and reasonable experimental data were obtained,[7] no animal to man kidney transplants have been performed in the past 20 years. The widespread availability of artificial kidney therapy and increasing availability of cadaver kidneys make further animal renal transplants both inappropriate and unlikely. On the other hand, the limited availability of a suitable artificial heart and the scarcity of human hearts for transplantation suggest the possibility of further experimental primate cardiac transplants as a bridge transplant pending availability of a human heart for transplantation.

Cadaver Donors

Cadavers are the sole source of human livers, hearts, and lungs for transplantation and the source of nearly 75 percent of the kidneys transplanted in this country for the past three years.

The following list includes the steps in procurement of cadaver organs. Each step has posed legal, moral, or ethical problems, several of which are currently under active debate.

1. Pronouncement of Death
2. Pronouncement of Legal Consent for Donation
3. Surgical Removal of Organ(s)
4. Preservation of Organs(s)
5. Identification of Suitable Recipient
6. Transportation of Organ(s)
7. Transplantation of Organ(s)

Pronouncement of Death

The Uniform Anatomical Gift Act of 1968 and the growing practice of cadaver organ transplantation focused attention on death pronouncement.

The pronouncement and certification of death are the responsibility of the physician. Traditionally, and in common law, death has been determined to be when respiration and circulation cease. Advances in technology, including respirators and circulatory assist devices, make it difficult if not impossible to apply traditional means of ascertaining death in many patients, notwithstanding any consideration of organ donation.

The ideal potential cadaver organ donor is a young person suffering sudden head trauma, usually as a result of a motor vehicle accident or gunshot wound. This potential donor must reach a hospital while the heart is still beating, circulation is maintained, and respiration continues or is artificially but adequately provided. Occasionally, cadaver donors suffer a natural death from a ruptured intracranial artery aneurysm or other natural event.

Early cadaver kidney transplants were achieved with organs obtained as soon as possible following respiratory and circulatory arrest and conventionally pronounced death. Frequently, the period of warm ischemia—the interval between death and cold perfusion of the isolated kidney at the surgical procurement— was so great that the organ was irretrievably damaged. The ability to discern irreparable damage to these organs was imperfect, and many organs were transplanted but never functioned, contributing to morbidity and mortality of the recipients of these organs. This experience led to the concept of the "heart-beating" cadaver and the use of brain death as the accepted criteria for death.

The acceptance of brain death criteria prevents the useless continuation of life-saving technologies after life has, in fact, ceased, but in the instance of potential organ donation, early determination of brain death offers potential life to others. There is, therefore, a basic conflict of interest. The interest of brain-injured persons, their families, and care teams is in doing everything possible to promote recovery; the interest of potential organ recipients, their families, and care teams is, *if in fact brain death has occurred*, to have death pronounced while the organs remain viable. To this end, an ad hoc committee of the Harvard Medical School examined the definition of brain death,[8] and the resulting criteria are now widely accepted and used. Briefly, these criteria include unreceptivity and unresponsiveness, no movements or spontaneous breathing, no reflexes, and a flat electroencephalogram in the absence of hypothermia or central nervous system depressant drugs.

Brain death pronouncement is critical to successful whole organ transplantation and to the practice of medicine with its current technologies. Sixteen states have enacted legislation recognizing brain death as a legal basis of death pronouncement. In other states, the courts have recognized brain death.[9] The house of delegates of the American Bar Association, in 1975, adopted the statement that, "For all legal purposes, a human body, with irreversible cessation of total brain function, according to usual and customary standards of medical practice, shall be considered dead."[10] In 1980 the National Conference of Commissioners on Uniform State Laws approved and recommended for enactment by all states a Uniform Determination of Death Act, which states, "An individual who has sustained either (1) irreversible cessation of circulatory and respiratory functions, or (2) irreversible cessation of all functions of the entire brain, including the brain stem, is dead. A determination of death must be made in accordance with accepted medical standards."[11]

Even in the absence of specific laws, brain death pronouncement and certification is practiced in virtually all states.

Procurement of Legal Consent for Donation

The Uniform Anatomical Gift Act of 1968 made it possible for an individual to express during life the wish to make an anatomical gift after death. This statute was adopted by all 50 states by 1970 and now appears in some form on the driver's license in many states as a convenience to encourage organ gifts. More than 20 million people in this country have completed organ donor cards. At least 18 other countries utilize organ donor cards.[12]

Organ donor cards, and an intense public education and awareness program conducted by the National Kidney Foundation and its 50 affiliates, have done much to encourage organ donation. A Gallup survey commissioned by the National Kidney Foundation in 1983 indicated that 72 percent of those polled would be very likely to grant permission for the donation of a loved one's kidneys after death.[13] However, only 40 percent of medically suitable donors come to the attention of transplant teams, according to a 1979 survey conducted by the United States Public Health Service Centers for Disease Control.[14] The same survey determined that consent was actually obtained 47 percent of the time when requested, and that actual organ salvage resulted in 81 percent of instances when consent was obtained, resulting in an actual retrieval rate of only 15 percent of medically suitable potential cadaver donors. The significant increase in cadaver kidney transplants from 3,422 in 1980 to 5,264 in 1984 suggests the success of recent efforts to increase public awareness of the scarcity of organs for transplantation.

Obviously, many patients who die in the hospital and would be medically suitable for organ donation are not brought to the attention of a transplant team. Family members are not being asked to consider organ donation. Since most potential donors are victims of a sudden and tragic event, it is understandably difficult to ask a family unprepared for the death of a loved one to consider organ donation. It may be inappropriate to make such inquiry before death has actually been declared, since this might suggest to the family that the care team would limit their efforts on behalf of the dying patient. The patient's physician and care team may be reluctant to accept the death of the patient, even after all criteria of brain death are met, if they interpret death of the patient as failure of their care despite overwhelming brain damage. Finally, it is surely easier simply not to become involved in, and spend the time necessary for, consideration of organ donation.

The shortage of cadaver organs for transplantation and the problem of failure to inquire have encouraged the concept of required inquiry or required request for consent.[15] At least 13 countries practice presumed consent to organ donation in the absence of objection by the decedent's family; and in the absence of any family members, a hospital official or coroner can provide consent in 12 countries.[16] In the United States, six states now require the hospital to ask family members if they will agree to donate a deceased's organs. The National Kidney Foundation has initiated a new public education campaign encouraging routine inquiry to request the "gift of life." France, under a law enacted in 1976 and effective in 1978, requires the living who do not wish to donate organs for transplantation after death to register a written refusal to do so, and abolishes the right of the family of the deceased to forbid organ donation.[17]

Surgical Removal of Organs

Removal of organs has not been the subject of significant controversy or ethical concern. However, in Arizona, a man convicted of first degree murder appealed to the state's supreme court claiming that the termination of life support systems just prior to organ removal for transplantation, not the gunshot wounds to his head and resultant brain death, was the cause of the victim's death. The Arizona Supreme Court ruled that the victim was legally dead before life support systems were withdrawn, despite the absence of a brain death statute in Arizona.[18]

Preservation of Organs, Identification of Suitable Recipient, Transportation, and Transplantation of Organs

Each of these are separate steps in the procurement and transplantation of a cadaver organ from the medical standpoint. However, the medical aspects of these steps change as technology advances and have only limited pertinence to the related moral and ethical questions.

Of the approximately 80,000 patients now on dialysis in this country, it is estimated that about 10,000 are on kidney transplant lists waiting for a cadaver organ. Thousands more die each year whose lives could have been prolonged if they could have received a cadaver liver or heart transplant. Therefore, from the moment of surgical removal, a cadaver heart, liver, or kidney is a precious resource donated as a gift to society for transplantation—a "gift of life." Donor cards specify the reason for the gift ("in the hope that I may help others"), and the purpose of the gift (transplantation, therapy, medical research, or education) but do not limit or specify an institution or recipient of their gift. Donation is, in fact, a gift of person to person.

Who, then, has the responsibility to keep this organ viable, to identify a suitable recipient, to see that the organ reaches this suitable recipient, and to transplant the organ into the recipient? Is the organ a local, state, regional, national, or international resource? Should only the true costs associated with each step of procurement become the cost of the organ transplanted, or should a profit be allowed at any step?

The advent of Medicare funding for kidney transplantation and donation in July 1973 led to both a substantial increase in renal transplantation in the 1970s and the establishment of certain requirements for approval of (and payment to) transplant centers. As a result, transplanting hospitals, alone and in cooperation with other transplanting hospitals, established systems for organ preservation, immunologic characterization of organs, match of organs with potential recipients at other hospitals and at free-standing dialysis centers, and transportation of organs between transplanting hospitals. In some instances, separate not-for-profit organ procurement centers were established to provide services ranging from simple computer matching of donor organs to a regional list of potential recipients, to organ removal, preservation, tissue and recipient matching, and organ transportation. Some organ agencies functioned principally within a single major city, some within a state or an ESRD network, and others within a significant region of the country.

Cooperation between transplant centers often extended only as far as necessary and practical to meet local objectives. There existed no national criteria for sharing of organs, no national system for sharing of organs, and no national registry of waiting recipients of organs. The local and regional systems served effectively during the 1970s, but by 1980 growth in cadaver renal transplants had stalled.

As the need for transplantation grew, and particularly as results of cardiac and liver transplantation improved in the early 1980s, the inadequacies and inequities of the existing organ procurement efforts became increasingly apparent. Charles Fiske's televised appeal before the 1982 convention of the American Academy of Pediatrics for a liver for his 9-month-old daughter Jamie poignantly demonstrated the scarcity of such organs for transplantation. Her subsequent operation suggested that media manipulation, in the absence of an organized national system of organ identification and distribution, was effective in organ procurement and transplantation. This event, and Barry Jacobs's establishment of the International Kidney Exchange, Ltd., in Reston, Virginia, to broker kidneys from unrelated living donors "both from the United States and worldwide,"[19] excited the media, all kidney-related organizations, the U.S. surgeon general's office, and members of the United States Congress. This interest extended to issues involving both cadaver and living donor organs.

In the ensuing months, television, newspaper, and magazine coverage was extensive. Science and medical writer Harry Schwartz wrote in the *Wall Street Journal*, "Why are we so afraid to use the simple capitalist technique of a reward? Why is there no societal agreement that when a potential donor is located, that donor's closest relatives will be paid a substantial sum if they agree in time to make his organs available?"[20] *Fortune* carried an article entitled "The Life-and-Death Question of an Organ Donor Market."[21] The *San Francisco Chronicle* trumpeted "Doctors Blast the Human Organ Brokers."[22] The *New York Times*, the *Washington Post*, the *Los Angeles Times*, *USA Today*, and the wire services all covered the issues. ABC's "Nightline" and "Good Morning America" devoted major time segments to the controversy on the sale of donor organs.

The National Kidney Foundation issued a press release stating that it "is firmly opposed to the sale of donor organs for both medical and ethical reasons. . . . We have encouraged and worked for a national health policy . . . for dialysis and transplantation for all, regardless of socio-economic status, [and] . . . the gift of cadaver organs on a *voluntary* basis. These organs have been used based on medical need and criteria without discrimination based on racial, sex, social, or economic factors." Its testimony to a Congressional committee said, "It is immoral, and unethical, to place a living person at substantial risk of surgical complication and a small risk of death for a cash payment." The International Transplantation Society, the American Society of Transplant Surgeons, and the American Society of Transplant Physicians "strongly condemn[ed] the recent scheme for commercial purchases of organs from living donors," and indicated that "removal of organs and transplantation of organs obtained commercially will not be handled by any member of the Transplantation Societies, and anyone doing so will be expelled." The American Association of Nephrology Nurses and Technicians stated: "We believe the solicitation of organs, procurement and/or transplantation of them for financial advancement, to be unethical." The National Association of Patients on Hemodialysis and Transplantation, Inc., testified to a Congressional committee in November 1983 that "the commercial sale of organs for transplantation should not be permitted."

The surgeon general convened the Solid Organ Procurement Workshop in Winchester, Virginia, June 7–9, 1983, which ultimately resulted in the formation of a multidisciplinary group called the American Council of Transplantation.

Representative Philip Crane (R-Ill.) introduced a bill to provide income and estate tax deductions for decedents who donate organs for use as transplants. Representative Albert Gore (D-Tenn.), Senator Edward M. Kennedy (D-Mass.), and Senator Orrin G. Hatch (R-Utah) all introduced legislation concerning organ procurement and transplantation in the summer and fall of 1983. President Reagan proclaimed National Organ Donor Awareness Week, 1984.[23] After extensive committee hearings and reconciliations concerning the Gore, Hatch, and Kennedy bills, the National Organ Transplant Act (PL 98-507) was signed by the president in November 1984. This act established the 25-member multidisciplinary Task Force on Organ Procurement and Transplantation; established funding for non-profit regional organ procurement organizations and an organ procurement and transplantation network, including a national registry of potential organ recipients and computer matching system; and prohibited organ purchases in interstate commerce.

The Task Force on Organ Procurement adopted the principle of a model organ procurement and transplantation network in October 1985. The regional organ procurement organizations (OPO) and national organ procurement and transplantation network (OPTN) created by the task force were being established in early 1986.

Unrelated Living Donors

A number of renal transplants from unrelated living donors were performed in the 1960s. Such transplants were usually from marital partners or very occasionally a very close friend of the recipient. Some potential recipients advertised in the local paper for a donor. Such ads invariably produced significant response, which seemed to include some of questionable mental stability, some who clearly expected a cash or other reward, and some with apparently altruistic motivation. I am not aware of any instance of actual transplantation of a kidney from a living donor solicited by a newspaper advertisement, though such may have occurred. I have personally received telephone calls from individuals, apparently speaking with sincerity, who wished to donate *both* kidneys and other organs as a living donor, even after the consequences of such a donation were carefully explained.

In the first half of the 1960s, the Denver transplant group utilized a number of kidneys obtained from inmates at the state penitentiary in Canon City, Colorado. These inmates granted "informed consent," including the understanding that they would not benefit in terms of earlier parole or commutation of their sentences. At a colloquium, published in 1967, Thomas Starzl said of this experience, "The penal volunteers had been accepted in our Colorado hospitals under conditions that it was thought would fully insure the protection of their individual rights and permit their complete freedom of choice, objectives that may [not] have been . . . realistic," and "The acceptance of criminal volunteers was permanently discontinued at the University of Colorado 1½ years ago." In the discussion that followed, he indicated, "I think [the penal donors] were all strongly motivated, most for . . . very high-minded social reasons. . . . We know for certain that there were certain others or at least one other who was . . . motivated by the thought that he would . . . more easily escape from the hospital than from the prison. This, in fact, he did." Starzl went on to say, "I think . . . that in the absence of their civil liberties they might not be really free to make a choice," and "I think we made a mistake in accepting prison volunteers. . . ."[24]

The increasing use of cadaver kidney transplantation, particularly for those patients with ESRD who did not have a suitable or willing related donor, and the demonstration that cadaver kidney transplantation was as successful as unrelated living donor transplantation, led to a virtual discontinuation of any unrelated living donor transplantation for many years. Recently, however, the relative shortage of cadaver kidneys has revived this issue.

The advocates of a free market approach to unrelated living donor transplants argue that paying a market-determined price for a kidney will increase the supply;

will permit timely performance of the transplant; will allow improved matching of a donor organ to the recipient; and should provide at least equal if not improved results compared with cadaver kidney transplantation with today's immunosuppressive drugs. Opponents find the " 'free market' sale of one's organs . . . morally offensive and ethically indefensible," and state "It is immoral to offer someone an incentive to undergo permanent physical damage."[25]

The Task Force on Organ Transplantation established by PL 98-507 issued the following statement in November 1985: "The Task Force is alarmed that even with a statute prohibiting the sale of human organs, certain transplant centers are reportedly brokering kidneys from living unrelated donors. The Task Force finds this practice to be unethical and to raise serious questions about the exploitation and coercion of people, especially the poor. The Task Force believes that transplanting kidneys from living unrelated donors should be prohibited when financial gain rather than altruism is the motivating factor." The statement, in an apparent effort to close any loopholes in the federal law, recommends that states prohibit the sale of organs from cadavers or living donors.

The Council of The Transplantation Society published guidelines for the donation of kidneys by unrelated living donors.[26] These guidelines state that "living unrelated donors should be used exceptionally when a satisfactory cadaver or living related donor cannot be found; that it must be established that the motives of the donor are altruistic and not self-serving or for profit; and that an independent donor advocate should be assigned to the unrelated donor to ensure that informed consent is made without pressure."

A recent Sounding Board article in the *New England Journal of Medicine* indicates, "It is now time to reevaluate the ethical and medical justifications for this policy" of rejecting living persons not related to the recipient as potential kidney donors.[27] This article espouses potential advantages to the recipient of a living unrelated donor versus a cadaver donor and finds that "the risks of nephrectomy to the donor are minimal." It defines the risks as a 0.03 percent incidence of death during the operation; 2–3 percent incidence of major morbid events including deep wound infections, pulmonary emboli, and hemorrhage requiring reoperation; and a 10–20 percent incidence of minor complications including superficial wound infections, pulmonary and urinary infections, pneumothorax, or other minor problems. They find that the possible long-term consequences of donor nephrectomy are of little or no concern. Others have referred to donor nephrectomy as "permanent physical damage."[28] I had personal experience with a number of marital donor-recipient pairs more than 20 years ago. Feelings of subtle coercion were sometimes expressed, often after the donation had occurred, and particularly if the transplant failed. These feelings approached those of frank resentment ("he or she took everything else I had and now has taken my kidney too"), and were expressed even though each donor was interviewed by a psychologist before donation and was told a medical reason could be provided for finding donation inappropriate if the donor so wished.

Related Living Donors

The principal ethical issue concerning related living donors is whether the benefits to the donor justify the risks to the donor. The benefits to the recipient are quite real. The timing of the transplant is facilitated and is sometimes possible without any prior dialysis therapy. The match between donor and recipient is likely to be better than can be achieved either with a cadaver or unrelated living donor transplant, both with regard to recognized and unknown factors contributing to the match. The improved match minimizes necessary immunosuppressive medication, and in the instance of identical twins, makes immunosuppression unnecessary. Finally, the short- and long-term survival of kidney and recipient are better with related living donor than with cadaver or unrelated living donor transplantation.

The benefits to the donor of donation to a first-degree relative are difficult to define and more difficult to quantify. The principal benefit is the gift of renewed life to a loved one. Donors have described donation as an intensely meaningful experience that has brought about substantial beneficial changes in themselves and in their lives.[29] It has been successfully argued that prevention of donation might be psychologically harmful.[30] A follow-up study an average of more than nine years after donation found that the early psychological and spiritual benefits of donation persisted, although such benefits tended to be greater among donors whose recipients were still alive.[31]

The risks of donation are more easily defined and quantified; they include both perioperative and long-term risks. The preoperative evaluation is of little medical risk except the small risk of injection of contrast media intraarterially for definition of the renal vasculature and renal anatomy. Donor nephrectomy, however, is a major procedure, frequently requiring rib resection and entry of the pleural space. It is associated with a complication rate of 14–47 percent, depending on different definitions of complications in the several reported studies.[32–35] Major perioperative complications have included death, myocardial infarction, pulmonary embolus, small bowel obstruction, acute kidney failure, pneumonia, and nerve injury. Minor complications include atelectasis, pleural effusion, ileus, and urinary tract infection. These complications extend hospitalization and, therefore, donor morbidity.

The long-term risks of renal donation are still a subject of debate. Following unilateral nephrectomy, the remaining kidney promptly increases in size and function. Within a few days, renal function increases to 70 percent of the two-kidney preoperative function.[36] It is known that rats normally develop progressive loss of the filtering elements (glomeruli) of their kidneys as they age, and that this process in their normal kidney is accelerated if one kidney is removed. This has been attributed to the increased work performed by the remaining kidney after unilateral nephrectomy. It has been postulated that the same effect might be seen in human kidney donors.[37] Over 750 living donors have now been studied between 10 and 20 years after unilateral nephrectomy. These donors demonstrate very low grade increased protein but not albumin in their urine; a trend toward a slight increase in blood pressure, still within the normal range, except in the number that would be expected in the general population; and preservation of the 70 percent of kidney function demonstrated shortly after nephrectomy.[38-42] It may be, however, that studies of these same donors 20–30 or more years after donation will reveal deleterious effects of increased work of the remaining kidney.

ALLOCATION OF ORGANS

Available kidneys, and especially livers and hearts, are critically short of the need for transplantation in this country and throughout the world. An old Scottish recipe for rabbit stew starts with "first catch your rabbit." How does, and how should, the waiting recipient "catch a rabbit?"

Health care has always been rationed, and it remains so today. Its allocation has characteristically been determined by wealth. Those less able or unable to pay are subjected to various delaying or denying tactics (long waits to see a physician or obtain medication, denial of access to specialists, provision of emergent care only). Access to organs for transplantation, particularly liver and heart transplants usually not funded by Medicare, continues to be limited by the ability to pay for treatment.

The National Organ Transplant Act of 1984 (PL 98-507) requires that Organ Procurement Organizations "have a system to allocate donated organs among transplant centers *and patients according to established criteria.*" However, as of this writing, no criteria are uniformly accepted or practiced for allocation to those in need.

Historically, whole organ transplantation has been allocated by:

- ability to pay (kidney transplants prior to 1973 [PL 92-603], liver and heart transplants today)
- clinical efficacy of the therapy (age and comorbid disease factors in kidney transplants, age in liver and heart transplants)
- age, even though medical evidence of inefficacy was or is lacking
- ethnic origin (the striking lack of non-Caucasians in the ESRD program prior to 1973)
- sex (the preponderance of male kidney transplant recipients prior to 1973)
- self-inflicted diseases (the reluctance to provide liver transplants to those with alcoholic cirrhosis as opposed to posthepatitis cirrhosis)
- public policy (the delay in governmental approval of liver and heart transplantation, or limitation of facilities approved to perform the procedures)

Criteria for acceptance for kidney, heart, and liver transplants vary widely and continue to depend significantly on organ availability as well as medical criteria. In March 1986, a 65-year-old man received a heart transplant at the University Medical Center in Tucson, Arizona.[43] The newspaper reported that officials at another university heart transplant center indicated they wouldn't even consider a heart transplant for a 65-year-old man, mainly because of the donor shortage. The transplant coordinator at UMC is quoted as explaining the decision on this patient: "He was a good candidate. He was nice, outgoing, had a positive attitude and was in relatively good shape, except for his heart disease." The donor of the heart was a local accident victim.

In September 1985, the National Kidney Foundation issued a statement concerning organ allocation, which indicated that "the distribution and assignment of organs must be made by medical criteria and cannot be influenced by any other considerations, such as political, special payment or favoritism."[44] In the same month, the Council of The Transplantation Society published guidelines for cadaver organ distribution, which included: "Organs should be transplanted to the most appropriate recipient on the basis of medical and immunologic criteria"; "Sharing of organs should only be arranged via national and/or regional organ sharing networks"; and "Priorities in the assignments of organs cannot be influenced by political considerations, gifts, special payments or by favoritism to special groups."[45] In November 1985, the Task Force on Organ Transplantation adopted these guidelines. It remains to be seen how they will be interpreted and whether they will be uniformly used.

EXPORTATION OF ORGANS AND IMPORTATION OF RECIPIENTS

In 1985 it became apparent that the practice of exporting kidneys to foreign nations and soliciting citizens of other nations for transplantation in the United States was expanding. Although firm numbers are not available, it is estimated that as many as 600 kidneys obtained in this country were exported in 1984,[46] sometimes with significant profit to the exporting group. It has also been estimated that 5 percent of whole organ transplants in this country involve transplantation of organs obtained in this country into foreign nationals, also sometimes involving substantial profit to the transplanting organization(s). Is, then, a scarce donor organ a national or an international resource? If profit results from an organ donation, is the concept of organ donation as a benefaction threatened? Will this practice establish a market price for a donor organ, and what will be the effect on the supply of organs?

In its letter of September 1985, the National Kidney Foundation stated, "There should be no shipment of kidneys to foreign countries . . . unless there is verifiable evidence that an attempt has been made to place these kidneys in recipients somewhere else in the United States,'' and ''The National Kidney Foundation opposes active recruitment of foreign nationals for the sole purpose of transplantation in the United States.'' The Council of the Transplantation Society adopted the resolution that ''No transplant surgeon/team shall be involved directly or indirectly in the buying or selling of organs/tissues or in any transplant activity aimed at commercial gain to himself/herself or an associated hospital or institute. Violation of these guidelines . . . may be cause for expulsion from the society.''[47] It also stated, ''When the less privileged can be exploited to improve the health of the more privileged, all in society are diminished.'' The Task Force on Organ Transplantation recommended ''that exportation and importation of donor organs be prohibited except when distribution is arranged or coordinated by the Organ Procurement and Transplantation Network,'' further indicated that ''documentation must be available to demonstrate that all appropriate efforts have been made to locate a recipient in the U.S. and/or Canada,'' and indicated that it had ''every expectation that these international organ sharing programs will be reciprocal.''

Advancing technology in organ procurement and transplantation, as in other medical fields, continues to pose challenging questions of right and wrong—of one's duty to another. It is increasingly apparent, however, first with Seattle's ''life-and-death'' committee and now with the Task Force on Organ Transplantation, that the evolving practices in this field that have commanded the fascination of society are the responsibility of the same society.

NOTES

1. J.P. Merrill et al., ''Successful Homotransplantation of the Kidney between Nonidentical Twins,'' *New England Journal of Medicine* 262 (1960):1251–1260.

2. U.S. Bureau of the Budget, Report of the Committee on Chronic Kidney Disease (Washington, D.C.: September 1967).

3. G. de Rosa, *Il Popolo* (Italian Christian Democrat newspaper), 1968.

4. T.E. Starzl, March 27, 1986: personal communication.

5. ''They Decide Who Lives, Who Dies,'' *Life* 102, Nov. 9, 1962.

6. T.E. Starzl et al., ''Renal Heterotransplantation from Baboon to Man: Experience with 6 Cases,'' *Transplant* 2 (1964):752–775.

7. D.A. Ogden, V. Sitprija, and J.H. Holmes, ''Function of the Baboon Renal Heterograft in Man and Comparison with Renal Homograft Function,'' *Journal of Laboratory Clinical Medicine* 65 (1965):370–386.

8. ''A Definition of Irreversible Coma: Report of the Ad Hoc Committee of the Harvard Medical School to Examine the Definition of Brain Death,'' *Journal of the American Medical Association* 205 (1968):85–88. ''Refinements in Criteria for the Determination of Death: An Appraisal. A Report by the Task Force on Death and Dying of the Institute of Society, Ethics, and the Life Sciences,'' *Journal of the American Medical Association* 221 (1972):48–53.

9. D. Margolick, ''New York's Highest Court Rules Life Ends When the Brain Dies,'' *New York Times*, Oct. 31, 1984; *State v. David Madrid Fiero,* Supreme Court of Arizona, No. 4271, Oct. 22, 1979.

10. Summary of Action of the House of Delegates Mid Year Meeting, American Bar Association (Chicago: American Bar Association, February 1975), 19.

11. National Conference of Commissioners on Uniform State Laws (Chicago: 1980).

12. F.P. Stuart, F. Veith, and R.E. Cranford, "Brain Death Laws and Patterns of Consent to Remove Organs for Transplantation from Cadavers in the United States and 28 Other Countries," *Transplantation* 31 (1981):238–244.

13. The Gallup Organization *Attitudes and Opinions of the American Public towards Kidney Donations*. Prepared for the National Kidney Foundation (GO 8305) (Washington, D.C.: 1983).

14. K.J. Bart et al., "Increasing the Supply of Cadaveric Kidneys for Transplantation," *Transplant* 31 (1981):383–387.

15. A.L. Caplan, "Ethical and Policy Issues in the Procurement of Cadaver Organs for Transplantation," *New England Journal of Medicine* 311 (1984):981–982.

16. Stuart, "Brain Death Laws."

17. "France Widens Authority for Transplants from Dead," *New York Times*, April 16, 1978.

18. *State v. Fiero.*

19. H.B. Jacobs, Letter to Dear Hospital Administrator, International Kidney Exchange, Ltd., Reston, VA, Undated (1983).

20. H. Schwartz, "Providing Incentives for Organ Donations," *Wall Street Journal*, July 25, 1983.

21. F.S. Chapman, "The Life-and-Death Question of an Organ Market," *Fortune*, June 11, 1984.

22. D. Perlman, "Doctors Blast the Human Organ Brokers," *San Francisco Chronicle*, October 22, 1983.

23. Proclamation 5163 of March 17, 1984: National Organ Donor Awareness Week, 1984. *Federal Register* 49:10533, 1984.

24. T.E. Starzl, "Ethical Problems in Organ Transplantation: A Clinician's Point of View," *Annals of Internal Medicine* 67 (1967):32–36, and Discussion, *Annals of Internal Medicine* 67 (1967):51–56.

25. C.B. Carpenter, R.B. Ettenger, and T.B. Strom, " 'Free-Market' Approach to Organ Donation," *New England Journal of Medicine* 310 (1984):395–396.

26. The Council of The Transplantation Society, "Commercialisation in Transplantation: The Problems and Some Guidelines for Practice," *Lancet* 2 (1985):715–716.

27. A.S. Levey, S. Hou, and H.L. Bush, "Kidney Transplantation from Unrelated Living Donors: Time to Reclaim a Discarded Opportunity," *New England Journal of Medicine* 314 (1986):914–916.

28. Carpenter, "Free-Market Approach."

29. C.H. Fellner and J.R. Marshall, "Twelve Kidney Donors," *Journal of the American Medical Association* 206 (1968):2703–2707. D.M. Bernstein and R.C. Simmons, "The Adolescent Kidney Donor: The Right to Give," *American Journal of Psychiatry* 131 (1974):1338–1343.

30. *Masden v. Harrison*, Mass. Supreme Judicial Court, Equity Number 68651 (1957).

31. J.R. Marshall and C.H. Fellner, "Kidney Donors Revisited," *American Journal of Psychiatry* 134 (1977):575–576.

32. I. Penn et al., "Living Related Kidney Donors: Complications and Long-term Renal Function," *Archives of Surgery* 101 (1970):226–231.

33. C. Buszta et al., "Kidney Donor Evaluation," *Dialysis and Renal Transplantation* 11 (1982): 296–300.

34. D.T. Vehling, G.H. Malek, and J.B. Wear, "Complications of Donor Nephrectomy," *Journal of Urology* 111 (1974):745–746.

35. S.C. Jacobs et al., "Live Donor Nephrectomy," *Urology* 5 (1975):175–177.

36. A.G. Krohn, D.A. Ogden, and J.H. Holmes, "Renal Function in 29 Healthy Adults Before and After Nephrectomy," *Journal of the American Medical Association* 196 (1966):322–324.

37. B.M. Brenner, T.W. Meyer, and T.H. Hostetter, "Dietary Protein Intake and the Progressive Nature of Renal Disease: The Role of Hemodynamically Mediated Glomerular Injury in the Pathogenesis of Progressive Glomerular Sclerosis in Aging, Renal Ablation, and Intrinsic Renal Disease," *New England Journal of Medicine* 307 (1982):652–659.

38. R.M. Hakim, R.C. Goldszer, and B.M. Brenner, "Hypertension and Proteinuria: Long-term Sequelae of Uninephrectomy in Humans," *Kidney International* 25 (1984):930–936.

39. F. Vincenti et al., "Long-term Renal Function in Kidney Donors," *Transplant* 36 (1983):626–629.

40. C.F. Anderson et al., "The Risks of Unilateral Nephrectomy: Status of Kidney Donors 10 to 20 Years Postoperatively," *Mayo Clinic Proceedings* 60 (1985):367–374.

41. S. Smith, P. Loprad, and J. Grantham, "Long-term Effect of Uninephrectomy on Serum Creatinine Concentration and Arterial Blood Pressure," *American Journal of Kidney Disease* 6 (1985):143–148.

42. D. Weiland et al., "Information on 628 Living-related Kidney Donors at a Single Institution with Long-term Follow-up in 472 Cases," *Transplant Proceedings* 26 (1984):5–7.

43. C. McLain, "65-year-old Given New Heart at UMC: Oldest Patient to Get Modern Transplant," *Tucson Citizen*, March 28, 1986.

44. R.W. Schrier, National Kidney Foundation Letter to Chairman, Task Force on Organ Transplantation, September 26, 1985.

45. Council of The Transplantation Society, "Commercialisation."

46. Ibid.

47. Ibid.

Chapter 8

Quality of Life As a Criterion for Allocation of Life-Sustaining Treatment: The Case of Hemodialysis

Carol Estwing Ferrans, PhD, RN

During the last 25 years, medical science has produced several modern miracles in life-sustaining technology: hemodialysis, heart-lung bypass machines, artificial hearts, and unprecedented success in kidney, heart, liver, and lung transplantation. However, these advances have raised unique ethical questions regarding their allocation. These issues are of primary importance because they form the basis for ultimate decisions regarding who will live and who will die. Dialysis provides an example of a technological innovation that has progressed from experimental stages to widespread use. As such, its history provides a model for examination of the ethical and practical issues involved in the allocation of life-sustaining technology.

SCARCE RESOURCE PHASE

The technology for long-term, intermittent hemodialysis first became available in 1960, when the permanent arteriovenous shunt was developed by Scribner and his colleagues. After its effectiveness was demonstrated, the allocation of hemodialysis occurred in two phases: the scarce resource phase and the open access phase. The scarce resource phase lasted approximately from 1960 to 1973, when the number of patients who needed dialysis for survival far exceeded the supply of treatment facilities. Those patients who were determined medically suitable were either treated on a first come first served basis or selected by physicians and committees. One typical committee consisted of a clergyman, a housewife, a banker, a labor leader, and two physicians.[1]

A nationwide study revealed that half of the dialysis centers had no explicit, written criteria for selection of patients,[2] so that committee members had only their own consciences to rely upon. The criteria most frequently used by the remainder of the dialysis centers were absence of disabling disease, age, future employment potential, social welfare, family cooperativeness, intelligence, and financial resources for treatment. Social worth and social class considerations were often given a great deal of weight,[3] which resulted in an inordinate number of white, middle- and upper-income, male patients on dialysis. For example, in 1967, 91 percent of patients on hemodialysis were white, 75 percent were male, and 41 percent were gainfully employed. In contrast, in 1978, when dialysis was freely available without selection by committee, only 63.7 percent were white, 49.2 percent were male, and 18.4 percent were employed.[4]

The justification for such selection on the basis of social worth is derived from utilitarian principles of justice, which emphasize the maximization of public and private utility. Society is viewed as investing a scarce resource in the selected patient and consequently is entitled to consider the probable return on the investment.[5] However, Edlund and Tancredi pointed out that in practice the problem with assessing social usefulness is that it has an "unknowable multiplicity of potential meanings. . . . People will quickly ascribe to the concept their own personal meanings and less frequently ask themselves if these meanings are really shared by others."[6] Hence, the situation became in many cases, as Sanders and Dukeminier characterized it, "the bourgeoisie sparing the bourgeoisie."[7]

Also skewing the selection of patients toward the middle and upper class was the fact that patients had to demonstrate their ability to pay for treatments, the most common method of rationing health care in the U.S. The options for funding fell into four basic categories: self-funding through personal assets; private funding from insurance or charity; public funding from governmental agencies; or no funding, in which case the patient simply died for lack of treatment. The latter option was the most prevalent.[8] In 1972 in-unit hemodialysis treatments cost approximately $30,500 per person annually,[9] which rapidly depleted personal funds and insurance policies. In fact, some patients chose to die rather than to wipe out their savings and put their families into poverty. An administrator of a dialysis center reported that

> there are lots of cases where patients just haven't showed up. Patients have been referred to private centers, say, where they demand a deposit of $10,000, and they just toss in the towel. One man I know of personally—thirty-seven years of age with three children and $19,000 in the bank—elected to die. He was perfectly frank. He said if he went into treatment he would destroy his family.[10]

The ethical justification for allocation of health care via the free market system (ability to pay) is basically drawn from libertarian theories of justice. Libertarian theories emphasize rights of social and economic liberty, in which individuals are free to engage in or withdraw from arrangements according to their personal interests.[11] Sade defended libertarian means for the distribution of health care by arguing:

> In a free society, man exercises his right to sustain his own life by producing economic values in the form of goods and services that he

is, or should be, free to exchange with other men who are similarly free to trade with him or not. The economic values produced, however, are not given as gifts by nature, but exist only by virtue of the thought and effort of individual men. Goods and services are thus owned as a consequence of the right to sustain life by one's own physical and mental effort. . . . Medical care is neither a right nor a privilege: it is a service that is provided by doctors and others to people who wish to purchase it.[12]

OPEN ACCESS PHASE

The inequities in access to dialysis treatment motivated Congress to pass Pub. L. No. 92-603, which extended Medicare coverage to almost anyone with end-stage renal disease (ESRD) who required dialysis to live. The ESRD program went into effect in 1973, marking the beginning of the open access phase in the allocation of hemodialysis. Equal access was the primary objective of the program, and its success was demonstrated by a shift of sociodemographic characteristics to those that more closely reflected the incidence of ESRD.[13] The ethical justification for the ESRD program is found in egalitarian theories of justice, which emphasize equal access to goods, regardless of wealth or social position.

Originally it was thought that the numbers of patients participating in the ESRD program would increase steadily for a time and then level off as supply met demand. However, since 1973 the number of patients on dialysis has increased by 5,000 to 6,000 per year,[14] until in 1985 there were approximately 72,000 dialysis patients in the United States.[15] This steady increase has prompted concern that profit-making motives by proprietary dialysis centers have resulted in the dialyzing of patients who are too old or sick to benefit.[16] A close examination of this concern is warranted, since the cost of the ESRD program in 1985 was estimated to be over $2 billion per year.[17] It would be unjust on utilitarian grounds to use resources to treat persons who are unable to benefit, since the greatest possible good would not be obtained from those federal funds. Such money would be better spent to ease the financial burden of other illness groups or to decrease the federal deficit.

To evaluate the validity of this concern, the concept of being "too old or sick to benefit" must first be examined. Essentially, the determination of whether some persons are too old or sick to benefit from dialysis requires an assessment of quality of life and a judgment regarding whether the quality of life is so poor that it is not worth living, since death is certain without dialysis. However, it is very difficult to define and measure quality of life and equally difficult to determine standard criteria for the judgment that life is not worth living.

DEFINITION AND MEASUREMENT OF QUALITY OF LIFE

The concept of quality of life has its roots in some of the oldest philosophical thought, such as Aristotle's *Ethica Nicomachea*. However, the term "quality of life" did not enter into common American vocabulary until the 1950s. It was used originally to emphasize that the good life required more than material affluence.[18] Since then quality of life has become an important concept for decision making in health care and social policy. Unfortunately, quality of life is very difficult to define, because its meaning varies from individual to individual, depending upon personal values and underlying motivations. Hence, there is no consensus regarding standards for life quality, even among members of the same group or profession. For example, Pearlman and Jonsen presented a case description of an elderly man with chronic pulmonary disease to 205 internal medicine and family medicine physicians. The physicians' perceptions of the patient's quality of life were found to vary markedly and to lead to diverse conclusions regarding whether to withhold or give additional treatment.[19] Because decisions based on quality of life ultimately depend upon how it is defined, the question of whose values should be used to define it in a given situation becomes an issue of critical importance.

Some of the most common definitions of quality of life focus on social utility, the ability to live a normal life, and happiness or satisfaction.

Definitions That Focus on Social Utility

Social utility definitions are those that focus on the ability to lead socially useful lives[20] or to attain attributes highly valued by society. Although the concept of a socially useful life has a potentially infinite variety of meanings, in practice its operational definition is typically determined by the sociopolitical orientation of those defining it. For instance, government policy makers generally use social utility definitions to mean contributions to the national economy,[21] as measured by income and occupation. Social utility definitions also may focus on the ability to function in socially valued roles, such as parent, scout leader, or Sunday school teacher.

One of the major weaknesses of social utility definitions of quality of life is that discriminating prejudices may be hidden below the surface of apparently benign criteria.[22] For example, when productivity is measured only by earned income, as in the assessment of "human capital," bias against homemakers and elderly, retired persons can result.[23] In the human capital approach, the value of a person's life is calculated from the projected earnings for his or her remaining lifetime. Homemaking is appraised at minimum wage, and retirees are assumed to lead minimally productive lives. Hence these persons are valued much lower than preretirement-aged men. In addition to objecting that discrimination is inherent in this approach, the validity of appraising the contributions of homemakers and retirees so cheaply must be questioned. Moreover, Avorn protested against such valuation of human lives without "the notions of compassion, rights, one's debt to one's parents and forebears, or any sense of altruism or equity."[24] It also must be questioned whether objective indicators, such as income and occupation, actually give an accurate indication of the experience of quality of life. For example, Campbell found that between 1957 and 1972 there was a steady decrease in the number of persons who reported themselves to be very happy, even though almost all objective socioeconomic indicators increased over that period of time. This trend was most pronounced among higher socioeconomic groups.[25]

Social utility definitions that focus on functioning in socially valued roles also may result in discriminating bias. During the scarce resource phase of dialysis allocation, committees often favored patients who had a record of public service, such as scout leader, Sunday school teacher, or Red Cross volunteer.[26] However, Sanders and Dukeminier pointed out that a middle-class suburban definition of public service was employed, ruling out creative nonconformists, who historically have made large contributions to America. They asked, "Were the persons who got themselves jailed in the South while working for civil rights doing a 'public service'?"[27]

Definitions That Focus on the Ability To Live a Normal Life

The second category of common definitions of quality of life focuses on the ability to live a normal life. These types of definitions may use such phrases as the ability to function at a level similar to typical persons of the same age or the ability to act in typically human ways. These definitions are appealing because they appear quite plausible initially. However, in practice they are difficult to put into measurable terms, because there are potentially as many conceptualizations of being "normal" as there are members of the population.[28]

One way to deal with this problem is to use each individual as his or her own standard of normalcy. This has been done by comparing physical activities for each patient before and after a treatment or onset of illness. For example, the number of physical symptoms, frequency of sexual intercourse, and number of hours worked have been compared before and after the onset of illness in numerous studies. In these comparisons it is assumed that the closer the activities are to the preillness level, the better the quality of life. This type of comparison does give an idea of changes in status due to treatment or illness. However, this approach fails to take into account the importance of these changes to the individual. Individuals differ in the importance they place on various aspects of illness and in their success in adaptation, which results in a differential impact on quality of life.[29] A disability that makes life not worth living to one person may be only a nuisance to another.

The concept of the "quality adjusted life year" is another example of an attempt to put this type of definition into measurable terms. Quality adjusted life years are used typically to bring quality of life considerations into cost effectiveness evaluations of health care programs. Using this approach the quality of a year of life with an illness or disability is compared with the quality of a year with perfect health. One number ranging between 0 (death) and 1.0 (perfect health) is assigned to each kind of illness.[30] An assignment of 0.5 would mean that the quality of a year of life with a certain illness would be worth one half of a year with perfect health. However, we must question the validity of assigning one number to represent the quality of life of all persons with the same diagnosis. Individuals vary with regard to severity of illness and accompanying disability. Individuals also differ in the importance they place on various aspects of illness, as was discussed previously. Avorn contended that an infinite range of outcomes would be needed to adequately account for differences among patients, which would correct "the concept of quality adjustment . . . out of existence."[31]

Definitions That Focus on Happiness or Satisfaction with Life

The third category of definitions of quality of life focuses on the patient's opinion of happiness or satisfaction with life as a whole or with various aspects of life. An example of this type of definition is "a person's sense of well-being, his satisfaction or dissatisfaction with life, or his happiness or unhappiness."[32] Another example is "a person's sense of well-being that stems from satisfaction or dissatisfaction with the areas of life that are important to him/her."[33] Although happiness and satisfaction are closely related concepts, satisfaction may be a better choice for defining quality of life, since in present English usage happiness implies short-term feelings or moods, whereas satisfaction suggests a somewhat more permanent state. In this respect satisfaction comes closer to the Aristotelian ideal of happiness, which was something permanent and not easily changed. In addition, satisfaction also is preferable because it suggests a cognitive, judgmental experience, which makes it fit better conceptually with the idea that quality of life is determined by judgment and evaluation of life's conditions.[34]

Measurement of quality of life using this type of definition depends upon patients' own descriptions of the quality of their life experience, something that definitions focusing on social utility or the ability to live a normal life typically do not. It generally is more difficult to devise reliable and valid instruments to measure such subjective assessments of happiness or satisfaction than strictly objective types of data. Nevertheless, Campbell argued that subjective evaluation is absolutely essential for the valid assessment of quality of life, and that objective indicators merely assess those things that influence it.[35] As stated by Neugarten et al., "the individual himself is the only proper judge of his well-being."[36]

VALUE JUDGMENTS REGARDING THE QUALITY OF LIFE

In addition to assessing quality of life, a judgment regarding whether life is so poor that it is not worth living is required to determine whether some persons are too old or sick to benefit from dialysis. This type of judgment, which moves from the assessment of quality of life to the value of life, requires ethical justification. However, recognize that the value of individual lives must be handled very carefully. Our own recent history warns us that this area is vulnerable to abuse—the most heinous example was the determination by Hitler's regime that the lives of entire categories of people were worthless or useless. This provided the ideological justification for mass extermination of the insane, poor workers, gypsies, Jews, Poles, and Russians under the label of "euthanasia."[37]

The value judgments made to select dialysis patients during the scarce resource phase differ fundamentally from those required to determine whether patients are too old or sick to benefit from treatment. In the latter case the value of each individual's life is determined by evaluation of his or her own quality of life alone. In contrast, during the scarce resource phase many patients were chosen because they were judged to be worth *more* than other potential patients. Sanders and Dukeminier object to such comparisons on the grounds that they fail to meet the constitutional command of equal protection under the law and violate the principle that man should not play God with human life.[38]

Consequentialist Ethic

Ethical justification for judgments on quality of life can be based on the consequentialist ethic. This holds that human life has value only because of the higher qualities that can result from it, such as happiness, satisfaction, or love.[39] Higher qualities in turn depend upon the presence of "humanhood qualities," such as rational function, ability to consciously experience, capacity for human relationships, and potential for a meaningful life.[40] In the absence of these humanhood qualities, there is no moral obligation to protect or preserve life, because no potential for happiness, satisfaction, or love exists.[41] Hence, persons without these qualities would be considered unable to benefit from dialysis and so could be allowed to die without it. Cost-benefit analysis would determine whether a person possessing humanhood qualities should be provided with dialysis. A positive balance of benefits over costs/harms would justify the preservation of life.[42] This analysis could be conducted from either a social or personalistic perspective.

The social perspective of the consequentialist ethic is based on the principle of utilitarianism: the greatest good for the greatest number.[43] This perspective considers the impact of sustaining the patient's life on all concerned parties, including the patient, family, community, nation, and human race.[44] In contrast, the personalistic perspective focuses the analysis on the costs and benefits for the patient alone.[45] The personalistic perspective is based upon the principle of the duty of nonmaleficence, which is basically the principle of doing no harm. This principle finds its roots in the Hippocratic Oath: "Neither will I administer a poison to anybody when asked to do so, nor will I suggest such a course . . . . I will abstain from all intentional wrong-doing and harm . . . ."[46] However, a modified version of the principle is needed to support the personalistic form of the consequentialist method: "Do no harm [e.g., by terminating a patient's life or maintaining it in a seriously defective condition] unless there is corresponding benefit to the patient."[47]

In order to make value judgments based on quality of life, one must decide whose criteria to use for the cost-benefit analysis: those of the patient or a proxy, such as family, physician, or society.[48] In the case of incompetent patients, judgments must be made by proxy, except when patients make their wishes known in advance, as in a living will. However, respect for the patient's autonomy strongly supports competent patients making judgments based on their own standards. Autonomy refers to the right of self-rule without constraints by others.[49] Legal support for this principle was found in the 1960 case of *Natanson v. Kline*, in which it was stated that:

> Anglo-American law starts with the premise of thoroughgoing self-determination. It follows that each man is considered to be master of his own body, and he may, if he be of sound mind, expressly prohibit the performance of lifesaving surgery, or any other medical treatment.[50]

A recent report of the Canadian Law Reform Commission also upheld the patient's right to refuse treatment even when it would lead to death.[51]

Objections to the Consequentialist Ethic

Many objections to the consequentialist method have been made, both on ethical and practical grounds. First, the consequentialist cost-benefit analysis assigns unequal value to various lives. This assignment is based on a merit theory of justice, which holds that "the right to life is earned by the accomplishments or the potential contribution of the individual."[52] Hence, the method violates the principle of equality of all human lives.

Second, the consequentialist notion that the right to life is earned also conflicts with the principle that all human beings have a right to life, regardless of their current or potential quality of life. Singer argues that the right to live is the most fundamental of natural rights, since without it all other rights are pointless.[53] Support for the right to life can be found in the principle of respect for patient autonomy, in that the greatest violation of this principle would be to take someone's life without his or her consent.[54] Strong legal support also exists for the idea that all have a right to life. An example is found in the ruling of David E.

Roberts, a Maine superior court justice, that "at the moment of live birth there does exist a human being entitled to the fullest protection of the law. The most basic right enjoyed by every human being is the right to life itself."[55]

Third, according to the consequentialist method the value of life is based upon variable qualities. This notion violates the principle of sanctity of life, which holds that human life has unique value regardless of the presence or absence of other qualities. This principle is based on the Judeo-Christian belief that human beings are made in the image of God and possess immortal souls.[56] Their spiritual nature and special relationship to God confer them with unique value. Hence, mankind has the moral responsibility to protect and sustain the lives of fellow humans.

Fourth, cost-benefit analyses depend upon the accurate prediction of future qualities and outcomes, which are difficult if not impossible to make. Childress argues that a person's potential contributions cannot be extrapolated from his present state of affairs.[57] Future accomplishments depend on social support and other contingent factors, which often cannot be foreseen. Moreover, it is also difficult to predict accurately what future societal needs will be.

Finally, implementation of cost-benefit analyses in practice results in excessive reductionism of human worth and oversimplification of complex ethical questions.[58] Excessive reductionism occurs in attempting to quantify relevant criteria, as in the use of IQ scores to represent the capacity for rational thought. Oversimplification occurs by focusing on a narrow range of concerns, such as social roles, family relationships, and occupational function. Childress argues that such reductionism "dulls and perhaps even eliminates the sense of the person's transcendence, his dignity as a person which cannot be reduced to his past or future contribution to society."[59]

QUALITY OF LIFE OF HEMODIALYSIS PATIENTS

To explore the validity of the concern that patients who are too old or sick to benefit may be receiving dialysis, studies that reflect the quality of life of in-center hemodialysis patients will be examined. A detailed cost-benefit analysis will not be attempted, due to lack of sufficient data and to the problems inherent in defining, measuring, and assigning value to a person's quality of life, which have been discussed.

Studies Reflecting Social Value and "Normal Life" Definitions

Studies of hemodialysis patients that focus on employment status and the ability to function reflect social value definitions of quality of life. In general, these studies have reported a fair to poor quality of life for the majority of patients. For instance, a 1985 study, whose sample was representative of the diversity of U.S. dialysis patients, found that only 37.2 percent of patients were able to work. Patients' mean physical functioning was rated a low 3.11 (1 = moribund, 10 = normal activity).[60]

Similar findings have been reported in studies focusing on the ability to live a normal life. Three major studies compared variables before and after the initiation of dialysis treatment. A 1978 nationwide study found that although 72.1 percent of patients were employed prior to dialysis, only 18.4 percent were employed after initiation of treatment.[61] Similarly, of the 795 nondiabetic men aged 21 to 59 years who were surveyed by Gutman et al., 97.0 percent were employed before dialysis and only 41.8 percent after.[62] Gutman's findings are particularly interesting, since they dealt with the most productive years of these men's lives. In addition, Gutman found that 45 percent of 2,191 nondiabetic patients were unable to perform any activity beyond caring for themselves. Bonney et al. found that although 90 percent of 136 patients had been employed before starting in-unit dialysis, only 33 percent were employed afterward.[63] Seventy-one percent of patients were capable of performing all usual activities before dialysis; this figure had dropped to 3 percent at the time of the study. Seventy percent had sexual intercourse twice weekly prior to dialysis, whereas only 17 percent continued at this rate. The authors concluded that there was substantial impairment in all of the quality of life parameters investigated. A fourth study used the quality adjusted life year to assess quality of life. It was found that dialysis patients considered one year of life on in-unit hemodialysis to be worth 0.52 years of perfect health.[64]

Studies Reflecting Happiness- or Satisfaction-Based Definitions

In contrast, in studies in which patients evaluated their happiness or satisfaction, quality of life has been reported to be relatively good—in many studies, similar to that of healthy persons. For instance, in ten studies patients have rated their overall satisfaction with life using Cantril's Self-Anchoring Scale.[65-74] The scale is a ten-point ladder that is anchored at either end by the best possible life (10) and the worst possible life (0). This allows the patient's own concerns, values, and perceptions to establish the end points. Patients indicate which number on the scale best represents their life at the present time. The means of the ratings reported in these studies ranged from 5.2 to 7.3, which were similar to the mean ratings of 6.0 to 6.6 reported for the general United States population by Watts using the same instrument.[75]

Hemodialysis patients also have evaluated their quality of life using the Index of Well-Being. This instrument combines a subjective life satisfaction question with an affect (happiness) score to produce a well-being score. Using this instrument, Johnson et al. reported a mean score of 9.7 (2 = low, 15 = high) for 39 hemodialysis patients.[76] Evans et al. reported a higher mean of 10.9 for a larger sample of patients (n = 634).[77] Both these means were just slightly lower than the national norm of 11.8 for the Index of Well-Being.[78]

The question remains: Why is there such a discrepancy between quality of life as measured by happiness/satisfaction and by more objective indicators, such as employment, physical functioning, and frequency of sexual activity. One possible explanation is that those who are dissatisfied may be deciding to stop dialysis for themselves, and that those who are too old or sick to benefit may be taken off dialysis. Neu and Kjellstrand reported that discontinuation of dialysis was a common mode of death, especially in elderly patients and those who had degenerative diseases.[79] They found that 22 percent of all deaths (n = 155) occurring within a group of 1,766 patients were due to discontinuance of treatment. The patients were mentally competent in half of the cases, all of whom made the final decision to withdraw from dialysis themselves. Medical complications preceded the decision in 39.4 percent of these patients. For all incompetent patients, new medical complications preceded the decision to withdraw treatment. The most frequent complications were dementia (28.3 percent), catastrophic acute illness (14.2 percent), and cerebrovascular accident (12.3 percent).

Another likely explanation is that the patients' happiness or satisfaction reflects successful adaptation to living with end-stage renal disease. Strauss and Glaser state that "the chief business of a chronically ill person is not just to stay alive or keep his symptoms under control, but to live as normally as possible despite his symptoms and disease."[80] In studies measuring the psychological adjustment to end-stage renal disease, hemodialysis patients have been found to be fairly well adjusted overall. Means of 34.4 and 49.5 (maximum score indicating inadequate adjustment = 135) have been reported from hemodialysis patients using the Psychological Adjustment to Illness Scale.[81,82] Similarly, Katz examined sociocultural and psychological characteristics of patients and found that the majority were relatively well adjusted.[83] The notion that adaptation is related to quality of life was supported by Murphy,[84] who found that better adjusted patients also enjoyed greater life satisfaction.

One of the ways that hemodialysis patients have been found to adjust to illness is to modify their life goals and values. Ferrans and Powers reported that 63 percent of patients changed their life goals after starting on dialysis treatment.[85] Their goals changed in the following ways: career and monetary goals decreased, goals related to personal independence decreased, family relationship goals increased, and goals changed to focus on living for today. Similarly, Goldberg found that a definite change in value structure occurred after patients started on dialysis: they valued their families more and the rewards of work, including money, less.[86] This shift in goals was typified by one dialysis patient's comment that "having been on dialysis eight years, I've come to terms with some aspects such as not being employed. Earlier on, employment was very important, but I've channeled my energy into other areas."[87] Another patient expressed the active struggle to adjust to end-stage renal disease by stating, "A dialysis patient has many mental and physical problems and life can be very black . . . but I'm fighting!!!"[88]

CONCLUSION

In summary, in the scarce resource phase of dialysis, patients were often selected to live on the basis of social value considerations and their ability to pay for treatment. This selection process resulted in an inordinate number of middle- and upper-income, white, male patients on dialysis. To provide equal access to dialysis, the ESRD program was established to supply federal funding for treatments. The success of the program was demonstrated by a shift in sociodemographics to those that more closely reflected the incidence of end-stage renal disease. However, the steadily growing number of patients on dialysis prompted concern that some patients were receiving treatment who were too old or sick to benefit. To examine the validity of this concern requires assessing quality of life and judging whether the quality of life of some patients is so poor that it is not worth living. However, it is very difficult to define and measure quality of life because its meaning varies from individual to individual, depending on personal values and underlying motivations. It is also difficult to determine standard criteria for the judgment that life is not worth living. A cost-benefit analysis using the consequentialist ethic has been proposed as a means to accomplish this. However, difficulties such as the inability to predict future outcomes, excessive reductionism of human worth, and oversimplification of complex ethical questions must be dealt with before confidence can be placed in the results of such analyses. Moreover, critics also object to cost-benefit analyses on the grounds that they violate the principles of equality of all human lives, right to life for all human beings, and sanctity of life.

Studies reflecting social value and "normal life" definitions of quality of life have reported a fair to poor quality of life for the majority of patients. These studies used objective measures of quality of life, such as employment and physical functioning. In contrast, studies in which patients evaluated their own happiness or satisfaction with life reported quality of life to be relatively good, in many cases comparable to that of healthy populations. One reason for the discrepancy between the results obtained using objective indicators and subjective measures of happiness/satisfaction may be that those who are dissatisfied and/or too old or sick to benefit from treatment are making the decision to stop dialysis for themselves. Another likely explanation is that the patients who continue on dialysis are adapting successfully to living with end-stage renal disease and hence are satisfied with their lives. Moreover, there is evidence that subjective evaluation provides a more valid assessment of life quality and that objective indicators merely assess those things that influence it. Therefore, we can conclude that the ESRD program has been highly successful in providing equal access to dialysis and in supporting the lives of people who are accommodating to their illness and are quite satisfied with life.

NOTES

1. D. Sanders and J. Dukeminier, Jr., "Medical Advance and Legal Lag: Hemodialysis and Kidney Transplantation," in *Ethics and Medicine*, eds. S. Reisner, A. Dyck, and W. Curran (Cambridge, MA: MIT Press, 1977), 606–612.

2. A. Katz, "Patients on Chronic Hemodialysis in the United States: A Preliminary Survey," *Social Science and Medicine* 3 (1970): 669–677.

3. R. Fox and J. Swazey, *The Courage to Fail* (Chicago: University of Chicago Press, 1974), 240–279.

4. F. Evans, C. Blagg, and F. Bryan, "A Social and Demographic Profile of Hemodialysis Patients in the United States," *Journal of the American Medical Association* 5 (1981): 487–491.

5. N. Rescher, "The Allocation of Exotic Medical Lifesaving Therapy," *Ethics* 79 (1969): 173–186.

6. M. Edlund and L. Tancredi, "Quality of Life: An Ideological Critique," *Perspectives in Biology and Medicine* 28 (Summer 1985): 598.

7. Sanders and Dukeminier, "Medical Advance and Legal Lag," 610.

8. B. Suczek, "Chronic Renal Failure and the Problems of Funding," in *Chronic Illness and the Quality of Life*, eds. A. Strauss and B. Glaser (St. Louis: C.V. Mosby Co., 1975).

9. R. Rettig, "The Politics of Health Cost Containment: End-Stage Renal Disease," *Bulletin of the New York Academy of Medicine* 56 (1980):115–138.

10. Suczek, "Chronic Renal Failure," 116.

11. T. Beauchamp and J. Childress, *Principles of Biomedical Ethics* (New York: Oxford University Press, 1983).

12. R. Sade, "Medical Care as a Right: A Refutation," *New England Journal of Medicine* 285 (1971): 1289.

13. Evans, Blagg, and Bryan, "A Social and Demographic Profile."

14. A. Relman and D. Rennie, "Treatment of End-Stage Renal Disease," *New England Journal of Medicine* 303 (1980): 996–998.

15. R. Freeman, "Treatment of Chronic Renal Failure: An Update," *New England Journal of Medicine* 312 (February 1985): 577–579.

16. Relman and Rennie, "Treatment of End-Stage Renal Disease."

17. Freeman, "Treatment of Chronic Renal Failure: An Update."

18. A. Campbell, *The Sense of Well-Being in America* (New York: McGraw-Hill, 1981).

19. R. Pearlman and A. Jonsen, "The Use of Quality-of-Life Considerations in Medical Decision Making," *Journal of the American Geriatrics Society* 33 (1985): 344–352.

20. Edlund and Tancredi, "Quality of Life."

21. Ibid.

22. Pearlman and Jonsen, "The Use of Quality-of-Life Considerations."

23. J. Avorn, "Benefit and Cost Analysis in Geriatric Care," *New England Journal of Medicine* 310 (1984): 1294--1301.

24. Ibid., 1297.

25. A. Campbell, "Subjective Measures of Well-Being," *American Psychologist* 31 (1976): 117–124.

26. Sanders and Dukeminier, "Medical Advance and Legal Lag."

27. Ibid., 610.

28. Edlund and Tancredi, "Quality of Life."

29. C.E. Ferrans and M. Powers, "Quality of Life Index: Development and Psychometric Properties," *Advances in Nursing Science* 8 (1985): 15–24.

30. Avorn, "Benefit and Cost Analysis in Geriatric Care."

31. Ibid., 1300.

32. N. Dalkey and D. Rourke, "The Delphi Procedure and Rating Quality of Life Factors," in *The Quality of Life Concept* (Washington, D.C.: Environmental Protection Agency, 1973), II-210.

33. C.E. Ferrans, *Psychometric Assessment of a Quality of Life Index for Hemodialysis Patients* (Doctoral dissertation, University of Illinois, 1985), 6.

34. F. Andrews and S. Withey, *Social Indicators of Well-Being* (New York: Plenum Press, 1976).

35. Campbell, "Subjective Measures of Well-Being."

36. G. Neugarten, R. Havighurst, and S. Tobin, "The Measurement of Life Satisfaction," *Journal of Gerontology* 16 (1961): 134.

37. A. Ivy, "Nazi War Crimes of a Medical Nature," *Federation Bulletin* 33 (1947): 133–146.

38. Sanders and Dukeminier, "Medical Advance and Legal Lag."

39. J. Gustafson, "Mongolism, Parental Desires, and the Right to Life," *Perspectives in Biology and Medicine* 16 (1973): 529–557.

40. W. Reich, "Quality of Life," in *Encyclopedia of Bioethics* (New York: Georgetown University Free Press, 1978), 829–840.

41. Gustafson, "Mongolism, Parental Desires, and the Right to Life."

42. Reich, "Quality of Life."

43. Ibid.

44. J. Fletcher, "Ethics and Euthanasia," in *To Live and To Die: When, Why, How*, ed. R. Williams (New York: Springer-Verlag, 1973), 113–122.

45. Reich, "Quality of Life."

46. *Hippocrates*, trans. W. Jones, in *Ethics in Medicine*, eds. S. Reisner, A. Dyck, and W. Curran (Cambridge, MA: MIT Press, 1977), 5.

47. Reich, "Quality of Life."

48. Ibid.

49. Beauchamp and Childress, *Principles of Biomedical Ethics*.

50. Ibid., 69.

51. W. Curran, "Quality of Life and Treatment Decisions: The Canadian Law Reform Report," *New England Journal of Medicine* 310 (1984): 297–298.

52. Reich, "Quality of Life," 837.

53. P. Singer, "Value of Life," in *Encyclopedia of Bioethics* (New York: Georgetown University Free Press, 1978), 822–829.

54. Ibid.

55. R. McCormick, "To Save or Let Die: The Dilemma of Modern Medicine," *Journal of the American Medical Association* 229 (1974): 172.

56. P. Singer, "Value of Life."

57. J. Childress, "Who Shall Live When Not All Can Live?" in *Ethics in Medicine*, eds. S. Reisner, A. Dyck, and W. Curran (Cambridge, MA: MIT Press, 1977), 620–626.

58. Reich, "Quality of Life."

59. J. Childress, "Who Shall Live When Not All Can Live?", 623.

60. R. Evans et al., "Quality of Life of Patients with End-Stage Renal Disease," *New England Journal of Medicine* 312 (1985): 553–559.

61. Evans, Blagg, and Bryan, "A Social and Demographic Profile."

62. R. Gutman, W. Stead, and R. Robinson, "Physical Activity and Employment Status of Patients on Maintenance Dialysis," *New England Journal of Medicine* 304 (1981): 309–313.

63. S. Bonney et al., "Treatment of End-Stage Renal Failure in a Defined Geographic Area," *Archives of Internal Medicine* 138 (1978): 1510–1513.

64. D. Sackett and G. Torrance, "The Utility of Different Health States as Perceived by the General Public," *Journal of Chronic Disease* 31 (1978): 697–704.

65. M. Bihl, *Stressors and Quality of Life of Hemodialysis and Peritoneal Dialysis Patients* (Masters thesis, University of Illinois, 1985).

66. C.E. Ferrans and M. Powers, "The Employment Potential of Hemodialysis Patients," *Nursing Research* 34 (1985): 273–277.

67. S. Hartmann, *A Comparative Analysis of the Life Satisfaction Among Patients Undergoing Home, Self-Care Center, and Full-Care Center Dialysis* (Master's thesis, University of Illinois, 1978).

68. P. Hatz and M. Powers, "Factors Related to Satisfaction with Life for Patients on Hemodialysis," *Journal of the American Association of Nephrology Nurses and Technicians* 1 (1980): 290–295.

69. M. Jackle, "Life Satisfaction and Kidney Dialysis," *Nursing Forum* 13 (1974): 360–370.

70. J. Laborde and M. Powers, "Satisfaction with Life for Patients Undergoing Hemodialysis and Patients Suffering from Osteoarthritis," *Research in Nursing and Health* 3 (1980): 19–23.

71. S. Murphy, *Factors Influencing Adjustment and Quality of Life of Hemodialysis Patients: A Multivariate Approach* (Doctoral dissertation, University of Illinois, 1982).

72. K. Schultz, *Adjustment of Older Persons to Hemodialysis* (Masters thesis, University of Illinois, 1983).

73. J. Serrahn, *Adjustment to Hemodialysis Following Kidney Graft Failure* (Masters thesis, University of Illinois, 1983).

74. J. Swanson, *Compliance and Coping in the Hemodialysis Patient* (Masters thesis, University of Illinois, 1981).

75. W. Watts, "The Future Can Fend for Itself," *Psychology Today* 15 (1981): 36–48.

76. J. Johnson, C. McCauley, and J. Copley, "The Quality of Life of Hemodialysis and Transplant Patients," *Kidney International* 22 (1982): 286–291.

77. Evans, Manninen, Garrison, et al., "Quality of Life of Patients with End-Stage Renal Disease."

78. A. Campbell, P. Converse, and W. Rodgers, *The Quality of American Life* (New York: Russell Sage Foundation, 1976).

79. S. Neu and C. Kjellstrand, "Stopping Long-Term Dialysis, an Empirical Study of Withdrawal of Life-Supporting Treatment," *New England Journal of Medicine* 314 (1986): 14–20.

80. A. Strauss and B. Glaser, *Chronic Illness and the Quality of Life* (St. Louis: C.V. Mosby Co., 1975), 58.

81. A. Kaplan De-Nour and J. Shanan, "Quality of Life of Dialysis and Transplanted Patients," *Nephron* 25 (1980): 117–120.

82. S. Murphy, *Factors Influencing Adjustment.*

83. A. Katz, "Patients in Chronic Hemodialysis in the United States: A Preliminary Survey," *Social Science and Medicine* 3 (1970): 669–677.

84. S. Murphy, *Factors Influencing Adjustment.*

85. C.E. Ferrans and M. Powers, "The Employment Potential of Hemodialysis Patients."

86. R. Goldberg, "Vocational Rehabilitation of Patients on Long-Term Hemodialysis," *Archives of Physical Medicine and Rehabilitation* 55 (1974): 60–65.

87. C.E. Ferrans, *Psychometric Assessment,* 104.

88. Ibid., 104.

Part III
Termination of Treatment

Chapter 9

Refusal of Treatment: Rights, Reasons, Responses

Robert L. Schwartz, JD

Of all the areas of health law, and of all the disciplines required in hospital management, few if any are as shaded with subtlety and prone to blurred distinctions as the issues relating to termination of treatment. To fail to understand the nuances is not to slide from one shade of gray to another but to slip from the red end of the spectrum through orange to yellow and green. While there is continuity, shading, and some blending of issues, there are also clear distinctions.

TERMINOLOGY AND EMOTION

Emotion plays a large part in the tendency to misunderstand the issues presented in refusal of medical treatment. The ethos of death: social, cultural, religious, psychological, legal, and so forth, makes all death-related issues seem similar—the end is the same. But a requested "No Code," a refusal of nutrients, and a disconnection of a respirator all raise different issues even though the end result is often the same.

The tendency to blur distinctions in this field is shared by physicians, judges, hospital administrators, and the public at large. Moreover, each may see a different overriding concern, or central issue, in the same set of circumstances. Phrases such as "pulling the plug" carry various intrinsic significance to each group, often preventing a meaningful dialogue and sometimes masking widely divergent preconceptions. Likewise, widely diverse circumstances are lumped together under a common heading and important distinctions are lost.

Terminology also fuels the emotional fires. Euthanasia—mercy killing—is generally considered homicide. It is a term packed with value judgment and made for shouting matches. Authors who have couched discussions of refusal of treatment in the language of euthanasia (active vs. passive?) may have a philosophical argument but have let emotion rather than reason dictate the dialogue.

For example, in commenting on court decisions allowing the withdrawal of artificial nutrition, John Willke, President of the National Right to Life Committee, said, "These decisions . . . are a direct movement toward widespread euthanasia and we will strenuously oppose that . . . under no circumstances will you starve this person to death."[1]

Couching his remarks in terms of euthanasia, this speaker raises emotional responses but avoids questions of consent to treatment, or the right to bodily self-integrity, or the right to privacy that form the basis of judicial analysis of these issues.

To describe withholding or refusing treatment as "passive euthanasia" similarly creates an emotional bias. To understand the existing legal framework for analyzing refusals of treatment, a useful analysis must avoid the word "euthanasia" and all its emotional baggage.

ETHICS COMMITTEES

Ethics committees, unfortunately, have also confused ethical issues. Ethics committees are not always disciplined in defining issues and, therefore, two ethical issues, if similar but slightly different, are often blurred.

Because ethics committees are often composed of broad constituencies, the terminology and blurred distinction problems are common. Unless an ethics committee is careful to clearly define the issues before it, and to agree in advance on workable categories of treatment decisions, it can encounter considerable frustration as its members debate broadly divergent issues couched in the same terminology, or a single issue mistakenly categorized by divergent preconceptions.

THE EVOLUTION OF LAW

The nature and evolution of new bodies of law is confusing. This is the case with refusal of treatment issues. New technologies, increased ability to maintain artificial life support, and changing public attitudes toward medicine have given rise to a whole new field of law in a relatively short time.

Fifty state courts have approached these issues fifty different ways. Legislators, presidential commissions, and an evolving body of literature also blur distinctions. In the courts, specifically, new law is prone to error. Lower court judges faced with novel issues may not fully understand them, yet their rulings get broad publication.

The appellate law process tends to be single issue oriented. Therefore, a reversal of a lower court is often based on issues not immediately appreciated by the industry press. What the courts say—and what the press says they say— are often quite different. This happens often in rulings on temporary injunctions. These procedural matters rarely deal with substantive legal arguments, but rather deal with limited procedural matters. Nonetheless, a temporary injunction requiring continued treatment of a patient until the suit is resolved can be reported by the headline, "Court Forces Treatment on Unwilling Patient."

DEFINITIONS

The purpose of this chapter is to guide health care managers in cases where medical treatment is refused by, or on behalf of, a patient. Much confusion has been caused by the attempt to distinguish "refusal," "withdrawal," "withholding," and "termination" of treatment. For this chapter the following definitions are used:

- *Refusal*: Any attempt by a patient or his representative to prevent the initiation or continuation of treatment. Refusal couches the discussion in terms of consent and constitutes the negative of consent to treatment.
- *Termination/Withdrawal*: The removal or discontinuation of previously initiated medical care. This may be the result of either a refusal or a determination of death.
- *Withholding*: The intentional denial or failure to initiate medical care. This may be the result of a refusal, a determination of inappropriateness, a rationing, or other *a priori* decision-making process.

These areas are not mutually exclusive. Much confusion is created by a misconception that the terminology constitutes an orderly taxonomy. To the contrary, the terms constitute various intersecting sets and subsets of related situations. This lack of usable taxonomy is a predominant source of confusion and misunderstanding in this field.

REFUSAL AND CONSENT

Mr. S comes to the hospital administrator seeking a dignified death for his wife of 30 years. She is being kept alive on a respirator in the hospital's ICU.

A woman in her fifties, Mrs. S has had multiple sclerosis for many years and is progressively degenerating. She is doomed to a slow progressive death. Her condition is unquestionably terminal. The respirator is only prolonging the instant of her death. Mr. S refuses further treatment for his wife and requests the removal of the respirator.

What should the administrator do?

Is this a classic case of third party refusal (withdrawal) of treatment?

The administrator calls the head nurse of ICU for a report on Mrs. S.

"What is her condition?"

"Stable."

"What is her mental status?"
"Alert and well oriented to person, place, and time."
"Can she communicate?"
"Very well."
"Has anyone consulted her about removing the respirator?"
"Goodness NO!"

The clear lesson from this case is this: Do not overlook anything—get the total picture about the patient from several sources.

A disturbing footnote to the case of Mr. and Mrs. S is that Mr. S had regularly signed all of the consent forms for Mrs. S. As a matter of convenience the hospital staff had always relied on Mr. S for consent—consent that under law for that state was totally invalid. Only when he sought discontinuation of life support was his authority challenged. It had been assumed (wrongly) that Mr. S could consent to treatment for his wife. Therefore he could not understand why he couldn't refuse treatment.

Clearly, Mrs. S, being a competent adult, was the only party whose refusal of further treatment could control (although even her refusal needs to be carefully examined).

In fact, during the entire course of treatment Mrs. S should have been asked for verbal consents, which she could competently give or refuse and which could then be duly recorded and even countersigned by her husband. Failure to seek routine consents from a competent adult had complicated an attempted refusal on her behalf. *Competent patients must speak for themselves.*

Competency and the Right To Refuse

The right to consent is the first indication of the right to refuse. Competent adults speak for themselves (except where a greater public interest intervenes).

Refusal of Treatment by a Competent Adult

The long-standing general rule has been that a competent adult has the right to refuse treatment. This dates back to at least 1914 when Judge Cardozo wrote, "Every human being of adult years and sound mind has the right to determine what shall be done with his own body . . . ."[2] As early as 1905 the Minnesota Supreme Court saw constitutional implications, stating "under a free government, at least, the free citizen's greatest right, which underlies all others—the right to the inviolability of his person . . . is subject to universal acquiescence, and this right necessarily forbids a physician . . . to violate, without permission, the bodily integrity of his patient. . . ."[3]

Both the traditional common law right to bodily integrity (against battery) and the constitutional right to privacy were applied in the landmark decision *Superintendent of Belchertown State School v. Saikewicz.*[4] There, in upholding a refusal of chemotherapy by a leukemia patient, the court said, "The value of life is lessened not by a decision to refuse treatment, but by the failure to allow a competent human being the right of choice."[5] A clearly articulated and demonstrable choice has also been upheld after the patient is no longer competent.[6]

Similarly, the courts have upheld refusals of amputations,[7] continued use of a respirator,[8] blood transfusions,[9] and other treatments.

The questions with regard to the validity of competent refusals (after the determination of competence) revolve around so-called "state interests."

The doctrine of state interest includes the concept *parens patriae*. The state in this role undertakes to act as "the general guardian of all infants, idiots, and lunatics."[10] Most often used in cases involving children and incompetents, the doctrine has also been used to protect the children of a patient from possible "abandonment"[11] and, most recently, a state interest in preventing suicide has been cited as authority to override a patient's refusal of nasogastric feeding.[12]

The refusal of feeding cases have raised the most serious doubts about the validity of a competent adult's refusal of treatment.

The most notorious of these is the case of Elizabeth Bouvia. Her 1983 attempt to force a hospital to allow her to starve to death was unsuccessful, primarily on the state interest argument. However, in April 1986 a California appeals court ruled that as a competent adult, Elizabeth Bouvia's refusal of nasogastric feeding must be respected.[13]

There are, however, contrary rulings and much debate. A Massachusetts court refused to remove a gastrostomy tube from a patient who, when competent, had stated a preference against such treatment.[14]

Given the controversy involving competent refusals of feeding, it is understandable that the removal of artificial feeding from incompetents has caused even greater concern.[15]

The lack of unanimity among the courts and the level of public controversy engendered by these cases clearly indicate that such actions should be approached carefully and that judicial resolution should be sought.

THE NEED FOR JUDICIAL RESOLUTION

Conservative lawyers say that no one ever lost a lawsuit by keeping someone alive—and even in losing no money would be lost. This argues strongly for any error to be on the side of life. But it fails to address the issues of patient rights and possible harm and continued patient suffering. Is it possible to respect a refusal of treatment with the same comfort level as doing nothing to jeopardize life without a court order? Is there any guidance for health care personnel who deeply wish to resolve these increasingly frequent issues without going to court? The safest legal advice of necessity is to leave decision making to courts and lawyers. Thus, some administrators might choose to adopt a policy never to remove, withdraw, or withhold life-sustaining treatment without a court order. *Liability* will be nil, but an institution will spend an enormous amount of time and money in court. This seemingly "safe" course of action will strain relations with patients, families, physicians, and possibly the administrator's conscience. Therefore, there are negative consequences from delegating all ethical decision making to the courts.

As refusal of treatment is a new and complex area of law, it does make sense to consult your institutional attorney. However, your attorney may not have any painless, simple answers.

Deciding To Go to Court

A number of issues or situations compel judicial resolution.

If it is possible to identify situations where going to court is clearly justified, we can then limit the scope of our inquiry and derive some operative, and perhaps further applicable, principles for situations that do not require court involvement.

Do not accept a refusal, withdrawal, or withholding of treatment without a court order in the following instances:

- Active dissent among interested parties
- Prior statements by the patient indicating a desire for unlimited treatment
- Cases where the patient is a minor or the parent of minor children
- Cases where the patient has never been competent
- Cases on the legal frontier

Active Dissent among Interested Parties

Some sources suggest that where the patient (if competent or if prior competent expression is known), the family, the physician, and the hospital ethics committee agree to terminate treatment, no legal intervention is necessary.[16] Without examining this theory in depth, note that when the converse situation exists (e.g., active dissent) judicial action is the most prudent course.

> Mary A comes to the hospital administrator's office claiming to be the wife of Mr. A, an 81-year-old comatose cancer patient being sustained on a respirator. Mary wants the respirator removed.
>
> Jane A soon appears, also claiming to be Mr. A's wife (of a prior undissolved marriage) and insisting that all measures be taken to treat Mr. A.

No other facts need be explored. It is not the hospital administrator's (or lawyer's) job to resolve this question. Mary and Jane are welcome to do battle in court (and probably will, regardless of the hospital's action). No one can know for sure who will win. Meanwhile, Mr. A should receive every available medical resource. Nothing should be withheld. This would be true if Mary and Jane were his two surviving daughters, his two sisters, his wife and daughter, and so on.

This case illustrates three principles:

1. Never withhold life-sustaining treatment without a court order if the parties are in dispute.
2. If you are going to end up in court, one way or another, it is best to go there first.
3. Always identify all interested parties.

Don't risk the appearance of an unhappy, previously unidentified family member. After the respirator has been removed is the wrong time to discover that the patient has an additional child who doesn't speak to those who consented to the removal of the respirator and who opposes it vehemently.

Assuming, for the sake of argument, that unanimous and harmonious families can authorize the removal of life support—contentious and embattled families cannot.

Prior Statements by Patient Indicating a Desire
for Unlimited Treatment

Mr. B had been on renal dialysis for three years. His list of diagnoses would require a full page. He is now terminally ill with cancer and had slipped into a coma. His physician and family want to discontinue dialysis as a futile extraordinary measure. They know that dialysis is prolonging a certain death. They are in full unanimous agreement that dialysis is merely prolonging the moment of death for Mr. B.

The family and physician consult the hospital attorney for guidance in implementing their decision to terminate dialysis treatments.

During his investigation the attorney encounters Mrs. C, the hospital social worker, who has worked with this family through the course of Mr. B's disease. She is very disturbed, because Mr. B had once said, "I want to live every minute I can; I do not mind machines."

Does Mr. B still feel the same way? What did he really mean? What would he say now that death is imminent?

None of these questions can be resolved by hospital personnel. But, regardless of the good intentions and unanimous agreement of family and physician, this patient's last known expression of choice was in favor of treatment.

This request for termination of treatment should be viewed as a "third party refusal." The family is acting on the patient's behalf, refusing consent to further treatment. The courts tend to use a "substitute judgment" standard—what would the patient do if competent. When the patient's last known expression of intent was clearly for unlimited treatment, it is unwise to accept contrary directions from anyone else. The patient must be treated until he or she, or a court, says otherwise.[17]

Cases Where the Patient Is a Minor or the Parent of Minor Children

Courts are prone to go out of their way to protect children. The best interest of a minor child is a question that has taken on "state interest" characteristics. While health care professionals may believe that parents can freely choose among alternative treatments for a child, some alternatives are disfavored by the courts. For instance, when parents try to exercise discretion and choose among treatments that offer "handicapped life" versus "certain death," courts may intervene. Courts typically will overrule a parent's refusal of treatment where treatment would allow the child to live extended periods (a normal life span) but it would be retarded or handicapped. The unique treatment of minors—and issues regarding their parents—often necessitate judicial guidance.[18]

Cases Where the Patient Has Never Been Competent

The patient who is a lifetime incompetent is very similar to a minor (who is legally incompetent as well). Such patients should be treated in the same way as minors. In most cases such a patient has a legal guardian or conservator. Because of this, court action is preanticipated. The guardian or conservator derives his or her authority from the court and preliminaries have already been addressed by this appointment. It is a simpler matter for such a guardian or conservator to seek the court's guidance in a treatment decision than to institute a new guardianship case. Because of this, and because of legal and philosophical problems with substitute judgment in such cases—*go to court.*

Cases on the Legal Frontier

What is the legal frontier? Any novel case involving unusual facts or circumstances would fall here. Clearly, cases involving deprivation of nutrients are extremely volatile today.

Also, in health care's current economic environment, any case that hints of rationing or contains any element of economic consideration is dynamite and *will* end up in court.

In writing his finding in patient Z's progress notes, Dr. Q, a neurologist, first noted brain death. Rather than order termination of treatment, Dr. Q's note continued for a full page on the philosophical issues of death and the *economics*, including the hospital's financial loss from DRG reimbursement for this patient.

Dr. Q's note lamented the great cost to the institution for maintaining artificial respiration and circulation for this patient whom he found "neurologically and clinically dead."

Dr. Q was counseled to avoid future progress notes of this sort. As the patient was "clinically dead" there was no need for more than a pronouncement and termination of treatment under this state's law. Clearly, the economic issues are irrelevant.

Termination of treatment cannot be an economic decision. Any hint of financial motivation will invite litigation.

Decision Making without Court Involvement

The previous section describes instances where judicial resolution is required. In many of those cases it can be determined early that, one way or another, a court will get involved. When such cases arise, suit should be initiated as early as possible to avoid undue suffering and uncertainty and to expedite settlement.

But if a case is not a clear-cut case for court decision, what is the next step? The cases and the literature suggest that the courts need *not* be consulted in every case.[19]

State law should be examined (or known in advance). This chapter does not discuss every state law, but you must know that some states have by statute or case law established more or less mandatory procedures (for example, New Jersey[20]), and some have established guidelines.

Other state laws may be confusing or ambiguous, causing more uncertainty for the health care decision maker than they resolve. For example, the Texas Natural Death Act provides that under certain circumstances the attending physician and family may remove mechanical means of life support if death is imminent.[21] Does this foreclose withdrawal of treatment where death is not imminent? Without further clarification, can this law provide any useful guidance?

DOCUMENTATION

Finally, there are several considerations in cases where treatment is withdrawn without litigation. For example, the patient is terminally ill and the respirator is prolonging the moment of death. The physician and family agree on the course of action. An ethics committee either agreed or never heard the case (there may not be an ethics committee). State legal sources have been consulted and present no impediment.

The physician must document all relevant considerations regarding the health of the patient: diagnosis, prognosis, mental state. The physician's note should also document discussions with the family. This may be countersigned by family members (and the ethics committee if appropriate).

A consent to removal of life-sustaining devices is signed by *all* immediate relatives. Such a consent should be carefully drafted by an attorney knowledgeable about the applicable state law. I prefer to couch such refusals in the terminology of consent. Documentation should establish that the patient, or persons with authority to consent on the patient's behalf, have made an informed decision to withhold, refuse, or revoke consent to treatment. By taking a clear consent approach the refusal is easily examined. Do the parties have the right to consent (therefore to refuse)? Have they been informed on the consequences? Is their decision subject to established challenges—i.e., contrary to the patient's stated interests, medically unjustified, jeopardizing the rights of minors or incompetents, or beyond established norms (e.g., refusal of nutrients)? At this point it seems that life-sustaining treatment may be removed.

SUMMARY

In summary, let me restate some general principles.

- The right to consent is the first indication of the right to refuse.
- Don't overlook the obvious.
- Never withhold life-sustaining treatment without a court order if the parties are in dispute.
- Always identify all interested parties.
- If the probability is good that you are going to end up in court—go there first.
- You must go to court in the following cases:
  1. Active dissent among interested parties.
  2. Any indication of prior statements by the patient indicating a desire for unlimited treatment.
  3. Where the patient has *never been* competent.
  4. Cases on the legal frontier.

Within the framework of these principles, health care personnel can legally, ethically, and morally confront some of the most difficult problems facing them every day.

NOTES

1. *Wall Street Journal*, June 9, 1986.

2. Schloendorff v. Society of New York Hospital, 211 N.Y. 125, 105 N.E. 92, 93 (1914).

3. Mohr v. Williams, 95 Minn. 261, 104 N.W. 12, 14 (1905).

4. Superintendent of Belchertown State School v. Saikewicz, 373 Mass. 728, 370 N.E.2d 417 (1977).

5. Id. at 426. *See also* Satz v. Perlmutter, 362 So.2d 160 (Ct. App. Fla. 1978).

6. Eichner v. Dillon, *rep. sub nom* Matter of Storar, 52 N.Y.2d 363, 438 N.Y.S.2d 266 (1981).

7. Matter of Quackenbush, 156 N.J. Super 282, 383 A.2d 785 (1978).

8. Matter of Storar, supra.

9. In re Osborne, 294 A.2d 372 (D.C.Ct.App. 1972).

10. Hawaii v. Standard Oil Co., 405 U.S. 251 (1972).

11. Application of President and Directors of Georgetown College, Inc., 118 App. D.C. 80, 331 F.2d 1000 (D.C. Cir. 1964). *reh'g en banc denied* 118 App.D.C. 90, 331 F.2d 1010 *cert. denied* 377 U.S. 978 (1964).

12. Bouvia v. County of Riverside, Riverside General Hospital, No. 159780 (Sup.Ct. of Cty of Riverside, CA, Dec. 16, 1983).

13. Bouvia v. Superior Court, No.B019034 (Ct.App., 2d App. Dist. Cal., Apr. 16, 1986).

14. Brophy v. New England Sinai Hospital, Inc., No. 85E0009-G1 (Mass. Dist. Ct., Oct. 21, 1985).

15. In the Matter of Conroy, 98 N.J. 321, 486 A.2d 1209 (1985).

16. In re Quinlan, 70 N.J. 10, 355 A.2d 647 (1976). President's Commission for the Study of Ethical Problems in Medicine and Biomedical and Behavior Research (*Deciding to Forego Life-Sustaining Treatment, 1983*).

17. Eichner v. Dillon, supra.

I have also applied this principle in support of refusal. A competent adult cancer patient repeatedly refused surgery, chemotherapy, or radiation treatment. Once the patient lost consciousness, his physician asserted the right to provide ''emergency'' life-saving measures, including surgery and radiation therapy. As hospital counsel, I argued that this competent patient's refusal of treatment will stand until overruled by the patient or a court.

18. *See* Custody of a Minor, 393 N.E.2d 836 (Mass. 1979); Matter of Jenson, 633 P.2d 1302 (Or. Ct. App. 1981); *Tate v. Perricone*, 181 A.2d 751 (NJ, 1962), *cert. den.* 71 U.S. 890 (1962). In re Phillips B, 92 Cal.App.3d 796, *cert. den.* 445 U.S. 949 (1979).

19. *See* Note 16.

20. In the Matter of Conroy, supra.

21. Vernon's (Texas) Ann. Civ. St. art. 4590h.

Chapter 10

Withdrawing or Withholding Treatment

Joseph W. Kukura, STD, MA, and Gary R. Anderson, PhD

Perhaps no dilemma is more unsettling and controversial for health care professionals than choosing to withhold or withdraw medical treatment. The right of the competent adult to refuse treatment is discussed in Chapter 9. This discussion will focus on withholding and withdrawing treatment in cases where the patient cannot make the choice because of age or incompetence.

PROPORTIONATE AND DISPROPORTIONATE CARE

Many illnesses that once resulted in death can be readily addressed or forestalled today. This ability to prolong life is of relatively recent origin and can be attributed to a number of factors, such as medical technology, medications, physician skill and knowledge, and quality of care in health institutions. The prolongation of life was also affected by the setting in which health care services are delivered. Patients treated in their own homes or in medically isolated communities in which medical technology is not as available as in larger or more urban environments might not have access to the equipment or services which would sustain life. Consequently, today's health care delivery possibilities have created dilemmas that would not have existed a short time ago to the extent that they do in the 1980s.

Through the centuries, reasonable health care has been judged an ethical imperative. A moral distinction was suggested between "ordinary" and "extraordinary" medical care. These terms were not understood as medical terms, nor did they coincide with "routine" or "unusual" from the standpoint of medical practice. Morally understood, ordinary means of treatment can be defined as all medicines, treatments, and operations that offer a reasonable hope of benefit and can be obtained and used without excessive pain or burden. Extraordinary means are medicines, treatments, and operations that cannot be used without excessive pain or burden or, if used, would offer no reasonable hope of benefit.

The distinction between ordinary and extraordinary includes an evaluation of not only the efficacy of the treatment or medication but also the consequences for the patient—the pain and disturbance caused by the intervention; in short, burdens and benefits. This definition can be realistic only if applied to the concrete circumstances surrounding an individual patient's life. This includes the family and life context of the patient, time of the illness, place of treatment, and available resources. So, treatments such as respirators, kidney dialysis, and blood transfusions that would be considered ordinary means of treatment in a crisis or short-term circumstance may be defined in some cases as extraordinary if used for long-term treatment.

The consideration of means of treatment, information concerning the patient, and benefits to the patient suggest that the goal of medicine is not simply and irrefutably to prolong life and postpone death. Evaluating the efficacy, risks, pain, and burden of treatment strategies as well as the patient's resources and circumstances leads to a considered judgment about what is proportionate or disproportionate in response to a patient's condition. This suggests a more complex decision that requires the analysis of individual case circumstances with a goal of decreasing or preventing pain and suffering but not necessarily preventing death. In addition, decision making concerning the withdrawal or withholding of treatment should consider the patient's choice concerning the means of treatment that he or she has actually expressed or implied in a certain life style.

AUTONOMY AND TREATMENT DECISIONS

The question of who shall choose which course of action—choosing among alternate treatments or choosing to forgo or withdraw from treatment—is difficult in paternalistic settings such as hospitals. Ethical principles would suggest that one's autonomy and the right to determine the course of action affecting one's own body are the primary considerations. Consequently, decisions about treatment should be made by the patient, after consultation with medical personnel. The value of the individual patient is always presumed, and the right to choose or reject treatment belongs to that patient.

However, this principle is not so easy in practice, particularly when family members, physicians, nurses, administrators, and other caring people disagree with the patient and with each other on the course which is in the best interests of the patient. The limits of autonomy can become an issue. Such would clearly be the case if the patient requested active assistance to end his or her life— active euthanasia. Freedom of choice is limited by ethical rightness or wrongness and the rights of others, including institutions, to follow their conscience. The refusal of the competent patient raises different issues than the refusal of the incompetent patient or the case of the newborn who is unable to formulate or express a viewpoint.

INCOMPETENT ADULTS AND WITHDRAWING TREATMENT

In the case of incompetent adults, the role of choice falls upon those family members or others who are legally designated and recognized as the guardians of the incompetent person. They should choose what the patient would want, or if that choice is unknown, what they judge to be in the best interests of the patient. These decisions are not easy and raise questions of paternalism and the role of medical personnel in decision making.

This complexity is best illustrated through case discussion. One of the most recent and important cases involving an incompetent adult and the withdrawal of treatment is Claire Conroy—a nursing home resident in the state of New Jersey.[1]

Claire Conroy was 84 years old at the time her legal guardian, her nephew, requested removal of her nasogastric tube, which had been inserted for feeding. Claire Conroy was suffering from diabetes, heart disease, hypertension, organic brain syndrome, ulcers, and urinary tract infections. She was seriously demented: her brain functioning was severely impaired and she was unaware of her surroundings. According to medical assessment there was no expectation that her condition would improve. She had always been single, lived in her childhood home, and had little contact with other people. In the summer of 1979 Conroy was legally judged to be incompetent and her only surviving relative was appointed her legal guardian.

The nephew, concerned for her welfare, placed his aunt in the Parklane Nursing Home in Bloomfield, New Jersey. In the summer of 1982, Claire Conroy was admitted to a local hospital, Clara Maas, because of a gangrenous leg. The nephew was advised that his aunt would need an amputation or else she would die. He refused consent, judging that this consent would be contrary to his aunt's wishes. There was no amputation, but Conroy survived; the gangrene was brought under control, although only temporarily.

While at Clara Maas, a nasogastric tube was inserted. This tube was removed in October but reinserted one month later to provide Conroy with needed nutrition. At this time the nephew asked for the removal of the nasogastric tube. The attending physician would not remove the tube, and shortly Claire Conroy was returned to the Parklane Home. The guardian again asked for the removal of the tube and was again refused.

He filed suit arguing that his aunt would prefer to die if she could say so. Contrary to the court-appointed guardian ad litem's disagreement, the court authorized removal of the tube. The court found that Conroy's intellectual capacity had been permanently reduced to an extremely primitive level and her life had become "impossibly and permanently burdensome."[2] However, upon appeal, the New Jersey Appellate Court ruled a few months later that the removal of the tube would be homicidal—causing death by the painful conditions of starvation and dehydration. The lower court's ruling was reversed.

This case went to the New Jersey Supreme Court, which decided to rule on the case even though Conroy died some months before the court's ruling. In January 1985 the court affirmed an individual's right to accept or reject any medical treatment and a guardian's right to decide for an incompetent patient under certain specified conditions.

The court made a number of rulings and established guidelines for cases such as Claire Conroy's (involving an elderly person in a nursing home with less than one year to live). One of the most significant opinions of the court was that there is no distinction between artificially feeding a patient and other medical treatment. If competent patients have the right to refuse any medical treatment then they also have the right to refuse feeding.[3] If a competent patient can request that any medical treatment be discontinued, and have that request respected, then a patient can request that feeding be discontinued. This opinion sets a high priority on the principle of patient autonomy in deciding treatment: the central consideration is the patient's choice with regard to initiating or stopping medical treatment, including artificial feeding. In addition to this opinion equating feeding with medical treatment, the court established a number of rules to guide decision making in cases such as Conroy (specifically, an elderly nursing home resident with less than one year to live) where the patient is incompetent, and the decision must be made by someone other than the patient herself. These rules included three tests:[4]

1. Subjective Test

If the formerly competent patient's wishes can be clearly ascertained, for example by durable power of attorney (powers that remain in effect after the individual has become incompetent) or in a written "living will" or a clear oral declaration to a family member or health care provider, those patient choices are given priority in decision making. The goal is to understand what decision the patient would have made if he or she had been competent. This test requires that the incompetent patient's surrogate decision maker be given as much medical information as would be expected to have been given to the patient if he or she had been competent to consent to or reject treatment.

2. Limited Objective Test

If the patient's wishes cannot be clearly ascertained, the court identified two "best interests" tests. Under the limited objective test, there must be some trustworthy evidence that the patient would have refused treatment, although this evidence may not be as clear as that under the subjective test. Evidence might include the patient's moral, ethical, or religious beliefs, or attempts to refuse hospitalization or physicians' care (which was the case with Claire Conroy). This test requires the patient's surrogate or guardian to be convinced that the burdens of the patient's life, continued because of the treatment, outweigh the benefits of continued life for the patient. This test also requires medical evidence concerning the patient's current and future pain and suffering, including evidence with regard to the duration, degree, and constancy of pain with and without treatment.

3. Pure Objective Test

The second best interests test, the pure objective test, not only weighs the burdens versus the benefits for the patient but also adds that continuing treatment could be construed as inhumane because of constant, unavoidable severe pain for the patient kept alive by the treatment. However, even in these cases, if the patient had previously expressed the desire to be kept alive, regardless of the pain, the court ruled that life-sustaining treatment should not be withheld or withdrawn.

In addition to these guidelines (respect for the patient's obvious wishes, the limited objective test, and the pure objective test) the court established procedures that must be followed in New Jersey before life-sustaining treatment can be withdrawn. These procedures, limited to nursing home patients, include:

1. A court must find that the patient is incompetent and incapable of making a medical decision.
2. A court must appoint a legal guardian for the incompetent patient, and this guardian is empowered to make the necessary medical decisions.
3. If this guardian believes it appropriate to withhold or withdraw treatment of the incompetent patient, based on the above described rules, the guardian must notify the New Jersey Office of Ombudsman (an office established to protect the institutionalized elderly).
4. The ombudsman must conduct an immediate investigation and must assume that the reported request is potentially a case of ''abuse.''
5. The ombudsman, as part of the investigation, should question the attending physician and nurses concerning the condition of the patient.
6. As part of the investigation, the ombudsman should appoint two physicians who are not associated with the nursing home to confirm the patient's condition and prognosis.
7. If the medical information gained in this investigation is consistent with any of the three tests, and the guardian, attending physician, and ombudsman agree, life support treatment may be withheld or withdrawn. All involved have legal immunity.
8. This authorization is qualified in that if the patient's wishes are not clearly known, requiring one of the two best interests tests, the patient's spouse, parents, and children, or in their absence any next of kin to the patient, must concur with the guardian's, physician's, and ombudsman's decision to withhold or withdraw treatment.

Although the court's ruling seems to establish some rules and procedures in a pioneering area of medical treatment and ethics, it is important to realize that the guidelines apply to elderly nursing home patients expected to die within one year. A number of criticisms of these judgments have been raised. Primary questions and objections have included:

- The procedures seem unnecessarily cumbersome, especially when there is clear evidence of what the patient would want.
- The procedures seem problematic, particularly with the assumption of "abuse" discouraging family members and requiring three physicians to report on the patient's condition.
- The concentration on pain as the principal criterion of judgment of what is appropriate or mandatory does not bring into consideration issues such as patient inconvenience and expense.
- Overall, the restriction to nursing home residents is limiting, considering that these residents are frequently transferred to hospitals when they require invasive medical treatment. In fact, important decisions about withdrawing treatment in the Conroy case took place at Clara Maas Hospital.[5]

Despite these shortcomings, the Claire Conroy case and the resulting court opinion provide some guidance on decisions concerning withdrawal of life-sustaining treatment. The court affirmed patient self-determination by valuing the previously competent patient's wishes concerning medical treatment and respecting written and oral declarations of the patient's desires. The court recognized the validity of a carefully considered judgment assessing the patient's condition, burdens and benefits, and pain. Although possibly ponderous, the procedures established for nursing home residents both allow for withdrawal and express a societal concern that withdrawing treatment does not become a cavalier decision. In fact, the procedures incorporating an ombudsman and outside physicians as well as those closest to the patient build in time and safeguards for the patient, physician, and family.

This guidance is not the last word concerning the withdrawal of treatment. A number of other cases involving withdrawal and withholding of treatment have yielded different standards and considerations than those raised in the Claire Conroy case.

The *Clarence Herbert* case (1983) involved a 55-year-old patient who suffered respiratory collapse caused by cardiac arrest after routine surgery in August 1981. He was resuscitated and given respiratory assistance but lapsed into a deep comatose state. The attending physicians told the family that the prognosis for Herbert's recovery was very poor, and with their consent the respirator was withdrawn. The patient continued to breathe spontaneously but showed no signs of improvement. Again after consultation with the family, the attending physicians ordered removal of the patient's IV feeding, nasogastric tube, and air mist. The patient died six days later.

A number of court actions followed to determine whether the doctors (Nejdl and Barber) had murdered the patient by depriving him of medical treatment. The California Court of Appeals in October 1983 dismissed criminal charges, ruling that to continue futile treatment under these circumstances would be disproportionate to the benefits to be gained from the burden imposed. Also the court ruled that guardianship proceedings were not required. One spouse should be able to make the decision to withdraw treatment if the other is unable to do so. Although there was no living will in this case the wife did remember her husband saying he did not want to be kept alive by machines to "become another Karen Ann Quinlan." Finally, the court ruled that without legislative instruction, there was no requirement of court approval before medical treatment was withdrawn under these circumstances.[6]

The *Severns* case (1980) in Delaware involved a patient who had been in a coma for one year after an automobile accident that caused upper brain death. A court appointed her husband as guardian and authorized him to refuse consent for reinsertion of tracheal feeding, refuse placing his wife on a respirator, refuse antibiotics to combat infection, and to authorize a "No Code" order. All family members agreed that such proposed treatment would be futile; the patient had expressed a wish, before she was incapacitated, not to live as a vegetable by using extraordinary medical means.[7]

The *Joseph Saikewicz* case (1976) involved a 67-year-old mentally retarded state ward who was terminally ill with leukemia. In this case, the Supreme Judicial Court of Massachusetts ruled that only a probate court could authorize the nontreatment of Saikewicz. In fact, the probate court had ruled the previous year that chemotherapy, the treatment of choice with painful side effects but the 30 to 50 percent chance of a 2 to 13 month remission, would not be used as Saikewicz would be "better off" without the treatment. The court also held that the basis for this decision should be the probate court's determination of what the patient would have chosen for himself if he had been able to make the decision himself. The patient died of bronchial pneumonia, a complication of leukemia, in September 1976.[8]

The *Karen Ann Quinlan* case (1976) involved a young New Jersey woman in a chronic vegetative state. The Supreme Court of New Jersey ruled that the guardian, family, and physicians could withdraw treatment, in this case a ventilator, allowing her to die, if they agreed there was no realistic probability she would ever return to a recovered cognitive state. The court suggested that a prognosis committee might be helpful in arriving at a good decision. At the time, experts thought that removing the ventilator would in fact allow Karen Ann Quinlan to die. After the ventilator's withdrawal she continued to live in a New Jersey nursing home until she died of pneumonia in June 1985.[9]

Another recent case of interest is *Brophy* (Massachusetts), one of the few examples in which the court ordered continued treatment (artificial feeding) although Brophy has been irreversibly comatose since March 1983. This decision was appealed and overturned in September 1986.[10]

The recent cases of Herbert and Conroy suggest that a benefit and burdens analysis can be used to make some determination about the advisability of continuing medical treatment, including feeding: "If nourishment is not reasonably anticipated to provide the patient with any benefits, or can only provide benefits to the patient that are outweighed by the burdens attendant, then nourishment is not proportionate treatment and should not be legally, medically, or morally required."[11] Determining benefits versus burdens should be done in consultation with qualified medical personnel; the agreement of the authorized decision maker is necessary to withdraw treatment; and there must be some determination that this withdrawal is consistent with the expressed wishes of the patient before incompetence or what the authorized decision maker believes the patient would want under the circumstances—with no evidence to the contrary.

From these cases it seems possible to conclude that treatment may be withdrawn where the patient's medical condition is one of irreversible coma with no reasonable possibility of cognitive recovery, or imminent, incurable terminal illness. This suggests a criterion of "futility."[12]

Each of the described cases involved court intervention, and usually more than one court at that. Many health care professionals object to the necessity of involving courts in deciding to withdraw treatment. The requirement of court involvement seems to be questioned by the recent cases of Herbert and Conroy; *Herbert* stated that all cases do not have to go to court and *Conroy* established a set of procedures involving the ombudsman but not the court system (except for the appointment of a guardian). One analyst suggests that decisions to withdraw futile life-sustaining treatment of a mechanical nature need involve only the patient, the family, the physician, and the concurrence of a second physician.[13] If there is doubt or disagreement, a referral to an ethics committee or some other review mechanism is suggested.

However, in cases involving the withdrawal of nourishment, referral to an ethics committee might be mandatory unless there is a legally recognized written statement of intent in which the patient, while competent, states his or her wishes concerning nourishment. Health care institutions and physicians may be reluctant to withdraw nourishment without some type of court affirmation, given the pioneering nature of the discussion and the variability among judgments as well as the risk of litigation.

WITHHOLDING TREATMENT FROM NEWBORNS

The court ruling on Claire Conroy specifically noted that its guidelines and procedures were not intended for neonatal decision making. The dilemmas involving care for newborns have centered on the cases of Baby Doe and Baby Jane Doe.

Concern about decisions to withhold treatment from newborns became widespread due to cases involving Down's syndrome children. The case of Baby Doe, in which an Indiana court ruled that parents of a severely disabled newborn had the right to withhold food and routine life-saving surgery, prompted the United States Department of Health and Human Services to notify hospitals that they could not discriminate against handicapped newborns in this way. Proposed federal regulations began a concerted debate about the role of the federal government in neonatal decision making, the scope of section 504 of the Rehabilitation Act of 1973, and definitions and prosecutions of child abuse in the hospital.[14]

An example of the conflict between government and family and physician was the 1983 New York case of Baby Jane Doe.[15] In the summer of 1986 the U.S. Supreme Court, discussing the *Baby Doe* case, ruled that the 1973 law barring discrimination against the handicapped did not give the federal government authority to intervene in sensitive parental decisions in consultation with their physicians. It also said that state agencies could not be drafted to investigate hospitals' alleged discrimination against handicapped newborns.[16]

These cases highlight issues similar to adult cases: the role of patients' burdens and benefits in decision making, the criterion of futility in prognosis and consequent decision making, and the rights of the parents (surrogate decision makers for the child) versus state and health care interests. In Baby Doe regulations, the government advocated the establishment of infant care review committees. The federal government had pictured these committees as aiding in enforcement and investigation of federal regulations. Others had suggested that a review committee could provide internal ethical review and serve to sensitize staff and give advice when requested.[17] As in the *Quinlan* case, this call for a hospital committee to play a role in difficult decision making stimulated the development of institutional ethics committees.

PRINCIPLES TO GUIDE DECISION MAKING

A number of principles can be advanced to guide the health care administrator in understanding and responding to possible cases of withdrawing and withholding treatment.

1. Unless proven incompetent, each patient has the right to participate in his or her plan of medical care, including the right to change or refuse any portion of that care at any time, within sound ethical parameters. This principle of self-determination is affirmed by the American Medical Association Council on Ethical and Judicial Affairs: ''Where the perform-

ance of one duty conflicts with the other (to sustain life versus relieving suffering) the choice of the patient, or his family or legal representative if the patient is incompetent to act in his own behalf, should prevail."[18]

2. When a patient is incompetent or lacks the capacity to make a responsible decision, it is the attending physician's responsibility to see that the family designate someone as the surrogate decision maker. Ordinarily this will be the patient's spouse, immediate family member, or a significant other. The patient may have designated someone in an official document (admission information form, living will, and so forth). If so, this choice should be honored. Only when determination of the surrogate is impossible or when there is family disagreement on who is the appropriate spokesperson should application be made to the courts for a legal guardian.

3. The patient should have access to necessary information including diagnosis, prognosis, risks and benefits, treatment options, and recommendations. The patient or surrogate's understanding of these options will often increase over time so decision making should be viewed as a process rather than a one-time event. Informing patients and surrogates should begin as early as possible.

4. When the patient cannot make his or her own decisions, decisions to terminate care made by surrogates on the patient's behalf should follow either the expressed or implied wishes of the patient or, if unknown, the best interests of the patient. The patient's wishes may have been clearly expressed in a recent living will or assignment of a durable power of attorney ("subjective test"). These wishes may have been expressed in informal conversations or in a certain life style ("limited objective test"). When the patient's wishes are unknown or unclear, a surrogate should decide what is in the patient's best interests, taking into account the principles of burden and benefit ("objective test").

5. Decisions to initiate or forego, to continue or discontinue life-sustaining measures, can be guided by consideration of the benefits and burdens of treatment. The patient should be considered holistically (that is, taking into account medical conditions as well as personal values, religious convictions, psychological resources, and so on).

6. Reasonable care must always be given. Treatment becomes ethically optional either when it is of no benefit to the patient or when the burdens resulting from treatment are disproportionate to the benefits that the treatment offers. Treatment is considered disproportionate when the burdens outweigh the benefits.

7. Although ordinarily it is proper to provide various forms of life-sustaining treatment in emergency situations, this treatment can be discontinued when it is judged by patient or family and responsible physician (with corroboration) to be futile.

8. A medical prognosis committee can be activated by the hospital administrator or his or her designee. The medical prognosis—whether there is a reasonable possibility of return to cognitive or sapient life—is a focal point in decision making. This committee, composed of competent medical personnel, should confirm or reject the patient's prognosis made by the responsible physician.
9. Any physician or other health care personnel may decline to be involved in the limitation or withdrawal of treatment.
10. An ethics committee, a multidisciplinary review panel, can be available for consultation to all concerned parties particularly in the event that there is doubt or disagreement between these parties.
11. Withholding or withdrawing useless or burdensome treatment does not mean abandoning the patient. In all cases, the patient's dignity, comfort, hygiene, and social, psychological, and spiritual support must be maintained.

CONCLUSION

The withholding and withdrawing of medical treatment poses numerous ethical dilemmas. Thoughtful and concerned professionals may have very different views on rationale and justifications for removing a ventilator or continuing nasogastric feeding. Several ethical principles ought to be considered in the decision-making process:[19]

Autonomy

A key concern and guide to decision making is the choice of the patient and the right of the patient to make decisions about what will or will not happen to his or her body. In cases where the patient is incompetent, the patient's statements and directions while competent should guide decision making. Where these directions are either nonexistent or questionable, other principles should be considered. If the patient is incompetent, family members and guardians are entitled to careful medical consultation and are usually capable of providing direction with regard to consent for treatment or withdrawing treatment.

Beneficence

Doing what is in the patient's best interests involves consideration of the patient's choices and viewpoint of his or her own interests and an assessment of the benefits of alternate medical choices. If there is no benefit to a course of action, such as continuing treatment, it is difficult to justify that action (unless the continued treatment was the patient's choice).

Nonmaleficence

Related to beneficence, this principle says that actions should do no harm. If withdrawing treatment results in pain and suffering for the incompetent patient, that pain and suffering should be relieved (either by continuing the treatment or some other means). If continuing treatment can be demonstrated to be harmful— imposing a burden that greatly outweighs any benefit of continued treatment— it is difficult to justify continuing treatment.

Justice

This principle questions the fair distribution of limited resources. In questioning court decisions, such as the Massachusetts decision on the *Brophy* case, Rev. John J. Paris asks, "How can we justify spending $13,400 a month, as is true in the case of Paul Brophy, to maintain a patient in a permanently unconscious state when, as a society, we allot less than $500 a month to support the total needs of a family of four on welfare?" He adds, "This reality is compounded when we realize that Karen Ann Quinlan's 10 year survival in such a state was by no means a record. That honor is held by a Florida woman, Elaine Esposito, who survived in a persistent vegetative state for 37 years, 111 days."[20]

These principles and consequent decision making require careful discussion and collaboration within the health care environment. Respect for patient autonomy is not an abdication of all medical authority. It is a call for clear and accurate communication among a patient, family members, physicians, and other health care providers. It requires informed consent from patient surrogates and family members and sharing of advice as far in advance as possible to allow consideration and the development of concurrence. Normally such decision making will involve the patient, family, and physician, with the confirmatory opinion of a second physician and possibly the advice and guidance of an ethics committee. Resolution of difficulties might be first attempted by institutional ethics committees; in some cases, such as the withholding or withdrawing of nutrition and hydration, committee review might be required. Patients should be counseled on establishing legally recognized written statements of intent anticipating the possibility of future incapacity. In cases with great doubt or disagreement, a timely approach to the court seems advisable.

Finally, to facilitate decision making it is essential for administrators and physicians to recognize that value differences can cause heated conflict contributing to further difficulty in understanding issues and resolving dilemmas. Uncertainty should be minimized through communication and the clear and accurate marshalling of relevant medical information. Consultants and committees should be used to help resolve differences.[21] An educational process should begin in hospitals to plan for difficult decisions before being confronted with disturbing cases that require thoughtful moral reasoning as well as medical competency.

150   HEALTH CARE ETHICS

NOTES

1. *In the Matter of Claire C. Conroy*, A-108 (N.J. Sup. Ct., Jan. 17, 1985).

2. Mary L. Ahern, "New Jersey Supreme Court Outlines Standards for Treatment Withdrawal," *Health Law Vigil* 8, no. 4 (February 22, 1985):4–6.

3. George J. Annas, "Fashion and Freedom: When Artificial Feeding Should Be Withdrawn," *American Journal of Public Health* 75, no. 6 (June 1985):685–688.

4. David Schwartz, ed., *Withholding and Withdrawing Care: Practical Strategies for Clinical Decision Making* (Atlanta, Georgia: American Health Consultants, Inc., 1986), 2,3.

5. Annas, "Fashion and Freedom."

6. John R. Connery, "The Clarence Herbert Case: Was Withdrawal of Treatment Justified?" *Hospital Progress* 65, no. 2 (February 1984):32–34. Also, *Barber v. Superior Court*, 147 Cal. App. 3d 1006, 195 Cal. Rptr. 484 (1983). And, John J. Paris and F.E. Reardon, "Court Responses to Withholding or Withdrawing Artificial Nutrition and Fluids," *Journal of the American Medical Association* (April 19, 1985):2243–2245.

7. David W. Meyers, "Legal Aspects of Withdrawing Nourishment From an Incurably Ill Patient," *Archives of Internal Medicine* 145 (January 1985):125–128.

8. George J. Annas, "Reconciling Quinlan and Saikewicz: Decision Making for the Terminally Ill Incompetent," *American Journal of Law and Medicine* 4, no. 4 (1979):367–396.

9. *In re Quinlan*, 355 A.2d 647 (N.J. 1976), *cert. den.*, 427 U.S. 1922 (1976).

10. J. Stuart Showalter, "Artificial Nutrition for the Terminally-Ill Patient—An Ethical Issue," *Health Law Vigil* 9, no. 15 (August 1, 1986):21–24. Also see David Schwartz, *Withholding and Withdrawing Care*, p. 5.

11. Meyers, "Legal Aspects of Withdrawing Nourishment," 127.

12. Ibid., 128.

13. Ibid.

14. See Cynthia Wallace, "Baby Doe Compromise Shifts Burden to State Protection Agencies," *Modern Healthcare* November 1, 1984, pp. 27,28; and George J. Annas, "The Baby Doe Regulations: Governmental Intervention in Neonatal Rescue Medicine," *American Journal of Public Health* 74, no. 6 (June 1984):618–620.

15. George J. Annas, "The Case of Baby Jane Doe: Child Abuse or Unlawful Federal Intervention?" *American Journal of Public Health* 74, no. 7 (July 1984):727–729.

16. " 'Baby Doe' Ruling is Another Setback for the White House," *New York Times*, Sunday, June 15, 1986.

17. American Academy of Pediatrics, *Guidelines for Infant Bioethics Committees* (Elk Grove Village, Ill.: American Academy of Pediatrics, 1984).

18. "AMA Approves Stopping Artificial Feeding for Hopelessly Comatose," *Hospital Ethics* 2, no. 3 (May/June 1986):12,13.

19. Judy Cassidy, "Withholding or Withdrawing Nutrition and Fluids: What are the Real Issues?" *Hospital Progress* (December 1985):22–25.

20. Ibid., 24,25.

21. William Winkenwerder, "Ethical Dilemmas for House Staff Physicians: The Care of the Critically Ill and Dying Patient," *Journal of the American Medical Association* 254, no. 24 (December 27, 1985):3454–3457.

BIBLIOGRAPHY

President's Commission for the Study of Ethical Problems in Medicine and Biomedical and Behavioral Research. *Deciding to Forego Life-Sustaining Treatment*. Washington, D.C.: U.S. Government Printing Office, 1983.

Chapter 11

The Definition of Death: Actions by States and Courts That Frame Decision Making

Karen Rose Koppel Kaunitz, JD, Andrew Moss Kaunitz, MD, and Barbara Sue Koppel, MD

> The times have been,
> That, when the brains were out, the man would die,
> And there an end.
> —Shakespeare, *Macbeth*, act III, scene IV

INTRODUCTION

Why define death? There are pressing medical, legal, and ethical reasons to declare the time of death with precision. Economic and emotional costs of maintaining life in vegetative patients place pressure on health care providers to define death in a manner that acknowledges the changes in critical care medicine that have occurred in recent decades. The need for precision in determining the time of death has been intensified by the growth of organ transplantation. Life-saving transplant operations would be jeopardized by deterioration of the donor's organs if pronouncement of death was delayed until the heart stopped.

For the law, determining the time of death may be crucial in cases involving homicide, taxation, inheritance, property rights, insurance claims, workers' compensation, and wrongful death.[1] Courts have even been forced to ponder arguments that the act of withdrawing life support systems from a homicide victim was an intervening cause of death, and thus the defendant should be relieved of criminal liability.

Death affects and changes many legal relationships.[2] The law has largely adopted the criteria and definition of death set forth by the medical profession. In fact, the law has always been that an individual is dead when a licensed physician pronounces him dead, so long as the physician makes the determination based on accepted medical standards.[3]

A formulation about death must consist of a concept or definition of what it means to die, operational criteria for determining that death has occurred, and specific medical tests to show whether the criteria have been fulfilled.[4] Under-

152

standing the currently held definition of death requires an analysis of both the medical and legal standards for the determination of death. This chapter traces medical and legal definitions from a historic perspective, culminating in an assessment of the current situation.

THE TRADITIONAL DEFINITION OF DEATH

In 1872 New York's high court stated that "death is the opposite of life; it is the termination of life."[5] Common law historically considers a person "alive until respiration stops and the heart ceases." Whenever a court was called upon to decide the question of death it applied the traditional definition found in *Black's Law Dictionary*, which defines death as "the cessation of life; the ceasing to exist; defined by physicians as a total stoppage of the circulation of the blood, and cessation of the animal and vital functions consequent thereon, such as respiration, pulsation, etc."[6] This commonly accepted definition was easily applied and ascertained.

THE NEED FOR A NEW DEFINITION

"A dead brain in a body whose heart is still beating is one of the more macabre products of modern technology."[7] As one court expressed it: "Now, however, we are on the threshold of new terrain—the penumbra when death begins but life, in some form, continues. We have been led to it by the medical miracles which now compel us to distinguish between 'death,' as we have known it, and death in which the body lives in some fashion but the brain (or a significant part of it) does not."[8] Another court stated, "Because of the current gap between technology and law, physicians and families of these unfortunate victims are called upon to make intensely painful decisions regarding their case without clearly defined legal guidelines."[9]

The use of mechanical support to maintain circulatory and respiratory function for indefinite time periods, well beyond the complete and irreversible cessation of brain function, has forced medical science to reexamine the traditional definition of death. The implications for both medicine and law have been profound. Questions regarding the dignity due the patient, the emotional and financial costs to the family, and the competing demands on scarce equipment and intensive care space are asked with increased frequency.[10]

An irreversibly comatose individual with intact cardiac function and circulation, according to the traditional legal definition, is alive. Growing clinical applications of organ transplantation, therefore, have increased pressure for a new definition of death. Traditional definitions of death likewise can expose physicians to wrongful death claims and charges of homicide when they shut off ventilators in comatose patients. These now obsolete definitions have even interfered with criminal prosecution. In *People v. Flores*, a California trial court acquitted a defendant charged with manslaughter. Because the decedent's organs were later harvested for transplant purposes, the court found that the defendant's actions could not have resulted in death.[11] Based on all of these concerns, the medical community, and following them, the law, recognized the advantages of defining death based on brain function in addition to circulatory and respiratory function.

CRITERIA FOR ESTABLISHING BRAIN DEATH

Once there was a consensus for the need for a new supplementary definition based on brain death, the debate shifted to determining diagnostic criteria to confirm that irreversible cessation of brain function had, in fact, occurred.[12] The history of brain-based tests begins with the 1959 description of "coma dépassé" (beyond coma) by two French neurophysiologists. All of the classical descriptions of brain death are found in this early report.[13] The ad hoc committee of the Harvard Medical School formulated in 1960 the first widely accepted criteria for defining brain death. The committee described two reasons for publishing its definition of irreversible coma:

1. Improvements in resuscitative and supportive measures have led to increased efforts to save those who are desperately injured. Sometimes these efforts have only partial success so that the result is an individual whose heart continues to beat but whose brain is irreversibly damaged. The burden is great on patients who suffer permanent loss of intellect, on their families, on the hospitals, and on those in need of hospital beds already occupied by these comatose patients.
2. Obsolete criteria for the definition of death can lead to controversy in obtaining organs for transplantation.[14]

The Harvard criteria soon became widely recognized and accepted. They were a landmark because they pointed out the need for recognition of brain death as an entity. The so-called "Harvard Test" argues that a permanently nonfunctioning brain could be accurately diagnosed on the basis of four criteria:

1. Unreceptivity and unresponsiveness. There is a total unawareness of externally applied stimuli and inner need and complete unresponsiveness— our definition of irreversible coma. Even the most intensely painful stimuli evoke no vocal or other response, not even a groan, withdrawal of a limb, or quickening of respiration.
2. No movements or breathing. Observations covering a period of at least one hour by physicians are adequate to satisfy the criteria of no spontaneous

muscular movements or spontaneous respiration or response to stimuli such as pain, touch, sound, or light. After a patient is on a mechanical respirator, the total absence of spontaneous breathing may be established by turning off the respirator for three minutes and observing whether there is any effort on the part of the subject to breathe spontaneously.

3. No reflexes. Irreversible coma with abolition of central nervous system activity is evidenced in part by the absence of elicitable reflexes. The pupil will be fixed and dilated and will not respond to a direct source of bright light. Ocular movement (to head turning and to irrigation of the ears with ice water) and blinking are absent. There is no evidence of postural activity (decerebrate or other). Swallowing, yawning, vocalization are in abeyance. Corneal and pharyngeal reflexes are absent.

4. Flat electroencephalogram. Of great confirmatory value is the flat or iso-electric EEG. At least ten full minutes of recording are desirable, but twice that would be better.[15]

The validity of such data as indications of irreversible cerebral damage depends on the exclusion of two conditions: hypothermia (temperature below 90° F) or central nervous system depressants, such as barbiturates. Later modifications of the guidelines provide for apnea testing to include passive oxygenation and a $PaCO_2$ of 60 to stimulate respiratory drive; allow purely spinal cord reflexes; require that pupils need be only unreactive, not dilated; and require that EEG should be at least 30 minutes and need be repeated only if the cause of coma is not known.[16]

The Harvard committee called for repetition of all the above tests after at least 24 hours without change. A report issued in 1977 based on a collaborative study conducted at nine clinical centers across the country, however, concluded that a 24-hour repetition was unnecessary. This report suggested that the following criteria must be present for a duration of 30 minutes at least 6 hours after the onset of coma and apnea: "coma and cerebral unresponsivity, apnea, dilated pupils, absent cephalic reflexes and electrocerebral silence."[17] In addition, a new confirmatory test was suggested for whenever an early diagnosis of brain death is desired. This new test evaluates blood flow through the cerebrum (the "bolus isotope technique").[18]

The Harvard committee also addressed the legal ramifications of the brain death concept and surveyed relevant case law, suggesting that:

no statutory change in the law should be necessary since the law treats this question essentially as one of fact to be determined by physicians. The only circumstances in which it would be necessary that legislation be offered in the various states to define "death" by law would be in the event that great controversy were engendered surrounding the subject and physicians were unable to agree on the new medical criteria.[19]

As one commentator observed, the report "made physicians into lawyers, lawyers into physicians, and both into philosophers."[20]

The Harvard committee report "touched almost all branches of medicine, opened up new areas of law, and posed new and difficult problems for theologians and ethicists."[21] Almost every legal entity has had to come to terms with this new concept of death, and most medical standards for death of the brain emerge from the criteria set forth in this article. Although the medically acceptable criteria for total and irreversible brain death have been refined and updated, the thrust of the Harvard report remains unaltered.[22]

REFINEMENTS OF THE BRAIN DEATH CRITERIA

In 1972, the Task Force on Death and Dying of the Institute of Society, Ethics, and Life Sciences issued a report entitled "Refinements in Criteria for the Determination of Death: An Appraisal" that continued to rely on the concept of brain death. The report issued the following guidelines for protocols used to determine death:

1. The criteria must be clear and distinct.
2. The tests should be simple and easily and conveniently performed and interpreted and depend as little as possible on the use of elaborate equipment and machinery.
3. The procedure should include an evaluation of the permanence and irreversibility of the absence of functions and a determination of the absence of other conditions (such as hypothermia and drug intoxication) that may be mistaken for death.
4. Multiple criteria should be used.
5. Brain death criteria should be compatible with traditional criteria (cessation of spontaneous heartbeat and respiration) in the vast majority of cases where artificial maintenance of vital functions has not been in use.
6. All individuals who fulfill either set of criteria should be declared dead by the physician.
7. The criteria and procedures should be easily communicable, both to laymen and physicians, and acceptable by the medical profession as a basis for uniform practice.
8. The reasonableness and adequacy of the criteria and procedures should be vindicated by experience and autopsy findings.[23]

The task force report concluded that the criteria of the Harvard committee met the formal characteristics of "good criteria" and that experience to date suggests them to be reasonable and appropriate. In addition, the report viewed with concern proposals to place exclusive reliance on electroencephalography to determine death and urged that the more rigorous combined clinical and laboratory criteria of the Harvard report be adopted.

BRAIN DEATH VERSUS COMMON LAW

As the concept of brain death became accepted, disparity developed between current, accepted biomedical practice and the common law. The medical profession currently considers permanent cessation of brain function as important as cessation of cardiac and respiratory functions in determining death. However, evolution of these new medical criteria did little to change traditional common law definitions in many states.

With the progressive acceptance by physicians of the concepts of brain death, clinicians grew increasingly concerned about the lack of legal acceptance of this concept. As Joynt noted, "Although judicial opinion generally accepted this concept, there were numerous cases citing medical personnel as the proximate cause of death and seeking to dismiss charges against the assailant who was responsible for the final injury."[24] In addition, some lower courts had trouble accepting brain death in cases involving organ donations. These early contradictory trial court decisions added impetus to the efforts to avoid the case-by-case approach of common law. Since 1970, laws that included brain death criteria for determining death were enacted in more than two-thirds of the states.

STATUTORY RECOGNITION OF BRAIN DEATH

Recognition of brain death by state legislatures has not been consistent. State statutes fall into three groupings based on how they relate the brain-centered definition of death to the traditional heart-lung definition.[25] In 1970 Kansas was the first state to recognize brain death by statute. This legislation set forth the following alternative definitions of death:

Definition of death. A person will be considered medically and legally dead if, in the opinion of a physician, based on ordinary standards of medical practice, there is the absence of spontaneous respiratory and cardiac function and, because of the disease or condition which caused, directly or indirectly, these functions to cease, attempts at resuscitation are considered hopeless, and in this event, death will have occurred at the time these functions ceased; or

A person will be considered medically and legally dead if in the opinion of a physician, based on ordinary standards of medical practice, there is the absence of spontaneous brain function; and if based on ordinary standards of medical practice, during reasonable attempts to either maintain or restore spontaneous circulatory or respiratory function in the absence of aforesaid brain function, it appears that further attempts at resuscitation or supportive maintenance will not succeed, death will have occurred at the time when these conditions first coincide. Death is to be pronounced before artificial means of supporting respiratory and circulatory function are terminated and before any vital organ is removed for purposes of transplantation.

These alternative definitions of death are to be utilized for all purposes in this state, including the trials of civil and criminal cases, any laws to the contrary notwithstanding.[26]

This statute was greatly debated, widely praised, and criticized. Supporters viewed it as a well-written first step, protecting physicians who determine that resuscitation is not warranted. Critics felt it was too transplant-oriented and were concerned that it did not require two physicians, neither a member of the transplant team, to decide when the patient was dead. Detractors also noted the law provided for alternative definitions for determining death with no clear indication of when one definition or the other should be used. The critics argued that the Kansas approach might engender the mistaken impression that "there are two ways to die in Kansas"—that is, two different phenomena of death—and that a physician might, as a consequence, choose one definition if the patient were a prospective organ donor, while the patient would be alive according to the other definition.[27]

In 1977 the Supreme Court of Kansas, in the only brain death statute challenge, reaffirmed the provisions of its statute against several charges of unconstitutionality raised by a criminal defendant convicted of first degree murder.[28] Six other states (Maryland, New Mexico, Alaska, Virginia, Oregon, and Alabama) enacted statutes identical or similar to the Kansas model, basing death on absence of spontaneous respiratory and circulatory function or the absence of brain function.

In 1972 Capron and Kass criticized the Kansas statute and suggested a simplified definition. This proposed model brain death statute addressed itself to general physiological standards for a determination of death:

A person will be considered dead if in the announced opinion of a physician, based on ordinary standards of medical practice, he has experienced an irreversible cessation of spontaneous respiratory and circulatory functions. In the event that artificial means of support preclude a determination that these functions have ceased, a person will be considered dead if in the announced opinion of a physician, based on ordinary practice, he has experienced an irreversible cessation of spontaneous brain functions. Death will have occurred in the time when the relevant functions ceased.[29]

Six states (Michigan, West Virginia, Louisiana, Iowa, Montana, and Hawaii) followed this strategy. The supporters of this model applauded its definition of death as a single phenomenon that can be determined by brain-related criteria in situations in which an artificial support system precludes the use of the traditional standards. As Selby and Selby point out:

> Thus, it does not establish a separate kind of death called "brain-death." Rather it recognizes the fact that medical standards for pronouncing death may vary with circumstances, and unlike the Kansas statute it specifies under what circumstances each of the standards is to be used to measure different manifestations of this phenomenon.[30]

Some, however, have criticized the model for not requiring two physicians to participate in the pronouncement of death.[31]

A third group of states (California, Georgia, Illinois, Oklahoma, Tennessee, and Idaho) have followed the definition drafted by the Law and Medicine Committee of the American Bar Association (ABA) and approved by the ABA House of Delegates. This definition is based on the irreversible cessation of "total" brain function rather than the cessation of the heartbeat:

> For all legal purposes, a human body with irreversible cessation of total brain functions, according to the usual and customary standards of medical practice, shall be considered dead.[32]

Critics of the ABA model argue that by adopting cessation of brain function as the sole standard for determining death, it fails to recognize the still reasonable and common practice of pronouncing death based on cessation of heartbeat and respiration.[33]

State statutes defining brain death vary as to: (1) whether their use is mandatory or optional, (2) the criteria to be applied, (3) the procedure to be followed, (4) the time of death, (5) the relationship to the traditional death criteria, and (6) the circumstances in which the statute applies.[34] See Appendix 11-A for summaries of state definition of death statutes. The lack of uniformity among state statutes may lead to confusion "due to the lack of rigorous separation and ordered formulation of three distinct elements: the definition of death, the medical criterion for determining that death has occurred, and the tests to prove that the criterion has been satisfied.[35]

CALL FOR UNIFORM DEFINITION OF DEATH

After the 1975 ABA model was proposed, the American Medical Association (AMA) created its own Model Determination of Death Statute in 1979. On

August 3, 1978, in an effort to clear up the legal ambiguity, the National Conference of Commissioners for Uniform State Laws (ULC) created the Uniform Brain Death Act (UBDA), adopting the following definition based on the prior work of the ABA:

> For all legal and medical purposes, an individual who has sustained irreversible cessation of all functions of the brain, including the brain stem, is dead. Determination of death under this section must be made in accordance with "reasonable medical standards."[36]

The ULC assumed that the traditional criteria would stand automatically alongside the brain death standard described in the UBDA, so the criteria were not mentioned in the act itself. The omission proved confusing for states attempting to adopt comprehensive brain death legislation.[37]

Favoring a uniform definition of death that would address the inconsistencies between the medical and legal perceptions, on July 9, 1981, the President's Commission for the Study of Ethical Problems in Medicine and Biomedical and Behavioral Research recommended that the states endorse the concept that human life ends when the brain stops functioning. After hearing testimony from a variety of experts including philosophers, theologians, and neurologists, the President's Commission reported that "state by state variation is not justified on a matter that is so fundamental and . . . rests on biological facts of universal applicability."[38] It was viewed as unconscionable for matters of life and death to be treated differently in different jurisdictions. Furthermore, the consensus of the commission was that "the definition of death should be the same for criminal law (murder), tort law (wrongful death), family law (status of spouse and children), property and estate law, insurance law (payment of life insurance benefits), and tax law. Calling a person dead for one purpose and 'alive' for another is problematical."[39] The commission report was hailed as a landmark document in society's attempt to deal with bioethical dilemmas resulting from recent advances in medical technology.[40]

THE UNIFORM DETERMINATION OF DEATH ACT

The commission urged all 50 states to accept a simple, uniform law that defined death as "irreversible cessation of all functions of the entire brain including the brain stem."[41] The model Uniform Determination of Death Act (UDDA) was finalized in 1980 at a meeting of the AMA, the ABA, and the National Conference of Commissioners on Uniform State Laws, replacing the confusing UBDA. The UDDA is based on a ten-year evolution of statutory language on the subject. The new UDDA states,

An individual who has sustained either (1) irreversible cessation of circulatory and respiratory function; or (2) irreversible cessation of all functions of the entire brain, including the brain stem, is dead. A determination of death must be made in accordance with accepted medical standards.[42]

The UDDA sharpens the distinction between life and death. According to the prefatory note to the definition:

Part (1) codifies the existing common law basis for determining death—total failure of the cardio-respiratory system. Part (2) extends the common law to include the new procedures for determination of death based upon irreversible loss of all brain functions. The overwhelming majority of cases will continue to be determined according to part (1). When artificial means of support preclude a determination under part (1), the Act recognizes that death can be determined by the alternative procedures. Under part (2), the entire brain must cease to function, irreversibly. The "entire brain" includes the brain stem as well as the neocortex. The concept of "entire brain" distinguishes determination of death under this Act from "neocortical death" or "persistent vegetative state." These are not deemed valid medical or legal bases for determining death.[43]

The presidential panel deliberately avoided specifying how cessation of the brain function should be determined, leaving it to the medical community and acknowledging the ever-changing nature of biomedical knowledge, diagnostic tests, and equipment. It sets the general legal standard for determining death, not the medical criteria for doing so. The UDDA has been endorsed by the ABA, the American Academy of Neurology, the American EEG Society, the AMA, and the National Conference of Commissioners on Uniform State Law, as well as the President's Commission.

Since 1970, 38 states have adopted determination-of-death laws, usually by statute but sometimes by court decision. Among these at least 22 states and the District of Columbia have adopted the UDDA in total or in part:

Arkansas	Indiana	Montana	Tennessee
California	Kansas	Nevada	Vermont
Colorado	Maine	Ohio	Washington
District of Columbia	Maryland	Pennsylvania	Wisconsin
Georgia	Mississippi	Rhode Island	Wyoming
Idaho	Missouri	South Carolina	

What if the goal of uniform brain death legislation is not successful? One commentator responded: "Will this raise the specter (one that worries many commentators) that a person may be legally dead in one state, but all of a sudden become legally 'alive' when the ambulance crosses into another? Although a theoretical possibility such a result is unlikely."[44]

JUDICIAL DECISIONS ADOPTING BRAIN DEATH IN STATES WITHOUT STATUTES

Surprisingly, there have been few court decisions in which the concept of brain death was at issue. To date, these cases have found either that judicial intervention was unnecessary before removing life support devices from a brain-dead patient, or that the removal of such devices was not an intervening cause of death. A measure of the judicial system's acceptance of the brain death concept is that each court that has examined relevant cases has agreed that brain death is a legally proper determination for a physician to make, whether or not there is a state statute on the subject. The common law definition now clearly includes brain death.

States where the brain death rule has been approved judicially include Arizona (where the Harvard test was adopted as the definition of death), Indiana, Massachusetts, Nebraska, New Jersey, and Washington. In New York the Court of Appeals ruled in two consolidated cases that "death means an irreversible cessation of breathing and heartbeat or, when the functions are artificially maintained, an irreversible cessation of the functioning of the entire brain." Most of these cases involved criminal prosecutions in which defendants argued unsuccessfully that the termination of support systems by attending physicians or the removal of organs (for transplant) caused the victims' death.[45]

STATES WITHOUT BRAIN DEATH STATUTES OR JUDICIAL DECISIONS

In states without statutes or court decisions on the issue, law and medicine may be out of sync.[46] For example, in Minnesota, which has no statute, the most recent relevant court decision is a 1933 car accident case that defines death as "the cessation of all bodily functions." Due to the absence of a modern law, Minnesota hospitals and physicians could theoretically find themselves in a legal no-man's-land when, for instance, they harvest organs for transplant.

In practice, however, brain death pronouncement can be made in the absence of statute, since it has been accepted by the medical community and the courts.[47] Hospitals and physicians in states without updated laws should use the brain death definition, following accepted medical practice for determining death as incorporated in carefully drafted written hospital policies. No modern court has ever refused to recognize a definition of death based on brain death, and in fact, most courts may be reluctant to intervene in what they consider a medical determination. Hence, if the hospital and physicians follow reasonable medical procedures and standards in declaring a patient dead, exposure to liability will be negligible.

HOSPITAL DEATH POLICY AND DOCUMENTATION

All hospitals should have policies defining death in accordance with applicable state law. The policy should outline the criteria to be used in determining if a patient is brain dead and the medical record documentation necessary prior to removing life support from brain-dead patients.

Some states, in fact, specifically address requirements for recordkeeping. California requires "complete patient medical records," Hawaii requires "signed statements" from the physicians, and Virginia requires that the determination must be "recorded in the patient's medical record and attested by the aforesaid consulting physician."[48] It is always wise to document the clinical findings and diagnoses carefully in these situations.

TIME OF DEATH

For a variety of legal purposes, it is important to establish the actual time of death. The criminal laws of all jurisdictions require, for instance, a demonstration that the victim is dead as a prerequisite to a successful homicide or manslaughter prosecution. Partnerships dissolve upon death. Life insurance policies often pay double indemnity only if the insured dies within 90 to 120 days of the accident date. As one commentator summed it up, "Double indemnity, murder, life tenancy and taxation, conflicts of interest, speedy trial, double jeopardy—these legal issues and many more that appear to be unrelated to medicine are inextricably tied to what doctors do."[49]

State laws differ as to whether the time of death should be when all tests are completed or when cessation of spontaneous brain function is first observed.[50] The original Harvard committee report advocated using the time when all tests are completed because it is the first time when the diagnosis, including irreversibility, can be confirmed. The following four alternatives are often cited:

1. Some states provide that death *may* be pronounced before life support mechanisms are removed.
2. Several states provide that death *must* be pronounced before any life support mechanisms are removed.
3. At least two states provide that death is to be pronounced before any vital organ is removed for transplant.
4. The majority of states do not address the issue of when death is to be pronounced.[51]

In states that do not address the issue it would be prudent to note the time of death as the time when all tests are completed.[52]

CONCLUSION

The definition of death will continue to evolve as the legal system incorporates medical advances. In fact, it has been suggested that the emerging consensus over brain death may be only temporary. This opinion contends that death occurs not when the brain is wholly inactive but whenever the "higher cerebral functions" of the brain, including consciousness and cognition, are absent.[53] Thoughts of liberalizing definitions of brain death raise ethical as well as neurological concerns: could an overzealous insurance company pressure a physician to declare death prematurely in a borderline case? One commentator warns "these new concepts of death have opened Pandora's box, releasing the wild winds of doubt about man's life and death."[54] At present, however, medical science has not identified a reliable means of establishing the irreversible loss of higher cerebral functions. It is reassuring that the currently acceptable criteria for brain death described in this chapter allow little flexibility in their application.

Current legal and medical opinions uniformly support the use of brain death as the definition of death. Practitioners and providers should familiarize themselves with state law, taking comfort that in those states without statutes or precedents, brain death criteria are uniformly accepted as the basis to determine death. If hospitals and physicians follow reasonable procedures and standards in declaring a patient dead, exposure to liability will be negligible.

NOTES

1. Martin R. Ufford, "Brain Death/Termination of Heroic Efforts to Save Life—Who Decides?" *Washburn Law Journal* 19 (1980):227.

2. Lawrence Grey, "Death and Dying: Medicine and the Law Collide," *Generics* 2, no. 1 (March 1986):20.

3. G.J. Annas, L.H. Glants, and B. Katz, *The Rights of Doctors, Nurses, and Allied Health Professionals* (Cambridge, Mass.: Ballinger Books, 1981):224–225.

4. Stuart J. Youngner and Edward T. Bartlett, "Human Death and High Technology: The Failure of the Whole-Brain Formulation," *Annals of Internal Medicine* 99 (1983):252.

5. Frances J. Flaherty, "A Right to Die? The Premier Privacy Issue of the 1980s," *The National Law Journal* 7, no. 18 (Jan. 14, 1985):1.

6. *Black's Law Dictionary*, Rev. 4th ed. (St. Paul, Minn.: West Publishing Co., 1968).

7. C. Pallis, "ABC of Brain Death: Reappraising Death," *British Medical Journal* 285 (Nov. 13, 1982):1409.

8. *Severns v. Wilmington Medical Center, Inc.*, 421 A.2d 1334, 1344 (Del. 1980).

9. *Barber v. Superior Court of Los Angeles County, Wejdl v. Superior Court of Los Angeles County*, 147 Cal. App.3d 1006, 195 Cal. Rptr. 484 (1983).

10. Leonard Isaacs, "Death, Where is Thy Distinguishing?" *The Hastings Center Report* 8, no. 1, (Feb. 1985):5.

11. No. 20190, Somona County Municipal Court, California, 1973. *Chicago Tribune*, December 6, 1973, Sec. 2, p. 9.

12. A. Earl Walker, *Cerebral Death*, 3rd ed. (Baltimore, Md.: Urban & Schwarzenberg, 1985).

13. P. Mollaret and M. Goulon, "Le Coma Dépassé (Mémoire Préliminaire)," *Revised Neurosurgery* 101, no. 3 (1959):3–15.

14. Ad Hoc Committee of the Harvard Medical School to Examine the Definition of Death, "A Definition of Irreversible Coma," *Journal of the American Medical Association* 205, no. 6 (Aug. 5, 1968):85.

15. Ibid, 85–86.

16. "Guidelines for the Determination of Death," *Journal of the American Medical Association* 246, no. 19 (Nov. 13, 1981):2184–2186.

17. "An Appraisal of the Criteria of Cerebral Death (A Summary Statement, a Collaborative Study)," *Journal of the American Medical Association* 237, no. 10 (March 7, 1977):982.

18. Ibid.

19. Ad Hoc Committee of the Harvard Medical School, "Definition," 87.

20. Robert J. Joynt, "A New Look at Death," *Journal of the American Medical Association* 252, no. 5 (Aug. 3, 1984):680.

21. Ibid.

22. Isaacs, "Death Where Is," 6.

23. Task Force on Death and Dying of the Institute of Society, Ethics, and Life Sciences, "Refinements in Criteria for the Determination of Death: An Appraisal," *Journal of the American Medical Association* 221, (July 3, 1972):49.

24. Joynt, "A New Look at Death."

25. Isaacs, "Death Where Is," 7.

26. Kansas Statute Ann. Sec. 77-202 (1970).

27. Isaacs, "Death Where Is," 7.

28. *State v. Shaffer*, 574 P.2d 205 (Kan. 1977).

29. A.M. Capron and L.R. Kass, "A Statutory Definition of the Standards for Determining Human Death," *University of Pennsylvania Law Review* 121, no. 1 (Nov. 1972):87–118.

30. Roy and Marilyn T. Selby, "Status of Legal Definition of Death," *Neurosurgery* 5, no. 4 (1979):537.

31. Ibid.

32. Demere et al., Unpublished Report, 1975.

33. Selby, "Status," 537.

34. *Hospital Law Manual*, Attorney's Volume, "Dying, Death and Dead Bodies" (Rockville, Md.: Aspen Publishers, Inc.,) Sec. 3-7, p. 43.

35. J.L. Bernat, C.M. Culver, and B. Gert, "On the Definition and Criterion of Death," *Annals of Internal Medicine* 94, no. 3 (March 1981):389.

36. Uniform Brain Death Act, National Conference of Commissioners on Uniform State Laws, Chicago, 1978.

37. John M. McCabe, "Uniform Determination of Death Act," *Health Law Vigil* 8, no. 5 (March 8, 1985):21.

38. President's Commission for the Study of Ethical Problems in Medicine and Biomedical and Behavioral Research, *Defining Death, A Report on the Medical, Legal and Ethical Issues in the*

Determination of Death, Library of Congress, 81-6; 950 (Washington, D.C.: U.S. Government Printing Office, 1981), p. 60.

39. Ibid.

40. Howard R. Schwartz, "Bioethical and Legal Considerations in Increasing the Supply of Transplantable Organs: From UAGA to 'Baby Fae'," *American Journal of Law & Medicine* 10, no. 4 (Winter 1985):397.

41. Uniform Determination of Death Act, 12 U.L.A. 270 (Supp. 1985).

42. Ibid.

43. Ibid.

44. George J. Annas, "Defining Death: There Ought To Be a Law," *The Hastings Center Report* 13, no. 1 (February 1983):21.

45. *State v. Fierro*, 124 Ariz. 182, 603 P.2d 74 (1979); *Swafford v. State*, 421 N.E.2d 596 (Ind. 1981); *Commonwealth v. Golston*, 373 Mass. 249, 366 N.E.2d 744 (1977), *cert. denied sub nom Golston v. Massachusetts*, 434 U.S. 1039, 98 S.Ct. 777 (1978); *State v. Meints*, 212 Neb. 410, 322 N.W.2d 809 (1982); *State v. Watson*, 191 N.J. Super. 464, 467 A.2d 590 (1983); *In re Welfare of Bowman*, 94 Wash.2d 407, 617 P.2d 731 (1980); *People v. Eulo, People v. Bonilla*, 472 N.E.2d 286, 63 N.Y.2d 341, 482 N.Y.S.2d 436 (1984).

46. Flaherty, "A Right to Die?," 2.

47. Annas, "Defining Death," 21.

48. *Hospital Law Manual*, 45.

49. Grey, "Death and Dying," 24.

50. *Hospital Law Manual*, 46.

51. J. Horty, "The Right To Die," in *Hospital Law*, Chapter 5 (Pittsburgh: Action-Kit for Hospital Law, 1981): 2.

52. Ibid.

53. Youngner and Bartlett, "Human Death and High Technology," 252.

54. A. Earl Walker, "Editorial, Dead or Alive," *Journal of Nervous and Mental Disease* 172, no. 11 (Nov. 1984):641.

BIBLIOGRAPHY

Abram, Morris B. "Need for Uniform Law on Determination of Death." *New York Law School Law Review* 27:1187.

Alexander, Marc. "The Rigid Embrace of the Narrow House: Premature Burial and the Signs of Death." *Hastings Center Report* 10 (3):25–31.

American Medical Assn. Law Dept. "Death Definition and Diagnosis." *Journal of the American Medical Association* 208 (19):1759.

Annas, George J. "The Definition of Death: New Statutes, Old Laws." *American Medical News*, July 19, 1982, 12.

Bernat, J.L., Culver, C.M., Gert, B. "Defining Death in Theory and Practice." *The Hastings Center Report* 12 (1):5–9.

Bernat, J.L., et al. "Definition of Death" (letter). *Annals of Internal Medicine* 100 (3):456.

Bernstein, Arthur H. "Death with Dignity: Is Judicial Involvement Necessary?" *Hospitals* 56 (9):93–95.

Black, Peter M. "Clinical Problems in the Use of Brain-Death Standards." *Archives of Internal Medicine* 143:121–123.

Brennan, Susan L., and Delgado, Richard. "Death: Multiple Definitions of a Single Standard?" *Southern California Law Review* 54:1323.

Byrne, et al. "Brain Death—the Patient, the Physician, and the Society." *Gonzaga Law Review* 18:429.

Campos-Outcalt, Doug. "Brain Death: Medical and Legal Issues." *The Journal of Family Practice* 19 (3):349.

Capron, Alexander M. "Looking Back at the President's Commission." *The Hastings Center Report* 13 (5):7–11.

Coe, J.I. "Definition and Time of Death," in *Modern Legal Medicine, Psychiatry and Forensic Science*, eds. W.J. Curran et al. (Philadelphia: Davis, 1980).

Committees on Public Health and Medicine in Society. "Statement and Resolution on the Definition of Death." *Bulletin of New York Academy of Medicine* 60 (9): November 1984.

"Defining Death: Report on Medical, Legal and Ethical Issues in Determination of Death." *New York Law School Law Review* 27:1273.

"Definition of Death." *Journal of Medical Society of New Jersey* 80 (6):409.

Dornett, W. "How Does Your State Define Death?" *Legal Aspects of Medical Practice*, May 1980, pp. 19–23.

Dowben, C. "Prometheus Revisited: Popular Myths, Medical Realities, and Legislative Actions Concerning Death." *Journal of Health Politics, Policy and Law* 5 (2):250–276.

Eisner, J.M., Randell, L.L., and Tilson, J.Q. "Judicial Decisions Concerning Brain Death." *Connecticut Medicine* 46 (4):193–194.

Ethics Committee of the American Academy of Neurology. "Uniform Determination of Death Act." *Connecticut Medicine* 46 (5).

Flaherty, Francis J. "A Right to Die?" *The National Law Journal* 7 (18):1.

Goldowsky, Seebert J. "Uniform Determination of Death." *Rhode Island Medical Journal* 66:309–311.

Gorman, Warren F. "Medical Diagnosis versus Legal Determination of Death." *Journal of Forensic Sciences* 30 (1):150–157.

Gregory, Dorothy R. "A New 'Definition' of Death?" *Legal Aspects of Medical Practice* 9 (8).

Hoffman, Alan C. and Van Cura, Mark. "Death: A Medical Dilemma, a Legal Answer." *Legal Medical Quarterly* 3 (2):110–122.

Horan, D.J. "Definition of Death: An Emerging Consensus." *Trial* 16 (12):22–26.

Horty, John F. "Court Shares Burden with Doctors of Making Life-and-Death Decisions." *Modern Healthcare* 11 (8):144.

Jonsen, Albert R. "A Concord in Medical Ethics." *Annals of Internal Medicine* 49 (2):261–264.

Joynt, Robert J. "A New Look at Death." *Journal of American Medical Association* 252 (5):680.

Kaczynski, "We Find the Accused (Guilty) (Not Guilty) of Homicide: Toward a New Definition of Death." *Army Lawyer* 1.

Kaunitz, Karen. "Point of Law." *The Hospital Medical Staff* 10 (10).

Lappe, Marc. "Dying While Living: A Critique of Allowing-to-Die Legislation." *Journal of Medical Ethics* 4 (4):195–199.

Lynn, J. "The Determination of Death." *Annals of Internal Medicine* 99 (2)264–266.

McCabe, John M. "The New Determination of Death Act." *American Bar Association Journal* 67:1476.

Meyers, David. "Time of Death: Medicolegal Considerations." 16 *Proof of Facts 2d.*

Molinari, G.F. "Brain Death, Irreversible Coma, and Words Doctors Use." *Neurology* 32:400–402.

Pallis, C. "ABC of Brain Stem Death: The Position in the USA and Elsewhere." *British Medical Journal* 286.

Pallis, C. "ABC of Brain Stem Death: From Brain Death to Brain Stem Death." *British Medical Journal* 285.

Schenck, Brian. "Death and Prolonged States of Impaired Responsiveness." *Denver Law Journal* 58:609.

Showalter. "Determining Death: The Legal and Theological Aspects of Brain-Related Criteria." *Catholic Law* 27:112.

Sweet, David B. "Annotation: Homicide by Causing Victim's Brain-Dead Condition." 42 *ALR 4th* 742.

Task Force on Death and Dying of the Institute of Society, Ethics, and Life Sciences. "Refinements in Criteria for the Determination of Death: An Appraisal" *Journal of the American Medical Association* 221 (1):48–53.

"Tests of Death for Organ Transplant Purposes." 76 *ALR 3d* 913.

"The Citadel for the Human Cadaver: The Harvard Brain Death Exhumed." *University of Florida Law Review* 32 (2):275–307.

Thompson, W.T. "These Great Mysteries: Dying, Death, the Hereafter." *Virginia Medical* 107:69–71.

Trenker, Thomas R. "Annotation: Tests of Death for Organ Transplant Purposes." 76 *ALR 3d* 913.

Trenker, Thomas R. "Annotation: Tort Liability of Physician or Hospital in Connection with Organ or Tissue Transplant." 76 *ALR 3d* 890.

Ufford, Martin R. "Brain Death/Termination of Heroic Efforts to Save Life—Who Decides?" *Washburn Law Journal* 19:225–259.

Wershow, H.J., Ferris, J.R., and Alphin, T.H. "Physicians' Opinions Toward Legislation Defining Death and Withholding Life Support." *Southern Medical Journal* 74 (2):215–220.

Youngner, S.J., et al. "Psychosocial and Ethical Implications of Organ Retrieval." *The New England Journal of Medicine* 313 (5):321–324.

Appendix 11-A

State-by-State Analysis

Alabama. ALA. CODE tit. 31 sec. 22-31-1.
- No spontaneous cardiopulmonary function, or brain death (total and irreversible cessation of brain function).
- Two licensed physicians must make the brain death determination.
- Death may be pronounced before artificial life support is removed.

Alaska. ALASKA STAT. ANN. sec. 09.65.120.
- No spontaneous cardiopulmonary function, or brain death (lack of spontaneous brain function).
- Death may be pronounced before artificial life support is removed.

Arizona. There is no brain death legislation.
Brain death recognized in *State v. Fierro*, 124 Ariz. 182, 603 P.2d 74 (1970). Arizona Supreme Court rejected argument of accused murderer that removal of life support systems (rather than gunshot wounds to the head) was the actual cause of death.

Arkansas. ARK. STAT. ANN. sec. 82-537 to 82-538.
Uniform Determination of Death Act.

California. CAL. HEALTH AND SAFETY CODE sec. 7180 to 7183 (West).
Uniform Determination of Death Act.

Colorado. COLORADO REV. STAT. sec. 12-36-136.
Uniform Determination of Death Act.

Connecticut. CONN. GEN. STAT. ANN. sec. 19-139(i).
- Two physicians must make brain death determination (total and irreversible cessation of all brain function) in accordance with usual and customary standards of medical practice.

169

- Time of death determined by two physicians using generally recognized and accepted scientific and clinical means.
- Physicians who certify brain death shall not participate in transplant procedures.

Delaware. There is no statutory or judicial law dealing with brain death.

District of Columbia. D.C. CODE ANN. sec. 6-2401.
Uniform Determination of Death Act.

Florida. FLA. STAT. ANN. sec. 382.085 (West).
- Brain death (irreversible cessation of all brain functions, including the brain stem) or may use other medically recognized standards.
- Two licensed physicians, one of whom shall be board eligible or board certified neurosurgeon, internist, pediatrician, surgeon, or anesthesiologist, must make the brain death determination.
- Next of kin of patient must be notified as soon as practical of the procedure to determine brain death and efforts to notify next of kin should be reflected in the medical record.

Georgia. GA. CODE ANN. sec. 31-10-16.
Uniform Determination of Death Act.

Hawaii. HAW. REV. STAT. sec. 327C-1.
- Both traditional means and the brain death standard (irreversible cessation of brain function). The director of health must convene in every odd-numbered year a committee to report to the legislature a review of medical practice, legal developments, and other appropriate matters to determine the continuing viability of the statute.
- Two licensed physicians must make the brain death determination.
- Death must be pronounced before artificial means of life support are withdrawn and before any vital organ is removed for transplantation.
- Time of death shall be when the irreversible cessation of brain function first occurred.
- Physicians who certify brain death shall not participate in transplant procedures or in the care of any recipient.

Idaho. IDAHO CODE sec. 54-1819.
Uniform Determination of Death Act.

Illinois. ILL. ANN. STAT. ch. 110 1/2 sec. 302(b).
Only brain death standard (irreversible cessation of total brain function) provided for.

Indiana. No brain death statute.
The Indiana Supreme Court in *Swafford v. State*, 421 N.E.2d 596 (Ind. 1981) adopted, for homicide cases, the Uniform Determination of Death Act, holding that death may be established by proof of the irreversible cessation of the victim's total brain functions.

Iowa. IOWA CODE ANN. sec. 702.8.
• Both traditional means and brain death (irreversible cessation of spontaneous brain functions) are included.
• Two physicians must make the brain death determination.
• Death occurs at the time when the relevant functions ceased.

Kansas. KAN. STAT. ANN. sec. 77-204 to 77-206.
Uniform Determination of Death Act.

Kentucky. There is no statutory or modern judicial law dealing with brain death.

Louisiana. LA. REV. STAT. ANN. sec. 9:111.
• Spontaneous cardiopulmonary loss or brain death (irreversible total cessation of brain function).
• A licensed physician must make the determination.
• Death occurs when the relevant functions ceased.
• An additional licensed physician who is not a member of the transplant team must make the pronouncement of death in transplant cases.

Maine. ME. REV. STAT. ANN. tit. 22, sec. 2811 to 2813.
Uniform Determination of Death Act.

Maryland. MD. HEALTH–GEN. CODE ANN. sec. 5-201 to 5-204.
Uniform Determination of Death Act.

Massachusetts. No brain death statute.
The Massachusetts Supreme Court in *Comm. v. Golston*, 373 Mass. 249, 366 N.E.2d 744 (1977), *cert. denied*, 434 U.S. 1039, 98 S.Ct. 777 (1978) recognized the validity of the brain death concept, rejecting the accused assailants' argument that brain death did not satisfy the essential element of murder that requires proof of death.

Michigan. MICH. STAT. ANN. sec. 14.15 (1021) to 14.15 (1023).
- Both the traditional and the brain death standard (irreversible cessation of spontaneous brain functions) are included.
- A physician must make the brain death determination.
- Death must be pronounced before artificial means of life support are removed.
- Death occurs at the time when the relevant functions ceased.

Minnesota. There is no statutory or judicial law dealing with brain death.

Mississippi. MISS. CODE ANN. sec. 41-36-1 to 41-36-3.
Uniform Determination of Death Act.

Missouri. MO. ANN. STAT. sec. 194.005.
Uniform Determination of Death Act.

Montana. MONT. CODE ANN. sec. 50-22-101.
Uniform Determination of Death Act.

Nebraska. There is no statutory recognition of brain death.
The state supreme court in *State v. Meints*, 212 Neb. 410, 322 N.W.2d 809 (1982) held that "proof of brain death is sufficient as proof of the victim's death in a homicide case."

Nevada. NEV. REV. STAT. sec. 451.007, as amended by Assembly B No. 8 (New Laws 1985).
Uniform Determination of Death Act.

New Hampshire. There is no statutory or judicial law concerning brain death.

New Jersey. There is no brain death statute.
In *State v. Watson*, 191 N.J. Super. 464, 467 A.2d 590 (1983) the court held that in homicide cases brain death was "death in fact."

New Mexico. N.M. STAT. ANN. sec. 12-2-4.
- Absence of cardiopulmonary function or brain death (absence of spontaneous brain function) either because of a known disease or condition or when further attempts to restore brain function seem futile.
- A physician must make the determination.
- Death must be pronounced before artificial life support is removed and before any vital organ is removed for transplantation.

New York. There is no brain death statute.
The judiciary has recognized the validity of brain death. *People v. Eulo, People v. Bonillo*, 472 N.E.2d 286, 63 N.Y.2d 341, 482 N.Y.S.2d 436 (NY 1984), *In re Jones*, 433 N.Y.S.2d 984 (Supreme Court, Onondaga County, 1980) and *New York City Health and Hospital Corp. v. Sulsona*, 367 N.Y.S. 2d 686 (1975).

North Carolina. N.C. GEN. STAT. sec. 90-323.
• Brain death (irreversible cessation of brain function) or other medically recognized criteria.
• A licensed physician must make the brain death determination.

North Dakota. There is no statutory or judicial law dealing with brain death.

Ohio. OHIO REV. CODE ANN. sec. 2108.30.
Uniform Determination of Death Act.

Oklahoma. OKLA. STAT. ANN. tit. 63, sec. 1-301(g).
• Statute provides for brain death standard (irreversible total cessation of brain functions) and inability to resuscitate.
• Death is to be pronounced before artificial life support is removed and before any vital organ is removed for transplantation.
• Death occurs when the cessation of spontaneous circulatory or respiratory functions and the cessation of brain functions first coincide.

Oregon. OR. REV. STAT. ch. 146, sec. 146.001.
• Irreversible cessation of spontaneous respiration and circulatory function or irreversible cessation of spontaneous brain function.
• A licensed physician must make the determination.

Pennsylvania. PA. STAT. ANN. tit. 35, sec. 10201 to 10203.
Uniform Determination of Death Act.

Rhode Island. R.I. GEN. LAWS ANN. sec. 23-4-16.
Uniform Determination of Death Act.

South Carolina. S.C. CODE ANN. sec. 44-43-450, 44-43-460.
Uniform Determination of Death Act.

South Dakota. There is no statutory or judicial law dealing with brain death.

Tennessee. TENN. CODE ANN. sec. 68-3-501.
Uniform Determination of Death Act.

Texas. TEX. REV. CIV. STAT. ANN. Art. 4447t.
- Cessation of spontaneous cardiopulmonary or brain function (irreversible cessation of all spontaneous brain functions).
- A physician must make the determination.
- Death must be pronounced before artificial life support is removed.
- Death occurs at the time when the relevant functions ceased.

Utah. There is no statutory or judicial law dealing with brain death.

Vermont. VT. STAT. ANN. tit. 18, sec. 5218.
Uniform Determination of Death Act.

Virginia. VA. CODE. sec. 54-3257.
- Both the absence of spontaneous cardiopulmonary or the absence of brain function are included.
- Two physicians, one of whom is a specialist in the field of neurology, neurosurgery, or electroencephalography, must make the determination.
- Death shall be pronounced by the attending physician when the cessation of spontaneous circulatory or respiratory functions and the cessation of brain functions first coincide.
- The attending physician must record and attest to the pronouncement of death in the patient's medical record.

Washington.
Uniform Determination of Death Act adopted in judicial decision of *In re Welfare of Bowman*, 94 Wash. 2d 407, 617 P.2d 731 (1980).

West Virginia. W. VA. CODE ANN. sec. 16-01-1 to 16-10-3.
Statute provides only for the brain death standard (irreversible cessation of all brain functions).

Wisconsin. WIS. STAT. ANN. sec. 146.71.
Uniform Determination of Death Act.

Wyoming. WYO. STAT. ANN. sec. 35-19-101 to 35-19-103.
Uniform Determination of Death Act.

Part IV
The Right To Know

Chapter 12

Paternalism

Gary R. Anderson, MSW, PhD

The word "paternalism" may be used quite casually, but for the purpose of understanding and acting on ethical issues it is important to appreciate the term and its existence in medical settings. This chapter describes paternalism and offers guidelines for making decisions and minimizing paternalism.

PATERNALISM DEFINED

Two major moral principles clash in health care: respect for the choices of the patient (autonomy) and the professional desire to do what is most beneficial for the patient (beneficence). Often autonomy and beneficence are compatible: the patient's choice of treatment or nontreatment corresponds to the advice and judgment of the physician, nurse, or hospital administrator. But at times the health care professional believes that he or she knows what is best for the patient and acts on this belief without the patient's consent. Deciding for the patient is called paternalism.

There are various definitions of paternalism:

- "Acting upon one's own idea of what is best for another person without consulting that other person."[1]
- ". . . to guide and even coerce people in order to protect them and serve their best interests, as a father might his children. He must keep them out of harm's way, by force if necessary."[2]
- "Interference with a person's freedom of action or freedom of information, or the dissemination of misinformation, or the overriding of a person's decision not to be given information, when this is allegedly done for the good of that person."[3]
- "Paternalism occurs whenever a person's opportunities for deciding or acting, or her decisions about the conditions under which she shall or shall not decide, are interfered with, allegedly for her own good."[4]

These definitions have several common elements. First, a situation requires some type of action or decision. Second, at least two actors are aware of the need for this action or decision—the person who will be most affected by the decision and to whom the decision seems to be posed, and the second person who is an onlooker. In health care decision making this onlooker could be a nurse, social worker, administrator, physician, or member of the patient's family. This onlooker has an idea defining the best course of action for the patient, a degree of interest and concern for the patient that motivates the onlooker to want to spare the patient pain and harm, and the ability to make this decision, provide direction, or even override the patient's choice with respect to the decision.

> A patient is admitted to the hospital after an automobile accident. Her husband, the passenger in the car she was driving, was killed in the accident. The patient is beginning to recover from her extensive injuries but no one is sure how she would tolerate the news of her husband's death. One nurse believed it was unethical to withhold this information from the patient. The nurse noted that the patient had the right to know and was inquiring concerning her husband. Other nurses felt that this information would result in tremendous guilt and consequent regression in the patient's recovery.
>
> Susan's mother expressed her willingness to be a donor, but the medical team had reason to believe she did not really want to give Susan a kidney. The team noted that while the mother was being worked up she developed gastrointestinal problems and heart palpitations. As soon as she was told that she would not be the donor for her daughter, the mother's problems improved. Neither the mother nor the daughter was informed that the mother was turned down for psychological reasons. The medical team told the mother she could not be a donor because there was not a good tissue match with her daughter.[5]

These two cases illustrate five criteria that can be used to help health care professionals, and others, to determine whether a particular action is paternalistic:

1. In each case, the patient or family member thought *she knew what was best for herself*—in the first case the patient wanted to know about her husband; in the second case Susan's mother wanted to donate an organ.
2. The health care professionals *believed that they were justified* or had the right to act on the patient's behalf, whether or not the patient had given or ever would consent to such actions.
3. The health care professionals' actions involved *violating a moral rule*: in both cases there was deception, and in the second case the professionals clearly lied to the mother.

4. The health care professionals *believed that they were qualified* to act on the patient's and on the mother's behalf.
5. The health care professionals believed that their actions were *for the patient's and the mother's good* and benefit.[6]

This fifth criterion, the very well-intentioned aspect of paternalism, makes it both tempting and popular to health care professionals. In fact, imbedded in many other ethical dilemmas are paternalistic attitudes and actions. For example, sharing confidential information is done "for the good" of the person; medical treatment or hospital care decisions are made by experts without informing or involving the patient or the patient's family because the health care professionals "know" what is "best" for the patient. Consequently, an understanding of paternalism is crucial to recognizing and understanding a number of troubling ethical dilemmas.

REASONS FOR PATERNALISM IN HEALTH CARE

The nature and characteristics of patients, the identities and responsibilities of decision makers, the health care setting itself, and the type and intensity of decisions made by patients, families, and health care professionals all contribute to the paternalistic quality of health care.

Patient Competency

Certain characteristics of patients make them more vulnerable to paternalistic decision making and actions. These characteristics—age, cognitive ability, and "patient role"—question the patient's ability to make independent decisions.

In cases involving children or the elderly, concerned persons such as family members or health care professionals are more inclined to step in and assist in decision making. This tendency is particularly sanctioned with children. A father or mother is expected to guide a child's decisions and actions for the child's best interests and health.

People also act on behalf of someone else when they perceive that the person does not have the cognitive ability to make competent judgments. Competency requires the ability to understand the nature, extent, and severity of an illness, the rationale for recommended tests and medical procedures and the consequences of treatment alternatives and one's choices and actions.

Questions of patient competency are almost immediately raised by health care professionals when a patient chooses a course of action that may be harmful or deadly to the patient.

A 26-year-old man, horribly burned and blinded and battling almost overwhelming infection daily, requested discharge to his home, where he could not receive the daily Hubbard tank baths he needed to control infection. A psychiatrist was called to interview the patient. Prior to the interview he was given the impression that the patient was "irrationally depressed and probably needed to be declared mentally incompetent so that a legal guardian could be appointed to give the necessary permissions. . . ."[7]

A 75-year-old man, finding it difficult to wean from a respirator and tiring of frequent painful medical procedures, refused to cooperate with hospital personnel: "Although he had become less communicative, he remained alert and aware and in the opinion of the staff was fully competent. . . . 'I want to die,' he said."[8]

A 66-year-old man, acutely ill, refused all diagnostic procedures; a psychiatrist who evaluated the patient concluded that although he was obviously ill and had a degree of mental impairment manifested by poor memory, he was not mentally incompetent.[9]

In each case the patient refused recommended medical treatment. Health professionals interpreted this resistance as unreasonable and as evidence of cognitive dysfunction. In each case, upon more careful evaluation, the patients' competency was affirmed and, consequently, the patients' choices could not be disregarded.

The "patient role" or "sick role" is shaped by the expectations of how a hospital patient should act. These expectations include dependency, compliance with hospital rules and regulations, passive acceptance of decisions that are made for the patient by physicians or nurses, and abandonment of normal role responsibilities. As a result of these expectations, the patient who attempts to exert authority will be perceived negatively. In addition, a patient is involved in a special relationship with caregivers, whose own role definitions may promote the tendency to take paternalistic actions.[10]

Health Care Decision Makers

One of paternalism's primary qualities is that the person who is making choices or taking actions on behalf of another is motivated by good intentions: the best interests of the patient. It is perhaps this service quality that makes health care settings particularly paternalistic, as most health care professionals assume they are concerned about the best interests, health, and well-being of their patients.

This concern and service mentality is evident in professional hospital administration ethics codes: "Recognize that the care of the ill and injured is a prime responsibility and at all times strive to provide to all in need of health services quality care consistent with available resources."[11]

This commitment for physicians, like other professionals, is affirmed in the professional literature:

The doctor, by teaching and technique, through patient understanding and astute judgment, promotes the patient's good. . . . I do believe consideration of the condition of the individual patient's health, activity, and state of mind must enter these decisions if the decision is indeed to be for the patient's good. . . . The concern of the physician is the welfare of his patient.[12]

In addition to this strong and basic commitment to the good of the patient, providing the motivation for paternalism, there is also the authority of those providing services to the patient—providing the power and rationale for paternalistic acts. Describing the potentially curative powers of patient belief in "the power of the physician," one writer notes:

Since the client has no verifiable standard of evaluating either his doctor or his service, and since he must surrender his initiative and place himself entirely in the hands of the physician, the doctor will quite reasonably insist that the patient give him full 'confidence.'[13] In broad social relations and responsibilities as well as functionally specific technical competence the profession [medical practice] is blessed with a unique validation of its authority by the public.[14]

This combination of good will and authority possessed by hospital management, physicians, social workers, nurses, and other health care professionals provides the prerequisite conditions for paternalistic behavior.

Hospital Settings and Medical Decisions

The hospital setting is often characterized by processes and procedures that take away from individual identity and autonomy of patients. For example, visiting hours are restricted, mobility may be restricted, clothing and diet and personal care items may be limited or controlled by someone other than the patient, the ordering of one's schedule and day are in the hands of other people, and one's temperature and bathroom behavior may be objects of daily concern to others. Health care is organized to communicate that the patient is no longer in control of his or her own affairs.

Health care settings are also governed by legal and regulatory guidelines that limit the autonomy and control of the institution. Reimbursement and payment schemes shape hospitalization length, which may then affect discharge decision making. Sensitivity to medical malpractice litigation may prompt defensive decision making by health care professionals and institutions.

Finally, the types of decisions made in health care provoke the concern and the opinion of not only health care administrators and treatment providers but also the family and friends of the patient. If the only decisions were ones of menu, dress, or schedule, respecting the free and independent choice of the patient might come easily. However, when decisions include invasive and painful treatments and life-and-death alternatives it is more difficult, and perhaps inadvisable, to allow and accept the free choice of the patient.

JUSTIFICATIONS FOR PATERNALISM

There are two extreme views concerning paternalism. One readily excuses or allows making decisions for another person. The other supports total autonomy and self-determination. Most people would be slow to disregard self-determination, if for no other reason than they would want their own autonomy respected. Consequently, overriding self-determination requires justification. However, total freedom of choice in any situation is rarely advocated.

Protection against Harm

The primary philosopher who advanced autonomy and criticized paternalism, John Stuart Mill, allowed one reason for paternalistic actions:

> The sole end for which mankind are warranted, individually or collectively, in interfering with the liberty of action of any other of their number is *self protection*. That the only purpose for which power can be rightfully exercised over any member of a civilized community, against his will, is to *prevent harm to others*. . . .[15]

Consequently, if someone's decisions or actions were going to hurt someone else, choosing for that person or kindly thwarting the action was justified. For example, if a child needs a blood transfusion to live and the child's parents refuse to consent to such a transfusion for religious reasons, hospital and judicial personnel would typically order the transfusions over the objections of the parents for the good of the child.[16]

This principle of protection has been extended to include preventing self-harm, such as suicide. People who have made serious attempts to hurt themselves might find themselves hospitalized for supervisory purposes for their own good: to prevent suicide. Patients requiring some type of life-sustaining medical treatment might be given this treatment even over their own objections, for their own good: to preserve life. Prevention of harm is extended to nonlife-threatening situations. Buchanan describes a simple "prevention of harm argument" in three steps: (a) the physician's duty is to prevent harm; (b) giving the patient information X will do great harm to him or her; (c) therefore it is permissible for the physician to withhold this information from the patient.[17]

A similar justification for paternalism is that a person should not have the freedom to remove irretrievably the ability to be free. So, although paternalistic, it would be defensible to prevent people from selling themselves into slavery. There will probably be limited disagreement as to the justifiability of preventing harm to others, but preventing self-harm raises numerous and complex issues of a person's right to refuse treatment and a person's right to die. In fact, to describe refusal of treatment and choice to die as "rights" implies that they must be respected and their violation is a serious matter.

Special Populations and Implied Consent

Few people would question a parent's right to make decisions for his or her child based on the parent's perceptions of the best interests of the child. A parent would be expected to prevent a young child from jumping into deep and dangerous water; in fact, a parent's failure to act on behalf of a child is labeled "neglect."

One explanation of a parent's right to make decisions for the good of the child is "implied consent."[18] Implied, or future, consent means that when the child is older, and reflecting on the actions of the parent, the child would agree that the parent made a proper decision and would be grateful that the parent did not allow a harmful decision or action. Implied consent has been extended to adults. For example, it justifies treating a severe burn patient upon admission, even over protest by the patient, by arguing that treatment will allow the patient to make choices in the future. Also, when the patient is calm and reflects on the professionals' decision he or she would appreciate its merits.

Sissela Bok, in her discussion of paternalistic lies, notes that adults seem to be particularly inclined to lie to children to (a) shield the child from bad news; (b) present encouragement rather than an objective evaluation (for example, complimenting the child's first piano performance despite numerous missed notes); and (c) translate the truth to provoke a desired or appropriate response, such as telling a child that a required medicine "tastes good."[19] One might reasonably suggest that these paternalistic translations of the truth for the good of the subject are not limited to child subjects. For example, it has been observed that if a doctor is "optimistically biased" it ought to help a speedy recovery![20]

Paternalism is also justified in cases involving incompetent patients. Incompetence, or insanity or impaired mental capacity, implies that the patient does not understand what is in his or her best interests and another person must choose a course of action to protect the incompetent person from the consequences of an ill-formed or ill-understood decision.[21] Paternalistic actions are also excused if the patient is described as "irrational"—the patient is making a choice that a fully rational person would recognize as imprudent, harmful, and wrong. Because of the cognitive limits of incompetence and irrationality, not only *can* someone else make decisions for the patient but someone else *should*. Finally, some might argue that because of cognitive impairment, the incompetent or severely mentally retarded have no right to the truth as they have no "true liberty.'' This leads to a logical difficulty: if people have no liberty, it is not possible to abridge that liberty, and therefore it is not paternalistic to choose for them; in fact it is not possible to be paternalistic.

Influencing Circumstances

Aside from incompetency, it has been argued that paternalism is justified in cases where a patient's "harmful" choices were not the patient's true choices. The choice is disregarded because the medical professional perceives that it was:

1. not voluntary, but the result of some form of pressure or coercion;
2. not sincere, because it resulted from a temporary depression or disturbance, that clouded the patient's good judgment;
3. distorted by the effects of medication;
4. not truly a decision, but more accurately interpreted as a cry for help, control over one's life, or independence; or
5. ill-informed, so the patient didn't fully know the ramifications of a course of action.

Beneficence

A broader and more inclusive justification for paternalism is the principle of beneficence: the desire and the duty to do what is good for someone else. One of the schools of thought in philosophy—utilitarianism—argues that moral choices are made by weighing the consequences of alternate courses of action and then choosing that action that will optimize the happiness and well-being of those affected by the decision.[22] So, the primary consideration is the outcome of a decision—if it is most beneficial it is morally right. To justify paternalistic behaviors, the harm prevented by violating a person's autonomy must be greater than the harm that would have been caused by not violating the patient's rights.

This type of moral reasoning, appealing to beneficence, allows and promotes paternalistic actions by medical professionals; "a purely utilitarian model would justify most paternalistic acts."[23] Questioning health care's "new ethic's preoccupation with rights," two editorialists asserted, "medical interventions, including the sharing of information, are justified by physicians' knowledgeable determination of what will best minimize suffering and enhance health for their patients."[24]

Thus, paternalistic actions have a number of justifications: protecting the patient and others from harm, intervening to protect and guide those who because of age or cognitive handicap cannot make reasonable choices, overriding what is not the true choice or wish of the patient, and promoting what is best for all concerned. These choices are expected to be consistent with what the patient would choose if the patient were fully rational, in sound mind, or able to reflect back on the course of action chosen on his or her behalf. This reflection would be tinged with gratitude that someone else stepped in and did what was in the best interests of the patient.

In addition to philosophical defenses of paternalism, there are regulatory and legal considerations that shape a health care administrator's and medical person's response to patient decision making. In fact, the emphasis on patient rights and self-determination that were predominant in the past several decades must now be weighed against recent governmental and judicial interventions.

One such case involved a pregnant, competent adult Jehovah's Witness who ordered physicians not to give her blood even though she had a condition in which the placenta was improperly attached to the uterine wall and posed a danger of hemorrhage. Shortly after her baby was born, the woman began to hemorrhage. Her physicians had not ordered blood as they were respecting her order to not transfuse. As the woman became gravely ill the physicians asked for legal advice and were told to give the needed transfusions. There was an insufficient number of units of blood available; complications about ordered blood resulted in no more units than the two on hand. Administered too slowly, the woman died. Her husband, also a Jehovah's Witness, was awarded $1.25 million dollars by a New York State Supreme Court in 1984.[25]

Governmental intervention, on behalf of paternalistic decision making, is most clearly evident in the recent cases involving neonatal care for handicapped and ill newborns. Baby Doe regulations and the resulting case of Baby Jane Doe illustrate governmental efforts to supersede the parents' rights to determine the course of treatment for their child.[26] Establishing institutional infant care review committees, constructing a system for reporting cases of discrimination to child protective agencies, and challenging the hospital's, physician's, and parents' decisions in court impose another "voice" that says it speaks on behalf of the best interests of another person.

While ruling on the withdrawal of treatment in the case of Claire Conroy, the New Jersey State Supreme Court discussed patient autonomy. The competent patient's right to choose treatment was based on rights of bodily integrity, informed consent, and the constitutional right to privacy. However, the court stated that these personal rights are not absolute as they are limited by the interests of the state. Four commonly identified state interests were noted: (a) an interest in preserving life/the sanctity of life—"which usually gives way to the personal rights in cases involving competent patients"; (b) preventing suicide; (c) safeguarding the "integrity of the medical profession"; and (d) protecting innocent third parties.[27]

Consequently, administrators, physicians, nurses, or other health care professionals must confront the dynamic of paternalism not only in their own values and relationships with patients, but also in the legal, political, and economic environment in which health care is delivered.

THE LIMITS OF PATERNALISM

The basic argument against paternalism is that it is a violation of a human right: the right to autonomy and self-determination. Autonomy is in conflict with beneficence:

Many philosophers have insisted that the concept of a person as an autonomous agent must have a central and independent role in ethical theory . . . it provides a warrant for treating a person's own choices, plans and conception of self as generally dominant over what another believes to be in that person's best interests.[28]

In the end, individuals, when able, must be allowed to decide their own destiny, even that of death. When the patient decides that the future quality of life open to him is not worth the investment of pain and suffering to attain that future quality of life, that is a decision proper to the patient.[29]

Although few would argue in favor of total freedom to act as one chooses regardless of the harm done to others, violating the independence of another person is normally objectionable. It is generally accepted that people should be free to act as they choose unless they are not capable of acting in a voluntary or rational manner, as long as they are not harming others.

The previously cited justifications for paternalistic actions are brought into question:

- Although "harm" is a justification for paternalism, is it possible to define, measure, or predict harm precisely?
- How does one define "competence," "rationality," and "sanity" if these are criteria for choosing for another?
- With regard to implied or future consent, is it possible to assume future agreement or gratitude for actions taken on another's behalf?
- What degree of interference will be tolerated, and for how long?

Another question that provides some guidance for moral decision making is this: Are you willing to have your rationale and action generalized, to become law, for all cases? This is a version of the classic "golden rule": do unto others as you would have them do unto you. A 1960s study illustrates this principle: a study on what doctors tell cancer patients found a strong tendency to withhold information from cancer patients. In fact, 90 percent of the respondents indicated that they tend not to tell their patients the diagnosis of cancer. Reasons for not telling patients were paternalistic—the primary physician goal was to maintain hope. Withholding information was justified by saying it helped the patient have an optimistic outlook, however, withholding was found more accurately to reflect the physician's desire to deny the illness. However, responding physicians indicated they would not want information withheld from them if they were in the patient's position![30]

The defined motivation for paternalistic actions is that health care professionals are deeply and sincerely concerned about the patient's health and well-being. It is possible to question the purity of the paternalist's concern. Is this person solely concerned with and committed to the best interests of the patient, or is this commitment polluted with concerns for the self-interests of the health care professional or the interests of the health care institution? Is it simply easier to make the decision for the patient? One negative motive and result of paternalism is arrogance and disrespect for the patient as a person. One author described this as "professional narcissism."[31] Protection against the dangers of callousness, indifference, neglect, and unwarranted intrusion requires hospital personnel to assess the patient's condition from the patient's point of view.

Questions about the validity and strength of justifications of paternalism highlight the difficulty in decision making. This difficulty is particularly pronounced in health care when the issues are potentially as serious and as irreversible as life and death. Despite contradiction, uncertainty, and lack of precision, in this exploration concerning the proper place of paternalism some principles to guide the health care decision maker can be identified.

GUIDELINES FOR DECISION MAKING

The following guidelines are offered as a means of reconciling one's commitment to respect for the autonomy of patients with a professional purpose of healing and service.

As a general rule, there should be respect for the autonomy and self-determination of patients if the following conditions can be met:

First, the patient should have *adequate information* to make a decision. This does not mean perfect knowledge, but sufficient information to make a reasoned judgment about the alternatives available, the seriousness of risks, and the probability of various risky outcomes. The goal is an informed patient. For example, a 66-year-old man refused all diagnostic procedures to determine the cause of his acute illness; his physician spent two 45-minute sessions at his bedside and clearly explained the reasons for the procedures. The physician reported that, based on the patient's statements, the patient understood the gravity of his situation. Diagnostic procedures were not performed.

Second, related to being informed, the patient should *understand the consequences* of a chosen course of action. The abilities to anticipate and correctly weight consequences are aspects of rationality and competence in thinking. This second criterion for respecting patient autonomy is based on an assessment of the cognitive functioning of the patient. Questions of competence should be addressed by those professionals trained and designated to make this determination. Typically a competency decision would be made by a judge as incompetence would require appointing a guardian to act on behalf of the incapacitated patient. Decisions of competence typically involve psychiatric evaluation. To assume that all mentally retarded or mentally ill patients are incompetent is incorrect. For nonqualified health care professionals to make speedy judgments about the competency of patients is to open the door to an unjustified intrusion and denial of the rights of the patient to make decisions. In cases where the patient is accurately diagnosed as incompetent and a guardian has been appointed, it is the guardian's right to be informed about decisions and potential consequences.

Third, a patient's decision should be *voluntary* and not the result of undue sociological or psychological pressure. A guideline for assessing the sincerity and validity of a choice is to ask whether this decision is in accordance with the patient's preferences, desires, and personality. This is why cases involving Jehovah's Witnesses are such tests of respect for autonomy, because it can be demonstrated that the request not to receive a blood transfusion is very consistent with one's religious tenets and voluntary choice. Other examples of threats to sincerity have been mentioned, such as the effect of medication or a temporary acute psychological depression. To determine the voluntary nature of the decision a careful assessment of the patient and the patient's environment is necessary.

Fourth, a patient's choice *should not cause harm to another person*. On the surface this seems simple enough, but "harm" is not easy to assess. Again to use the case of the Jehovah's Witnesses: when the parent requesting no blood transfusion has minor children dependent on that parent for care, a judge has typically ordered a transfusion because of the economic if not psychological harm that would ensue if the parent died. A patient's choice to forgo life-sustaining treatment might be judged rational given the nature of an illness and the pain experienced while being treated, but is there a sense of "professional harm" for the health care professionals who don't believe in assisting a suicide?

These four criteria—informed choice, understanding the consequences (competence), voluntariness, and not harming others—may provide some guidance for health care providers responsible for the medical care and the medical setting in which a patient is treated. To assess these criteria fully it might be necessary to delay agreeing to a patient's choice, particularly if the decision would produce an irreversible change. This enforced waiting period would allow for an assessment of the patient's knowledge and understanding of the issues involved and provide an opportunity for any depression or nonvoluntary pressure to be identified and addressed.

So far this discussion has addressed the relationship of the patient to the medical care staff and the institutional staff. Another relationship to consider is the patient in the context of his or her family. Family members influence and shape the nature of the dilemma in a number of ways. They may be applying pressure to the patient. For example, one patient chose to forgo life-saving treatment, and it was determined that his motivation, rather than free choice, was a response to what he perceived to be neglect by his family. Family members may also serve as translators, assisting medical staff in communicating with a patient. This help in communication is very necessary if conditions of informed consent are going to be met and if an accurate assessment of knowledge of consequences is going to be made. This is especially necessary when the need for a translator is literal: when the patient speaks a different language or is from a different culture than the health care decision makers. There are two extremes to avoid: (a) speaking only with family members, treating them as the decision makers because they are pursuing the physician, or easier to talk to than the sick patient; (b) considering the patient an isolated individual. Although a family member's rights may not supersede the patient's right to autonomy, this risks a distorted and potentially harmful assessment of the patient.

MINIMIZING PATERNALISM

Respect for the patient's autonomy and right to make decisions concerning his or her treatment is a central ethical principle. Despite this primacy, these rights are not absolute—there are reasonable justifications for overriding autonomy and necessary conditions that should be considered in each case. However, exceptions do not negate the general principle. Health care professionals should work to prevent and minimize paternalistic decision making.

A variety of steps reduce the risk of paternalistic behavior. For instance,

- Careful communication with the patient and the patient's family increases the likelihood that the health care professional will know the patient's wishes and the reasons for patient requests and understand the patient's life circumstances. Dialogue between providers and patients will increase the patient's trust in the health care professional and increase the likelihood that decisions will be collaborative and respectful of the patient's desires. Consequently, health care professionals should be trained in communication with patients, and those skilled in interviewing, such as social workers and clergy, might be involved with the patient and family.

- Informed consent procedures should be carefully followed. Permissions and explanations should not be so hurried or truncated that informed consent is limited.

- Justifications for withholding information from patients, distorting information, or overriding expressed patient wishes should be identified and carefully scrutinized for their reasonableness, validity, and importance. Decisions about patient competency should be made by qualified professionals (generally psychiatric consultants).

Respect for patient rights and choices is compromised in numerous small incidents, not only in life-saving decisions. It is doubtful that any plan of action or set of procedures alone can suppress paternalism. A crucial ingredient is hospital administrators whose attitudes and actions set a moral tone for an institution. Their sensitivity to patients and patients' families, as well as to the health care professionals employed in the institution, affects the quality of care and decision making. As health care administrators, by example and instruction, provide moral as well as fiscal or administrative leadership, they should attempt to minimize paternalistic actions and attitudes. This leadership will communicate respect for patients' rights and will contribute to an environment appreciated by the hospital's service population.

NOTES

1. Ann Marchewka, "When is Paternalism Justifiable?" *American Journal of Nursing* 83, no. 7 (July 1983):1072.

2. Sissela Bok, *Lying: Moral Choice in Public and Private Life* (New York: Vintage Books, 1979), 215.

3. Allen E. Buchanan, "Medical Paternalism," in *Paternalism*, ed. Rolf Satorious (Minneapolis: University of Minnesota Press, 1984), 62.

4. Ibid., 62.

5. Bok, *Lying*, 222.

6. Bernard Gert and Charles M. Culver, "The Justification of Paternalism," *Ethics* 89 (January 1979):199–210.

7. Case Studies in Bioethics, "A Demand to Die," *The Hastings Center Report* 5, no. 3 (June 1975):9,10.

8. Case Studies, "Family Wishes and Patient Autonomy," *The Hastings Center Report* 10, no. 5 (October 1980):21,22.

9. Mark Siegler, "Critical Illness: The Limits of Autonomy," *The Hastings Center Report* 7, no. 5 (October 1977):12–15.

10. Edwin J. Thomas, "Problems of Disability from the Perspective of Role Theory," in *Families in Crisis*, ed. Paul Glasser and Lois Glasser (New York: Harper and Row, 1970).

11. American College of Healthcare Executives, *Code of Ethics*, February 1986.

12. Leon R. Kass, "Ethical Dilemmas in the Care of the Ill: What Is the Patient's Good?" *Journal of the American Medical Association* 244, no. 17 (October 24/31, 1980):1946–1949.

13. Wayne G. Menke, "Professional Values in Medical Practice," *The New England Journal of Medicine* 280, no. 17 (April 24, 1969):930–936.

14. Ibid., 936.

15. Gerald Dworkin, "Paternalism," in *Paternalism*, ed. Rolf Satorius (Minneapolis: University of Minnesota Press, 1983), 19–34.

16. Gary R. Anderson, "Medicine vs. Religion: The Case of Jehovah's Witnesses," *Health and Social Work* 8, no. 1 (Winter 1983):31–39.

17. Buchanan, "Medical Paternalism," 76.

18. Bok, *Lying*, 226.

19. Ibid., 216–220.

20. Menke, "Professional Values," 972.

21. For a discussion of legal criteria for competency see: Gary Hawk and Elissa P. Benedek, "The Forensic Evaluation in the Criminal Justice System," Chapter 27 in *Psychiatry* Vol. 3, ed. Kaplan and Sadock (Philadelphia: J.B. Lippincott Co., 1985), 4–6.

22. Fred Feldman, *Introductory Ethics* (Englewood Cliffs, N.J.: Prentice-Hall, 1978).

23. Marchewka, "Justifiable," 1073.

24. Roger Sider and Colleen Clements, "The New Medical Ethics: A Second Opinion," *Archives of Internal Medicine* 145, no. 12 (December 1985):2169–2171.

25. "A Verdict Against Doctors in a Jehovah's Witness Case," *The Hastings Center Report* 14, no. 3 (June 1984):2,3.

26. George J. Annas, "The Baby Doe Regulations: Governmental Intervention in Neonatal Rescue Medicine," *American Journal of Public Health* 74, no. 6 (June 1984):618–620.

27. Mary L. Ahern, "New Jersey Supreme Court Outlines Standards for Treatment Withdrawal," *Health Law Vigil* 8, no. 4 (February 22, 1985):4–6.

28. Bruce L. Miller, "Autonomy and the Refusal of Lifesaving Treatment," *The Hastings Center Report* 11, no. 4 (August 1981):22–28.

29. H. Tristram Engelhardt, Jr., "Case Studies in Bioethics: A Demand to Die," *The Hastings Center Report* 5, no. 3 (June 1975):10.

30. Donald Oken, "What to Tell Cancer Patients: A Study of Medical Attitudes," in *Ethical Issues in Death and Dying*, ed. Robert F. Weir (New York: Columbia University Press, 1977), 9–25.

31. Bok, *Lying*, 240.

BIBLIOGRAPHY

Beauchamp, Tom, and Pinkard, Terry, eds. *Ethics and Public Policy: An Introduction to Ethics.* Englewood Cliffs, N.J.: Prentice-Hall, 1983.

Satorius, Rolf, ed. *Paternalism.* Minneapolis: University of Minnesota Press, 1983.

Chapter 13

A Practical Approach to the Doctrine of Informed Consent

J. Phillip O'Brien, JD, Michael R. Callahan, JD,
and Jamie A. Savaiano, JD

INTRODUCTION

The doctrine of informed consent evolved from the simple notion that a person must give permission before a health care practitioner renders treatment.[1] Consent can be granted in many ways, the simplest of which is "implied" consent. For example, if a person voluntarily offers an arm to a physician who is administering a vaccine, the person can be presumed to have given consent to receive a vaccine. However, this simple requirement of consent to medical treatment becomes more complicated: such consent might not be valid if the person in reality expected to have his or her blood pressure taken. Thus, the requirement for consent is further complicated by the notion that such consent must be informed.

Perhaps the most complex issue in informed consent is the sufficiency of the information provided to the patient before consent is given. The legal community disagrees on the appropriate standard to judge whether or not the information furnished to the patient was sufficient to allow the patient to make an informed decision.[2]

In addition, with the growing complexity of the health care industry, determining who should be responsible for obtaining consent has also become more complicated. It is unclear whether a hospital and the hospital personnel who admit the patients, prepare them for treatment, and obtain signed consent forms indicating consent to treatment have a responsibility to ensure that the patients understand the nature of the treatment involved.[3]

Finally, there is the issue of documentation and the role it plays in the informed consent process. The drafting and use of consent forms must be given particular attention.

All of these aspects are important to the final determination of whether or not the defendant in a lawsuit met the duty to obtain such consent and, if not, whether he should be held liable for the plaintiff's damages suffered as a result of the lack of informed consent.

With regard to hospitals in particular, the informed consent issue may not seem one of primary concern because the duty has generally been placed directly on the treating physician. Nevertheless, some legal responsibility has been placed on the hospital in a number of jurisdictions, and it is likely that this trend will continue. Moreover, many hospitals have taken on the responsibility of drafting consent forms and making them available to the medical staff. In addition, some hospitals have imposed a requirement that such forms be signed prior to treatment and have required hospital personnel to make sure that the forms are signed. These actions may impose some duty on the hospital to ensure that informed consent is obtained.

Furthermore, a hospital can be held liable for failing to properly supervise its employees or independent physicians, especially where the hospital had reason to be aware of the practitioner's failure to obtain informed consent. Finally, some courts have even suggested that hospitals may have a direct duty to patients to ensure that they are not treated unless they have given their informed consent. In any event, hospitals should be aware of the indirect informed consent requirements and potential duties imposed upon hospitals and on treating practitioners to understand their duties under this doctrine.

RATIONALE—WHY INFORMED CONSENT?

In simple terms, the legal doctrine of informed consent emanates from the recognized right of every competent adult person to decide what will be done to his or her own body. As stated by one commentator: "To deprive a person of the right to make decisions regarding his or her own medical care is to treat that human being as an object, not as a person."[4] Therefore, the law has long recognized that an individual's right to self-determination or autonomy, when it comes to medical care, must be protected.[5] To protect this right, the law has required that medical practitioners obtain the oral or written consent of any person upon whom they intend to perform most types of medical treatment.

In order to obtain such consent, the practitioner must first disclose sufficient information regarding the nature of the person's illness, the details of the procedure, the potential risks and benefits of the procedure, the alternatives available, if any, and the risks and benefits of the alternatives. When this information is disclosed, a person can make an informed choice regarding the recommended procedure and therefore maintain control over his or her own destiny.

Research has revealed that additional benefits to obtaining informed consent, other than protecting the individual's right to self-determination, further support the existence and continuation of the doctrine.[6] For example, informed consent can benefit the overall physical and psychological well-being of the patient while enhancing the physician's decision-making process. Studies also have shown that information disclosure prior to treatment can improve a patient's ability to recover from a procedure.[7]

Furthermore, the requirement for disclosure can act as a check against unnecessary or inappropriate procedures. In some instances a physician may recommend a minimally beneficial procedure because of the financial rewards to the physician. An informed patient may reject this recommended but unnecessary procedure because the benefits do not outweigh the risks involved.[8] Finally, the informed consent process can enhance the quality of a physician's decision making by forcing the physician to consider alternatives and innovative treatment he or she might otherwise have ignored.[9]

In summary, the rationale behind the informed consent doctrine is more than the traditional notion of individual autonomy; justification extends to recognizable benefits that result from a more knowledgeable and educated patient population.

HISTORICAL DEVELOPMENT

Traditional Approach—Assault and Battery

The common law concept of assault and battery was the legal theory upon which the doctrine of informed consent was first based. The touching of another without his or her express consent is a battery, whereas placing a person in fear of being touched is an assault.[10]

Following this theory, a series of cases in the early 1900s established a civil cause of action for battery where a physician performed a procedure without the patient's consent.[11] To establish a claim for battery, it is necessary to prove that a physician performed a particular procedure without the patient's consent. The plaintiff need not prove that actual harm resulted from the failure of the physician to obtain consent. Consent actions on the basis of assault or battery have been successful where treatment was more extensive[12] or was performed on a different part of the patient's body than the patient authorized.[13]

As the informed consent doctrine evolved, the case law began to focus on the quality of consent rather than the unauthorized contact or nature of the treatment. Patients sued physicians alleging lack of consent when permission was in fact given but without a true understanding of the procedure to be performed. The assault and battery theory of consent was not an adequate basis for a claim where the patient consented on the basis of inadequate information, because there was no unauthorized touching. Some courts attempted to reason that lack of sufficient information to support the consent invalidated the consent, resulting in a battery.[14] However, this approach generally has been abandoned in favor of a negligence theory.

Modern Approach—Negligence Theory

The negligence theory of informed consent is based on a practitioner's breach of his or her duty to disclose relevant information regarding the nature of a patient's illness and the risks, alternatives, and benefits of the procedure recommended. Most states recognize the negligence theory of informed consent either by case law or by statute.[15]

Under the negligence theory, a physician can be held liable for failing to obtain informed consent even when express consent is given by the patient for the procedure. The basic criteria necessary to prove lack of informed consent under the negligence theory are that:

1. A patient-physician relationship existed.
2. The provider had a duty to disclose relevant information.
3. The provider failed to provide this information and the failure cannot be excused.
4. If the provider had furnished the patient with the undisclosed information, the patient would not have consented to treatment.
5. The plaintiff's injury and damages claimed were a reasonably foreseeable consequence of the inadequate information, i.e., the proximate cause.[16]

DOCTRINE OF INFORMED CONSENT

Who Has the Duty?

The negligence theory of informed consent evolved from the fiduciary relationship between the patient and the health care provider that gives rise to the duty to disclose adequate information. A treatment relationship must exist before the duty to disclose arises. Consequently, it is the duty of the person who is to perform a diagnostic, surgical, or medical intervention to obtain a patient's authorization for treatment.[17]

However, the treating physician is not always the physician who originally diagnosed or recommended the particular treatment in question and often delegates the responsibility to obtain informed consent to other health care personnel. These deviations from the traditional physician-patient relationship create more complex problems regarding compliance with the informed consent doctrine.

Another important issue regarding the informed consent duty is the potential liability of health care facilities when a physician or other practitioner fails to obtain informed consent or when the hospital has taken on the duty to ensure that informed consent is obtained.

Delegation of Responsibility

The doctrine of informed consent imposes the duty on the treating physician to disclose adequate information to the patient before treating the patient. Thus, the treating physician cannot relieve himself from liability by delegating the function of actually obtaining informed consent to another health care professional.[18] The case law and statutory law are unclear, however, with respect to whether a treating physician can satisfy that duty by delegating the act of obtaining informed consent to another person as long as he or she follows up with the patient to resolve any questions prior to the procedure in question.[19] If the case law or statutes do not expressly preclude delegation of the act of obtaining informed consent, it is likely that delegation is permissible as long as informed consent is obtained. Some commentators have suggested that it may be in the patient's best interest if the duty is delegated to persons who are specifically trained in communicating this type of information and who have the time and interest to do so.[20] Other commentators have argued vehemently against a physician delegating this important responsibility.[21] A Michigan study found that 22.1 percent of the hospitals studied used nurses to obtain informed consent, 31.8 percent used physicians other than the treating physician, and only 36.3 percent required the treating physician to obtain consent.[22]

There may be some room for compromise in jurisdictions where case law or statutory law does not prohibit delegation of the informed consent duty. The initial responsibility for disclosing necessary information can be delegated to a health care professional trained in communication skills and possessing a workable knowledge of the medical concepts involved. It still is the treating physician's duty to review the information with the patient, ascertain the patient's knowledge regarding the procedure and its alternatives, and inquire whether the patient has any remaining questions or concerns before the patient finally signs the consent form. However, the use of a trained professional can decrease the time a treating physician would be required to spend with the patient and increase the patient's understanding of the information.

In any case, the treating physician should realize that delegation of the act of obtaining consent is a risk that the physician will bear in the event that the informed consent process is challenged and found lacking. Therefore, even if the treating physician delegates the responsibility for disclosing the relevant information, it is essential that the physician makes sure that any consent given is fully informed and voluntary. A hospital should be put on notice that if the person to whom the task of obtaining consent has been delegated is a hospital employee, the hospital takes on a direct duty to the patient. Therefore, the hospital should give careful consideration before approving such an arrangement.

Duty of Referring Physician

Often, the physician who examined the patient will refer the patient to a specialist, a consulting physician, or a surgeon for further examination, diagnosis, or particular treatment. Under any referral situation, it is still the treating physician's duty to obtain informed consent and therefore he or she cannot rely on the referring physician to obtain the necessary consent.[23] Case law on the duty of the referring physician holds that a treating physician can be held liable where treatment is provided without informed consent even though the referring physician obtained the initial consent of the patient.[24]

Duty of the Health Care Facility

A majority of the jurisdictions that have addressed the issue of the hospital's responsibility in this area have held that a hospital does not have a duty to obtain consent from patients treated in the hospital.[25] At least one jurisdiction has indicated that a hospital may have a greater duty to the patient. In *Magana v. Elie*, an Illinois Appellate Court stated:

> Whether the standard of care which defendant Hospital must meet to satisfy its duty to its patients provides that the Hospital require physicians to whom it grants use of its facilities to advise their patients of risks attendant to treatment therein cannot be determined as a matter of law.[26]

The trial court had dismissed the patient's cause of action alleging that the defendant hospital had such a duty. The appellate court reversed and indicated that a hospital's failure to take affirmative steps to require the physician to disclose the requisite information could constitute negligence depending on the standard of care involved.[27]

In a New York case, the court stated that a hospital could be held liable where it knew or ought to have known that a doctor had not obtained a patient's consent.[28] In a common scenario that may give rise to such a duty, the hospital requires nurses or other hospital personnel to obtain patients' signatures on consent forms. In the event that the signature is not obtained or the patient expresses uncertainty or concern about signing the form, the hospital will have been put on notice of insufficient disclosure.[29] A failure to rectify the situation may subject the hospital to liability.

In general, there are two theories on which health care facilities can be held liable for the negligent or intentional misdeeds of physicians working in the hospital. These theories are the doctrines of respondeat superior and corporate negligence.

Under the doctrine of respondeat superior, a hospital can be held liable for the acts of a physician because it is the physician's employer or master and thereby controls the acts of the physician. Thus, if an employment relationship exists and the physician-employee has a duty to the patient to obtain informed consent and fails to do so, the hospital can be held liable. For the most part, however, the physician is not considered an employee but an independent contractor of a hospital and therefore not under the hospital's control.[30] In this case, the hospital will not be liable for the independent contractor's negligent or intentional failure to obtain informed consent.

However, some of the more recent cases have been reluctant to hold the hospital blameless and in fact have suggested that in some situations the physician can be treated as an agent for tort purposes.[31] Some courts have justified this unique position based on the position that the patient views the hospital as responsible for the physicians within its facility.[32]

The doctrine of corporate negligence imposes a duty on the hospital to exercise due care with respect to the treatment of its patients as it relates generally to (1) selection, retention, and supervision of physicians, (2) maintenance of grounds, and (3) maintenance and selection of equipment.[33] A claim of corporate negligence usually surfaces in a medical malpractice action in which the plaintiff claims that the hospital knew or should have known that the defendant physician was providing substandard medical care and that the hospital's failure to supervise the physician and take appropriate corrective action renders it liable to the patient. Using this theory, a plaintiff could easily maintain that through its supervisory duties the hospital knew or should have known that the treating physician did not obtain the informed consent of the patient or improperly delegated this task to an unqualified individual.

As a result of the common law theories of respondeat superior and corporate negligence, there are three potential ways in which a hospital can be held liable for the negligent or intentional acts of independent physicians. These are:

1. where the provider is deemed to be an employee or agent
2. where the hospital is deemed to have a direct duty to review the patient's treatment
3. where the hospital knew or should have known of a provider's failure to obtain informed consent

A provider will not generally be deemed an agent except where the provider is in fact an employee of the hospital.

Hospitals have generally not been found to have an independent duty to obtain informed consent. Nevertheless, it is possible that as the informed consent duty develops and as the role of hospitals changes, they will be deemed to have a separate and direct duty to require that informed consent be obtained from patients prior to treatment in the hospital.

A hospital could be held liable if it knew or should have known that informed consent was not obtained from a patient before treatment was provided by a physician in that hospital. Many hospitals take on the responsibility of developing informed consent forms or other informational media, while others make hospital personnel responsible for ensuring that informed consent is obtained prior to treatment. In this situation, it is possible that failure to carry out these self-imposed standards will be treated as an act of negligence if, as will be discussed later, the patient suffers some type of resulting damage or injury.

Elements of a Valid Consent

The three elements necessary for a consent to be valid are: (1) communication of sufficient information to meet the applicable standard of disclosure, (2) to a person with the capacity to understand the information and to fairly decide whether to consent to the treatment, in which (3) consent is given freely and voluntarily.[34] If any of the above criteria is not met, then consent is not valid.

Standard and Content of Disclosure

A primary component of informed consent is the physician's duty to disclose "adequate" information to allow the patient to make an informed choice. Some courts initially suggested that full and complete disclosure of *all* the risks, benefits, and alternatives was necessary in order to obtain truly informed consent.[35] It soon became apparent that full disclosure unduly burdened the physician, the patient, and the entire medical community. Consequently, courts have attempted to establish a standard for disclosure. Two approaches have developed to define the nature and extent of a physician's disclosure obligation.

However, some courts recently have concluded that the standard of disclosure should be determined not by a reasonable physician but rather by a reasonable patient; that is, the information that a reasonable patient would need in order to make an informed choice.

Professional Disclosure Standard. Under the professional disclosure theory, the physician's duty is governed by the standard of a reasonable medical practitioner practicing in the same or similar community and under the same or similar circumstances. Expert medical testimony is essential to establish the sufficiency of the physician's disclosure in a particular case.[36] This traditional approach reflects the criteria used in most types of medical malpractice lawsuits.

Therefore, the patient must present expert testimony that persuades the trier of fact that the physician's disclosures as to the nature of the procedure, risks, consequences, and alternatives were not sufficient in comparison with disclosures that would have customarily been made by physicians in the same or similar circumstances. In this way, the medical community establishes the professional standard of disclosure by which members of the community are judged.

The professional disclosure theory has been adopted by courts in a majority of those states that have considered the standard for disclosure, and it is preferred in legislative enactments.[37]

Reasonable Patient Standard. A minority of jurisdictions have adopted the reasonable patient theory, which is viewed as the "modern trend."[38] According to this view, a physician "owes to his patient the duty to disclose in a reasonable manner all significant medical information that the physician possesses or reasonably should possess that is material to an intelligent decision by the patient whether to undergo a proposed procedure."[39] Courts that have adopted this criterion argue that the reasonable physician standard does not necessarily protect a patient's right to self-determination because the standard for disclosure is unrelated to a patient's need for information.

Because the trier of fact, whether judge or jury, is deemed to be a "reasonable person," expert testimony is *not* required to establish whether the physician has met the duty of disclosure under the reasonable patient theory. The trier of fact will listen to testimony regarding the treatment and nature of the disclosure and then will be asked to determine whether, in light of the facts and circumstances, the disclosure was sufficient to allow the patient to make an informed choice.

A minority of those jurisdictions that focus on the patient's need for information go one step further by basing the determination on a subjective patient standard rather than the reasonable patient standard. Under the subjective patient standard, the physician must disclose risks that are material to the particular patient's treatment decision.[40] The trier of fact must determine whether this patient would have consented to the procedure if he or she had known all of the risks.

Hybrid Standard. In a recent article a commentator discussed jurisdictions that have appeared to blend the disclosure standards in order to achieve equitable results. This result has been designated the "hybrid standard."[41]

The Minnesota Supreme Court combined the professional physician, the reasonable patient, and the subjective standards, thereby requiring that a physician disclose "serious" risks, risks that a skilled practitioner of good standing in the community would reveal, and risks not generally considered serious enough by the medical profession to require disclosure, if the physician is aware that the patient attaches particular significance to such risks.[42] Similarly, the Colorado Supreme Court stated that if a reasonable medical practitioner knew or should have known that a particular risk would be significant in the patient's decision making, that risk must be disclosed by the physician.[43]

Finally, the Massachusetts Supreme Judicial Court also decided a case in which it rejected the professional disclosure standard to the extent that it required a physician to disclose only such information as is customarily revealed to the patient. The court required the physician to disclose all significant medical information that a physician reasonably should possess, as well as information "material" to the patient's decision to consent to treatment.[44] Under this standard, expert testimony is required to establish what a reasonable physician would disclose; however, the extent to which information is "material" can be established by lay persons.

The trend toward a reasonable patient or subjective patient standard and away from the traditional reasonable physician standard has significant consequences for the medical community. Under the traditional theory, a physician's burden was met as long as he or she acted like the typical physician in the same circumstances. It was often difficult for a patient to get physicians to testify against their peers, usually easy for a physician to get peers to testify on his or her behalf. Furthermore, the reasonable physician standard is generally insufficient because studies have shown that physicians have traditionally tended to underdisclose.[45]

But when the physician's duty depends upon a patient's need, a physician must give careful consideration to what information is "material," regardless of whether it would normally be disclosed by other health care practitioners. The information sought by a patient may not always be readily available to a physician and it will require more effort of physicians and all health care providers to gather such information and present it in a clear, understandable way.

Although the standard of adequate disclosure varies depending on whether the jurisdiction has adopted the reasonable physician, reasonable patient, subjective patient or a hybrid standard, there is a general consensus among the states regarding the general categories of information that should be disclosed.[46] Some states have enacted legislation to govern such disclosure while for other states it has been established by case law.[47]

According to these authorities, a provider is generally required to disclose (1) the nature of the procedure, (2) the risks and benefits associated with the particular procedure, (3) reasonable alternatives to the procedure, and (4) the risks and benefits of the alternatives.

Risk-benefit Information. With regard to risk-benefit information, the amount of disclosure required will vary from state to state depending to a large extent upon the standard recognized in that state. Generally, states that follow the physician disclosure standard require less risk information because it has been the custom in the medical community to underdisclose risks.[48]

On the other hand, in a state where a reasonable person or subjective person standard is applied, a physician could be required to disclose very remote risks if the patient would deem such a risk material. Thus, it is likely that a small incidence of a serious consequence must be disclosed even if a reasonable physician would not ordinarily disclose a risk of such minor incidence.

Under either standard, however, a provider can only be held accountable for disclosing risks and other treatment information that was reasonably foreseeable at the time of disclosure. Similarly, even in a subjective person jurisdiction, remote risks need not be disclosed unless the physician is aware that such a risk would be material or significant to that specific patient.[49]

Alternatives. Another important aspect of disclosure is the availability of reasonable alternative procedures. The only basis for not disclosing an alternative is (1) if the alternative is not reasonable, or (2) if disclosure would adversely affect the patient. This second reason for nondisclosure, referred to as the "therapeutic privilege," must be based on a reasonable expectation that the patient will suffer some real physical or mental injury and not merely because the physician believes that the patient will simply refuse to consent to treatment.

Similarly, for a practitioner to determine whether an alternative is so unreasonable that it need not be presented, he or she will often have to know more about the individual patient and also be able to support the decision with fact if it is later challenged.[50]

As with risks and benefits, the reasonable alternative standard for disclosure will usually be higher in a jurisdiction that has adopted the reasonable patient or the subjective patient standard.

Patient's Condition. A final important aspect of disclosure concerns information on the patient's medical condition obtained from examinations or test results. As a general rule, it is obviously important to inform the patient of his own medical condition. Therefore, except where special circumstances exist or where the physician decides not to disclose based on the "therapeutic privilege," information about the patient's medical condition should be disclosed.[51]

Capacity To Consent

The second element required for a valid informed consent is that the patient has the requisite capacity to consent to or refuse treatment. This topic is discussed in greater detail in other chapters of the book.[52] Generally, however, valid consent can be given by a person who is legally and mentally capable of (1) understanding the information communicated by the physician or other health care professional and (2) reaching an intelligent decision regarding the course of treatment.[53]

Coercion and Undue Influence

Another component of obtaining valid consent is that the patient's decision be voluntary. Due to the imposing nature of health care facilities and personnel, a patient might feel reluctant to ask questions or express doubts. In a majority of cases, however, a patient's uncomfortable feelings will not be sufficient to support a lawsuit claiming that the consent was invalid. In order for a patient's consent to be considered coerced or involuntary, the pressures must be very strong or the individual very susceptible to such pressures.[54] In any event, it is in the best interest of the physician, hospital, and hospital personnel to be receptive to the patient's concerns and willing to respond to questions so that a patient will feel comfortable enough to express any questions or hesitations he or she may have regarding the treatment.

The ethical concerns regarding a valid consent are obvious. A person cannot protect individual autonomy unless he or she has the ability to make decisions freely and intelligently.

From a legal standpoint, the physician's increased burden of disclosure as a result of a recent trend toward the reasonable or the subjective patient standard may seem unduly cumbersome. Understandably, medical practitioners and hospitals are concerned with the potential liability that arises from these higher standards of disclosure. Nevertheless, from an ethical standpoint, it is not unreasonable for a person to expect to be told of *all* the factors that he or she and the physician should consider in making a decision regarding medical care.

Physicians and hospitals should be aware of the disclosure standard in the jurisdiction where they are providing services. They also should give careful consideration to the content of their disclosures and make certain that the information they discuss is comprehensive and detailed enough to allow patients to truly understand the nature of their illness and all aspects of the treatment recommended so the patient can make an informed choice.

Causation Element of a Negligence Cause of Action

The fact that there was no valid informed consent where the practitioner had a duty to obtain consent does not necessarily mean that the practitioner will be liable to the patient for any damages resulting from the treatment involved. If the consent is not valid a practitioner can be held liable but only for injuries actually and proximately caused by the lack of consent.

As one of the fundamental elements of a cause of action for negligence, the plaintiff must prove that he or she would not have consented to the treatment if fully informed, and that the injury and damages were a reasonably foreseeable consequence of the physician's failure to inform the patient. Two theories of causation have developed: (1) the objective or the prudent patient standard, and (2) the subjective or individual patient standard.

Objective Standard

The objective patient approach has been adopted by a majority of jurisdictions.[55] The determination of causation is based on whether a reasonable or prudent person, in the patient's position, would have submitted to the medical procedure or course of treatment if properly informed of the risks. The focus is on the reasonable person rather than the patient-plaintiff.

The trier of fact must weigh such factors as the necessity of the medical procedure or course of treatment, the incidence of risk involved, and the severity of potential injury if not performed.[56] Based on these factors, the trier of fact must decide whether a reasonable person in the patient's position would have chosen to forgo the particular procedure because of the risks involved or would have consented regardless of the known risks. The testimony of the individual patient is relevant to determine what was disclosed, but it will not control with respect to the objective patient standard.[57]

Subjective Standard

Under the subjective standard, in order to prove causation, the individual patient must establish that he or she would have decided not to have the medical treatment if the undisclosed information actually had been provided. Although this approach on the surface would create the most correct result, it is often criticized because the standard encourages the patient to make self-serving assertions. Nevertheless, those few jurisdictions that have adopted the subjective standard assert that it is the only appropriate means of protecting the patient's right of self-determination.[58]

Exceptions or Excuses for Failure To Obtain Informed Consent

Negligent failure to obtain informed consent requires proof that the practitioner failed to meet the applicable standards of disclosure and that his or her failure to do so is not justifiable. In situations that fall within recognized exceptions a physician will be relieved of liability.

One such exception occurs when an emergency renders disclosure and informed consent impractical.[59] Thus, when a patient is unconscious or otherwise incapable of consenting and harm from a failure to treat is imminent and outweighs any harm threatened by the proposed treatment, consent is not required. Courts will imply consent on the assumption that a reasonable person in the patient's position would have consented to the treatment.[60]

Another exception is when the physician determines that full or even partial disclosure is not in the patient's best interests. This is referred to as the physician's "therapeutic privilege."[61] The physician's claim of therapeutic privilege must be based on provable fact and not merely the physician's feeling that the patient might be reluctant to proceed if informed of all the risks.[62]

Exceptions from the disclosure requirements are affirmative defenses, which the defendant may use to dispute an initial claim of lack of valid informed consent. If the patient is unable to disprove the defendant's affirmative defense, the patient's claim will be unsuccessful.

DOCUMENTING INFORMED CONSENT

Authorization for treatment may be given in several forms. The consent may be express or implied. Express consent may be given orally or in writing. Implied consent is usually taken from the surrounding facts and circumstances and the patient's own actions.[63] However, the fact that consent is given does not automatically establish that the consent was informed. Express or implied consent must be given after the patient has received sufficient information to make an informed choice.

From a legal standpoint, any form of consent, oral or written, is usually sufficient as long as the practitioner can prove that the consent was obtained. Nevertheless, from a practical standpoint it is much easier to establish that consent was given if the consent is in writing or at least was obtained in the presence of a third person who can testify that consent was given. Similarly, although the provider's oral disclosure is legally sufficient, as a practical matter it is much more difficult for a provider to dispute a patient's claim that he or she was not advised of a particular risk if there is no written evidence in the medical records, progress notes, or other document to establish the contents of disclosure.

It is important to remember that consent is a process, not a document. The document merely codifies and reflects the culmination of the process. Written consent alone without true disclosure and an opportunity for dialogue between the provider and the patient is generally inadequate.[64]

Consent Forms

Consent forms were developed primarily as a means of establishing that informed consent did in fact occur. However, such forms have been recognized as an important component of the process, as many states mandate that consent forms be used as a part of the decision-making process. Furthermore, such forms by their very nature are more readily adaptable for review by the physician, patient, and the courts, so that much of the investigation into the content of disclosure and consent relies on consent forms and other types of tangible consent.

Development of Consent Forms

Generally, when a patient brings a claim for negligence under the doctrine of informed consent, the patient alleges that the physician's improper failure to warn of specific risks or consequences led to consent to treatment that resulted in a harm he or she would have chosen to avoid if warned of the risks and their probable occurrence. The physician in defense will claim that (1) the patient was warned of the risks, (2) the risk was not significant enough that a reasonable physician would have disclosed it or that a reasonable patient would have thought it material, or (3) the patient would have decided to go ahead with the procedure even if he or she had been warned. Typically, this debate leads to a "testimonial contest" between the patient and the physician regarding the content of disclosure. Consent forms were developed in response to these contests as documentation of the content of disclosure and the fact that consent was given.[65]

Content of Consent Forms

A recent Michigan study revealed that although there is some variance in style and wording, the "average" hospital consent form[66] submitted by the participants contained the same general clauses. These clauses consisted of (1) an authorization clause, authorizing the physician and/or assistants or designees to perform the procedure(s) listed therein; (2) an extension clause, authorizing the treatment of unforeseen conditions as an extension of the procedures authorized if deemed necessary or advisable by the physician; (3) a no-guarantee clause, wherein the patient acknowledges that there are no guarantees regarding the results of treatments or examinations; (4) an anesthesia clause, consenting to the administration of necessary or advisable anesthetics with designated exceptions; (5) a disclosure clause, indicating that the nature, purpose, risks, possible complications, and alternatives to treatment, including the risks of such alternatives, have been explained to the patient; (6) a photography clause, consenting to photographing the procedures for medical purposes; (7) a tissue disposal clause, authorizing the hospital to retain and use or dispose of any tissue taken from the patient's body; (8) a patient understanding clause, indicating that a form has been explained to or read by the patient and that the patient understands its contents; and (9) a signature clause, requiring a patient to sign the form and often requiring the witness to verify the signature.[67]

Criticisms of Traditional Hospital Consent Forms

There has been substantial criticism of traditional consent forms in the recent past. The criticisms pertain to the inability of the forms to communicate a wealth of information in an understandable way, as well as the inadequacy of the health care system to prepare and use consent forms in the appropriate fashion to obtain the maximum degree of understanding. Three aspects of consent forms particularly affect their legal significance and contribution to the informed consent process. These are: (1) content, (2) readability, and (3) circumstances surrounding the signing of the form.[68]

Content. The main criticism of hospital consent forms is that they are too broad and ambiguous to help the patient understand or satisfy the legal requirements of informed consent.

The extension clause is often criticized in particular. An extension clause in general allows a physician to do whatever is "necessary and advisable" during the course of the procedure. This may be construed by a patient as merely authorizing additional procedures where an emergency occurs during the treatment. To the contrary, the common law already implies consent for a health care provider to act in the patient's best interest in the event that an emergency occurs during treatment and the patient is incapable of giving consent. Extension clauses, on the other hand, apply to unforeseen conditions that are not emergencies but of which the patient was unaware at the time of consent. Because they are so broad and ambiguous, some courts have construed such clauses to be meaningless.

The disclosure clause is also criticized for being overly broad and ambiguous. Often this clause merely states that the nature, purpose, risks, complications, and possible alternatives have been explained to the patient. The usefulness of such a clause is minimal for the patient, the provider, or the legal system in attempting to determine whether sufficient disclosure was made. By failing to list the specific contents of the disclosure, the clause becomes useless, and the court must again resort to the testimonial contest between provider and patient that the consent forms were designed to avoid.[69] Providers do not benefit or protect themselves by failing to detail the contents of disclosure—instead they subject themselves to the whim of the jury. A detailed disclosure clause will minimize the need for testimonial evidence to establish its content and will allow the provider to consider the contents seriously and prepare a document that reflects this carefully considered disclosure.

Readability. Many studies have investigated the readability of consent forms. The general consensus is that the readability level exceeds the reading level of the general population, directed toward undergraduate or graduate school students.[70] Therefore, the majority of the persons who execute consent forms are incapable of reading, let alone understanding, the forms.

The unfamiliarity of medical terms can significantly affect the patient's ability to understand. Complex descriptions and medical terms may increase the patient's apprehension because the patient is likely to view the procedure and the illness as serious. Studies have shown that when risks or side effects of a particular drug are described in both lay and medical terms, the risks or side effects are interpreted as less serious than when the medical term is used alone.[71]

The language used to explain the nature of the procedure and the risks, benefits and alternatives can also significantly affect the patient's understanding of the information conveyed. A particular word can have unintended connotations that disrupt the patient's concentration and understanding of the communication. Words that elicit an emotional response, unlike purely descriptive terms, may distract from the patient's comprehension. For example, the word "baby" as opposed to "fetus" has been documented to elicit a more emotional response in most people, which makes them less able to make an objective choice.[72]

Therefore, providers should consider the emotional effect of words and their familiarity before conveying information to patients either orally or in written form. One commentator suggests that the present disclosure standards be replaced by a comprehension standard that focuses on whether "the physician: (1) inquire[d] of the patient's understanding of the risks, (2) encourage[d] the patient to ask questions, and (3) repeat[ed] risk information to ensure the patient assimilate[d] it."[73]

Circumstances of Signing. The legal significance of any consent depends on the circumstances surrounding it. In the context of consent forms in particular, issues affecting the validity of the form are: (1) When was the consent form signed? (2) Was someone available to answer questions when the patient read and signed the document? (3) Who actually obtained the signature? (4) How much time was spent in obtaining consent? (5) What was the patient's physical and mental state when consent was obtained?

Allowing sufficient time for the patient to consider all of the information conveyed by the provider can significantly improve the informed nature of a patient's decision.[74] Where no emergency is involved, there is usually a delay between the time that the physician informs the patient of a diagnosis and recommends the treatment and the time that the patient receives the treatment. In this time the patient can review the information presented orally and in written form by the provider.

Many studies have demonstrated that the time it takes to assimilate information is directly related to the complexity of the information.[75] Therefore, in most cases, it will take the patient some time to assimilate complex medical information conveyed by the physician. Nevertheless, patients will usually never see a consent form until just prior to the time for treatment. At this point, the patient's high anxiety level and the pressures of time reduce the patient's ability to read and comprehend the information and to make an informed decision. Furthermore, the patient will be reluctant to reconsider the decision, feeling that he or she has already committed to the treatment.

A good example is when a woman enters a hospital for delivery. Because she is usually in labor, this is an extremely difficult time for her to make decisions regarding the method of anesthesia or other aspects of delivery. Nevertheless, these important aspects often are not discussed until the time she enters the hospital, and therefore the woman will often permit the physician to make these decisions on her behalf. To the contrary, where possible, these issues should be discussed with the patient in the doctor's office long before she enters the hospital. In addition, she should also be provided with the appropriate consent forms at the same time so she has adequate time to read and assimilate all of the information. Then, when the woman enters the hospital for delivery, she will have had the opportunity to carefully consider the options and will be prepared to give consent.

In line with this theory, one writer suggests that informed consent statutes should impose a mandatory delay between the time a patient receives information and consent forms and the time treatment is given.[76] A Michigan study found that an average of 8.5 minutes was spent obtaining a patient's consent to surgery. Obviously, this is insufficient where new and complex medical terms and procedures are involved.[77] All of the circumstances surrounding the signing of consent forms cannot be reviewed in detail. However, it is important for practitioners and others responsible for obtaining informed consent or ensuring that such is obtained to consider carefully all of the aspects surrounding the signing of consent forms to facilitate the patient's clear decision making.

Legal Status of Hospital Consent Forms

Although 47 states and the District of Columbia recognize some form of the doctrine of informed consent either by case law or statute,[78] only 16 have ruled on the legal validity of hospital consent forms.[79] Eight of these states provide by statute that a written consent form signed by the patient creates a rebuttable presumption of consent.[80] This presumption may be rebutted by proof that consent was not given fully or was induced by fraud or misrepresentation. Two other states hold that a consent form signed by a legally competent patient is prima facie evidence that the patient gave informed consent to the treatment.[81] In the remaining six states, the status of the signed consent form has varying legal consequences.[82] In two states the effect of consent forms has been determined by case law.

The Maryland Court of Appeals held that written consent is not proof of informed consent "unless a person has been adequately apprised of the material risks and the therapeutic alternatives incident to a proposed treatment. . . ."[83]

The Supreme Court of North Dakota upheld jury instructions on the relevance of hospital consent forms in a malpractice case. These stated that the fact that the patient signed a consent form is relevant and material to the determination of whether informed consent had been given but not binding on the patient if the patient does not have the necessary information to make an informed consent.[84]

Nevertheless, the large majority of states have no law on the status of a written consent. Generally, where there is no express law on the subject, the consent form will be considered merely part of the evidence on the patient's consent but will not be binding if the patient was not adequately informed.

Audiovisuals as Alternatives and Supplements to Consent Forms

Because of the criticisms of the insufficiencies of written consent forms, it is apparent that there is room for improvement in the present composition and usage of these documents. The forms can be improved by increasing their clarity and understandability and by specifying the content of disclosure. Furthermore, the effect of the forms can be enhanced by paying attention to the time, place, and manner in which the forms are presented.

Nevertheless, one of the major obstacles to physicians' obtaining informed consent is lack of adequate time for dialogue and follow-up. Physician's professional lives are often complex and fast-paced, leaving little time to engage in lengthy discussions with their patients. Furthermore, depending on the patient's general background knowledge of medicine and anatomy and physiology, true informative disclosure often would take a substantial amount of background for the patient to understand the details of the information about his or her medical condition.

Consequently, hospitals have recently begun to aid the physician by establishing educational programs for patients.[85] Generally, these have developed in the form of audiovisuals. These teaching tools have generally been found to have very positive effects in (1) increasing the patient's understanding of the problem and the treatment or procedure involved, (2) decreasing anxiety, (3) facilitating communication between the patient and provider or staff, and (4) encouraging questions by patients.[86] Furthermore, audiovisuals decrease the testimonial battles that occur when a patient brings a cause of action for inadequate disclosure, because the videos can be presented to the trier of fact to establish the content of disclosure.[87]

SUMMARY

The documentation of consent is a very important aspect of the informed consent process. The primary significance is not, as may be expected, the use of documentation to aid the evidentiary process. To the contrary, consent forms are most useful because they help to avoid litigation altogether. If properly drafted and used, consent forms can help significantly in the patient's ability to understand the information conveyed and in the practitioner's ability to portray the information necessary to obtain informed consent.

Consequently, it is essential that drafters pay close attention to the content of consent forms, avoiding overly broad and ambiguous clauses and assuring that the language in the form is understandable to the average or even below average reader. Forms should be drafted so that they encourage the patient to consider every aspect of the consent and require the patient to demonstrate his or her understanding of the disclosure. Finally, it is important that persons involved in the process of obtaining informed consent be acutely aware of the circumstances that surround the signing of the consent form so that it will be most conducive to allowing the patient to obtain maximum understanding of the information.

Finally, health care providers should consider the alternative means of conveying information, such as audiovisuals, so as to decrease the burden on physicians and increase the quality and uniformity of information conveyed. If such consideration is given to all the aspects surrounding documentation of informed consent, the process will be greatly improved and correspondingly the instances of litigation surrounding lack of informed consent will likely decrease.

NOTES

1. This chapter uses the terms "medical practitioner," "health care practitioner," "practitioner," and "physician" interchangeably to refer to persons who provide medical treatment to individuals.

2. *See* the section "Standard and Content of Disclosure," infra.

3. *See* the section "Who Has the Duty," infra.

4. Curran, *Foreword* to F. Rozovsky, Consent to Treatment a Practical Guide at XXXV (1984).

5. *See* Schloendorff v. Society of New York Hospital, 211 N.Y. 125, 129–130, 105 N.E. 92, 93 (1914).

6. Andrews, *Informed Consent Statutes and the Decisionmaking Process*, 5 J. of Legal Med. 163 at 164–71.

7. *Id.* at 165–68.

8. *Id.* at 168–70.

9. *Id.* at 170–71.

10. F. Rozovsky, Consent to Treatment a Practical Guide, at 4 (1984).

11. Andrews, *supra* note 6, at 175, n. 63.

12. Perry v. Hodgson, 168 Ga. 678, 148 S.E. 659 (1929).

13. Mohr v. Williams, 95 Minn. 261, 104 N.W. 12 (1905).

14. *See, e.g.*, Salgo v. Leland Stanford, Jr., University Board of Trustees, 317 P.2d 170 (Cal. App. 1957).

15. A presidential study in 1982 indicated that there were only 3 states with no statutory authority or case law on the subject of informed consent. 3 Presidential Comm'n for the Study of Ethical Problems in Medicine & Biomedical & Behavioral Research, the Ethical and Legal Implications of Informed Consent in the Patient Practitioner Relationship, app. L at 246, 248, 250. The states were Connecticut, South Carolina, and West Virginia. There are presently 23 states that have statutes requiring informed consent. For the citations to these statutes, see Andrews, *supra* note 6, at n. 83.

16. F. Rozovsky, *supra* note 10, at 60.

17. *Id.* at 60 n.5.

18. *See, e.g.*, Liera v. Wisner, 171 Mont. 254, 557 P.2d 805 (1976); Gray v. Grunnagle, 423 Pa. 144, 223 A.2d 663 (1966).

19. Andrews, *supra* note 6, at 204.

20. *Id.* at 204–05.

21. *Id.*

22. Note, *Informed Consent and Hospital Consent Forms: Paper Chasing in a Video World*, 61 J. OF URB. L. 105, at 119 and n. 105.

23. F. Rozovsky, *supra* note 10, at 647–48.

24. Liera v. Wisner, 171 Mont. 254, 557 P.2d 805 (1976); Gray v. Grunnagle, 423 Pa. 144, 223 A.2d 663 (1966).

25. *See, e.g.*, Roberson v. Menorah Medical Center, 508 S.W. 2d 134 (Mo. Ct. App. 1979); Cooper v. Cuny, 92 N.M. 417, 589 P.2d 201 (1978); Garzione v. Vassar Bros. Hospital, 36 A.D. 2d 340, 320 N.Y.S. 2d 830 (1971).

26. 108 Ill. App. 3d 1028, 439 N.E.2d 1219, 1322 (1982).

27. *Id.* The case was remanded for reconstruction by the trial court and appears to have been ultimately settled by the parties.

28. Fiorentino v. Wenger, 19 N.Y. 2d 407, 280 N.Y.S.2d 373, 227 N.E.2d 296 (1967).

29. F. Rozovsky, *supra* note 10, at 649–50.

30. *See, e.g.*, Schloendorff v. Society of New York Hospital, 211 N.Y. 125, 105 N.E. 92 (1914).

31. Bing v. Thunig, 2 N.Y.2d 656, 143 N.E.2d 3, 168 N.Y.S.2d 3 (1977); *See also*, Southwick, *Hospital Liability: Two Theories Have Been Merged*, 4 J. Legal Med. 1, 7 (1983).

32. Grewe v. Mt. Clemens General Hospital, 404 Mich. 240, 273 N.W.2d 429 (1978).

33. Southwick, *supra* note 31, at 17. *See also*, Darling v. Charleston Community Memorial Hospital, 33 Ill. 2d 326, 211 N.E.2d 253 (1965).

34. F. Rozovsky, *supra* note 10, at 8–9.

35. Salgo v. Stanford University, 154 Cal. App. 2d 560, 317 P.2d 170 (1957).

36. *See, e.g.*, Fuller v. Starnes, 597 S.W. 2d 88 (Ark. 1980); Robinson v. Mroz, 433 A.2d 1051, (Del. App. 1981); Karp v. Colley, 493 F.2d 408 (5th Cir. [Tex.] 1974); Buckner v. Allergan Pharmaceuticals, 400 So. 2d 820 (Fla. App. 1981); Searcy v. Manganhas, 415 N.E.2d 142 (Ind. App. 1981); Zeigert v. South Chicago Community Hospital, 425 N.E.2d 450 (Ill. App. 1981); Natanson v. Kline, 350 P.2d 1093 (Kan. 1960); Woolley v. Henderson, 418 A.2d 1123 (Me. 1980);

Rice v. Jaskolski, 313 N.W.2d 893 (Mich. 1981); Cress v. Mayer, 626 S.W.2d 430 (Mo. App. 1981); Collins v. Itoh, 503 P.2d 36 (Mont. 1972); Folger v. Corbett, 394 A.2d 63, 287 S.E.2d 892 (N.C. 1982); Dewes v. Indian Health Service, 504 F. Supp. 203 (D.S.D. 1980); Cunningham v. Yankton Clinic, 262 N.W.2d 508 (S.D. 1978); Rush v. Miller, 648 F.2d 1075 (6th Cir. [Tenn.] 1981); Roark v. Allen, 633 S.W.2d 804 (Tex. 1982); Ficklin v. MacFarlane, 550 P.2d 1295 (Utah 1976) [*but see* Nixdorf v. Hicken, 612 P.2d 348 (Utah 1980), *cf.* Reiser v. Lohner, 641 P.2d 93 (Utah 1982)]; Dessi v. U.S., 489 F. Supp. 722 (E.D. Va. 1980); and Bly v. Rhoads, 222 S.E.2d 783 (Va. 1976).

37. Of the 23 states that mandate informed consent by legislation, 12 have adopted a professional disclosure standard: DEL. CODE ANN. tit. 18, §6852(a)(2) (Supp. 1982); FLA. STAT. ANN. §768.46(3)(a) (West Supp. 1983); IDAHO CODE §39-4304 (1977); KY. REV. STAT. §304.40–320(1) (1981); ME. REV. STAT. ANN. tit. 24, §2905(1)(A) (Supp. 1983–84); NEB. REV. STAT. §44-2816 (1978); N.H. REV. STAT. ANN. §507-C:2(II)(a) (1983); N.Y. PUB. HEALTH LAW §2805-d(1) (McKinney 1977); N.C. GEN. STAT. §90-21.13(a)(1) (1981); OR. REV. STAT. §677.095 (1981); TENN. CODE ANN. §29-26-118 (1980); VT. STAT. ANN. tit. 12, §1909(a)(1) (Supp. 1983). Three impose a reasonable patient standard: PA. STAT. ANN. tit. 40, §1301.103 (Purdon Supp. 1983–1984); TEX. REV. CIV. STAT. ANN. art. 4590i, §6.01–.07 (Vernon Supp. 1982–1983); WASH. REV. CODE ANN. §7.70.050(2) (Supp. 1983–1984). Eight statutes are silent on the standard of disclosure: ALASKA STAT. §09.55.556(a) (1983); HAWAII REV. STAT. ANN. §671–3(b) (Supp. 1982); IOWA CODE ANN. §147.137(1) (Supp. 1983–84); LA. REV. STAT. ANN. §40:1299.40(A) (West 1977); NEV. REV. STAT. §41A.110 (1981); OHIO REV. CODE ANN. §2317.54 (Page 1981); R.I. GEN. LAWS §9-19-32 (Supp. 1983); UTAH CODE ANN. §78-14-5 (1977).

38. The seminal case is Canterbury v. Spence, 464 F.2d 772 (D.C. Cir. 1972). *See also,* Truman v. Thomas, 165 Cal. Rptr. 902 (Cal. 1980); Willard v. Hagemeister, 175 Cal. Rptr. 365 (Cal. App. 1981); Crain v. Allison, 443 A.2d 558 (D.C. App. 1982): Flannery v. President and Directors of Georgetown College, 679 F.2d 960 (D.C. Cir. 1982); Henderson v. Milobsky, 595 F.2d 654 (D.C. Cir. 1978); Hartke v. McElway, 526 F. Supp. 97 (D.D.C. 1981); LePelley v. Grefenson, 614 P.2d 962 (Idaho 1980); Rogers v. Brown, 416 So. 2d 624 (La. App. 1982); Zeno v. Lincoln General Hospital 404 So. 2d 1337 (La. App. 1981) [*but see*, Hanks v. Drs. Ranson, Swan & Burtch, Ltd., 359 So.2d 1089 (La. App. 1978)]; Harnish v. Children's Hospital Medical Center, 387 Mass. 152, 439 N.E.2d 240 (1982); Sard v. Hardy, 379 A.2d 1014 (Md. 1977); Creasey v. Hogan, 617 P.2d 1377 (Ore. App. 1980); Salis v. U.S., 522 F. Supp. 989 (M.D. Pa. 1981); Cooper v. Roberts, 286 A.2d 647 (Pa. Super. 1971); Wilkinson v. Vesey, 295 A.2d 676 (R.I. 1972); Nixdorf v. Hicken, 612 P.2d 348 (Utah 1980) [*but see*, Ficklin v. MacFarlane, 550 P.2d 1295 (Utah 1976), apparently followed in Reiser v. Lohner, 641 P.2d 93 (Utah 1982)], and Cross v. Trapp, 294 S.E.2d 446 (W. Va. 1982).

39. Harnish v. Children's Hospital Medical Center, 387 Mass. 152, 439 N.E.2d 240, 243 (1982).

40. *See, e.g.,* Scott v. Bradford, 606 P.2d 554 (Okla. 1979). *See also,* Truman v. Thomas, 27 Cal. 3d 285, 611 P.2d 902, 165 Cal. Rptr. 308 (1980) where the California Supreme Court ostensibly applied the reasonable patient standard but arguably in reality applied the subjective standard; Boland, *The Doctrines of Lack of Consent and Lack of Informed Consent in Medical Procedures in Louisiana,* 45 LA. L.R. 1, 11–13 (1984).

41. Le Blang, *Informed Consent—Duty and Causation: A Survey of Current Developments,* in Personal Injury Deskbook 335, 342–44 (Notes and Axelrod eds. annot. 1984).

42. Kinikin v. Heupel, 305 N.W.2d 589, 595 (Minn. 1981). *See also,* Plutshack v. University of Minnesota Hospitals, 316 N.W.2d 1 (Minn. 1982) and Cornfeldt v. Tongen, 295 N.W.2d 638 (Minn. 1980).

43. Bloskas v. Murray, 646 P.2d 907, 913 (Colo. 1982).

44. Harnish v. Children's Hospital Medical Center, 387 Mass. 152, 439 N.E.2d 240, 243 (1982).

45. Studies indicate that physicians have a tendency to underdisclose based on criteria such as (1) the patient's inability to understand the medical terminology, (2) the patient's inability to cope with pertinent information, (3) the seriousness of a patient's illness, and (4) a patient's apparent lack of desire for information. Andrews, *supra* note 6 at n.42 and accompanying text.

46. *See, e.g.*, IDAHO CODE §39-4304 (1975); KY. REV. STAT. §304040-320 (1976); NEB. REV. STAT. §44-2816 (1976); PA. STAT. ANN. tit. 40, §1301.103 (Purdon 1976). Under these statutes if the requisite information is disclosed, informed consent is given. *See also*, ALASKA STAT. §09.55.556 (1967); DEL. CODE ANN. tit. §6852 (1976); FLA. STAT. ANN. 768.46 (West 1975); UTAH CODE ANN. §78-14-5 (1976); VT. STAT. ANN. tit. 12, §1909 (1976). These statutes impose additional criteria before informed consent is proved.

47. *See, e.g.*, F. Rozovsky, *supra* note 10 at 43 n.3.

48. See, *supra* note 47.

49. F. Rozovsky, *supra* note 10, at 45.

50. *Id.* at 47–48.

51. Id. at 49–51. *See generally*, Le Blang, *Tort Liability to Nondisclosure: The Physician's Legal Obligations to Disclose Patient Illness and Injury*, 89 Dick L. Rev. 1 (1984).

52. Chapters 9 and 10.

53. *See generally*, F. Rozovsky, *supra* note 10, at 13–21.

54. *See generally*, Id. at 9–12.

55. Le Blang, *supra* note 41 at n.25 and cases cited therein.

56. *Id.* at 345.

57. *Id.*

58. *Id.* at 346–47.

59. *See, e.g.*, Canterbury v. Spence, 464 F.2d 772 (D.C. Cir.), *cert. denied*, 409 U.S. 1064, 93 S. Ct. 560 (1972); Pratt v. Davis, 222 Ill. 300, 309–10, 79 N.E. 562, 565 (1906); Sard v. Hardy, 281 Md. 432, 379 A.2d 1014 (1977); Crouch v. Most, 78 N.M. 406, 410, 432 P.2d 250, 254 (1967); Holt v. Nelson, 11 Wash. App. 231, 523 P.2d 211 (1974).

60. *Id. See generally*, F. Rozovsky, *supra* note 10, at 88–95, and Andrews, *supra* note 6, at 206–208.

61. *See, e.g.*, Roberts v. Wood, 206 F. Supp. 579 (S.D. Ala. 1962); Green v. Hussey, 127 Ill. App. 2d 174, 262 N.E.2d 156 (1970).

62. F. Rozovsky, *supra* note 10, at 98–103. *See also*, Andrews, *supra* note 6, at 211–15, and Boland, *supra* note 34, at 18.

63. F. Rozovsky, *supra* note 10, at 31–32.

64. Some state statutes create a rebuttable but conclusive presumption of valid consent if evidenced in writing. FLA. STAT. ANN. §768.46 (West 1975); OHIO REV. CODE ANN. §2317.54 (Baldwin 1977).

65. Note, *supra* note 22, at n. 20 and accompanying text.

66. *Id.* at 108–110.

67. *Id.*

68. Note, *supra* note 22, at 115–21.

69. Note, *supra* note 22, at 116.

70. *Id.* at 116–19.

71. *Id.* at 183–85.

72. Andrews, *supra* note 6, at 182–83.

73. *Id.* at n. 126.

74. *See generally*, Andrews, *supra* note 6, at 198–201.

75. *Id.*

76. *Id.* at 201.

77. Note, *supra* note 22, at 120.

78. *Id.* at n. 15 and accompanying text.

79. *Id.* at n. 44 and accompanying text.

80. *Id.* at n. 45 and accompanying text.

81. *Id.* at n. 47 and accompanying text.

82. *Id.* at nn. 48–71 and accompanying text.

83. Sard v. Hardy, 281 Md. 432, 438 N. 3, 379 A.2d 1014, 1019 (1977) (citations omitted).

84. Wasem v. Laskowski, 274 N.W. 2d 219, 226 (1979).

85. *See generally*, Note, *supra* note 22, at n. 115.

86. *Id.* at 122–25.

87. *Id.* at n. 125 and accompanying text.

Chapter 14

Confidentiality of Patient Record Information[*]

William H. Roach, Jr., MS, JD, and Susan N. Chernoff, MBA, JD

The extent to which health care institutions protect the confidentiality of their patient care records is a matter of growing importance. Patients increasingly are unwilling to trust health care providers to safeguard patient records from unauthorized and inappropriate access. As a result, the law is likely to further restrict rather than expand access to confidential hospital records in the future.

OWNERSHIP OF THE MEDICAL RECORD

It is a generally accepted rule that the medical record is owned by the hospital, subject to the patient's interest in the information contained in the record.[1] This rule is established by statute[2] or regulations[3] in most states. A few courts have held that a medical record is hospital property in which the patient has a limited property right[4] and that even a physician may have a definable legal interest in the record.[5]

ACCESS TO THE MEDICAL RECORD BY OR ON BEHALF OF THE PATIENT

In the past, hospitals in many states could deny patients access to their medical records. Patients seldom challenged the hospital's refusal to release record information. In recent years, however, the trend has been toward greater accessibility for the patient, so that most jurisdictions now grant the patient or the patient's representative the right to examine and copy the medical record.[6] Today, the general rule governing access by or on behalf of the patient may be stated

---

*This chapter was adapted from *Medical Records and the Law* by W.H. Roach, Jr., S.N. Chernoff, and C.L. Esley, pp. 59–116, Aspen Publishers, Inc., © 1985; and *Topics in Hospital Law*, Vol. 1, No. 1, pp. 1–13, Aspen Publishers, Inc., © December 1985.

as follows: the medical record is a confidential document, access to which should be restricted to the patient, to the patient's authorized representative, and to the attending physician and hospital staff members who have a legitimate need for such access.

The broad confidentiality of the record has been established in some states by statute or regulation. Some statutes and regulations simply state that medical records are confidential and may not be disclosed except under the circumstances set forth in the statute or regulation.[7] Other statutes are more specific and prohibit release or transfer of records without the consent of the patient or the patient's authorized representative.[8] The courts in some jurisdictions have recognized a hospital's duty to maintain the confidentiality of its patient records.[9] The Joint Commission on Accreditation of Hospitals (JCAH) imposes strict standards of medical records confidentiality upon accredited hospitals.[10]

The courts in many states have recognized the right of patients or their authorized representatives to have access to their medical records, even in the absence of statutory authority. While granting access, however, some courts may establish restrictions, such as permitting only the patient's attorney to inspect the records under the supervision of the hospital and to have photostatic copies made of only those parts of the record that the hospital considers proper under the circumstances of the case, bearing in mind the beneficial interest of the patient in the records and the general purpose for which the records were maintained.[11] Other courts have found that patients have a common law right to gain access to their records.[12] In *Rabens v. Jackson Park Hospital Foundation*, the court found that a hospital had breached its common law duty to disclose a patient's medical data to him or his representative upon request.[13] It also concluded that the hospital had violated a state statute that required a hospital to allow a patient's attorney or physician to examine and copy hospital records.[14]

In some instances, a question may arise as to the identity of the patient's representative. In *Emmett v. Eastern Dispensary and Casualty Hospital*, for example, the son of a deceased patient requested access to his father's medical record for purposes of bringing a negligence action against the hospital. The hospital refused to release the records on the grounds that the son was not the father's administrator and therefore not the father's legal representative. The court held that the fiduciary relationship between the hospital and the patient requires disclosure of medical record information to the patient and that this duty of disclosure extends after the patient's death to the patient's next of kin.[15]

The question is frequently raised as to whether hospitals must allow patients to examine their records while they are still hospitalized.[16] In the absence of a statutory or common law right of access the hospital is not obligated to permit its patients to inspect their records during hospitalization. However, hospitals should consider whether a refusal to permit such an inspection will create unnecessary problems for the institution and its staff. Patients who are not allowed to examine their charts in the hospital may become hostile and more difficult to treat. Furthermore, they may be more likely to file a claim against the hospital if treatment ends in a poor result. Therefore, unless the patient's attending physician can establish a reasonable basis for an opinion that disclosure of the inpatient medical record would be harmful to the patient, the hospital should allow the patient to review the record. In some instances, a record review, coordinated by the patient's attending physician, can be used as a beneficial teaching device. If inpatients are allowed to examine their records, the hospital should employ its customary record security procedures.

Records of Mental Health Patients

In some states, the rules governing access to the medical records of mental health patients differ from those applicable to medical records generally.[17] In the past, mental health patients were not granted access to their medical records, even in states that granted a right of access to other patients. It was widely believed that authorizing such patients to review their records would be injurious to their health. Today, however, mental health patients in some states have the same right to inspect their records as other patients.[18]

The courts have followed this legislative trend toward greater patient access. Recent court decisions have recognized the right of mental health patients or their representatives to review their medical records,[19] except where the interests of a minor might be jeopardized by permitting such access.[20]

Records of Minors

The law provides little specific guidance concerning who may have access to or who may authorize the release of the records of minor patients. In the absence of statutory or common law authority on this point, the generally accepted rule is that a hospital may disclose the medical record of a minor patient only upon the authorization of one of the patient's parents, unless a legal guardian has been appointed for the minor, and on the condition that a minor's parents may be allowed access to such records on behalf of the patient.

A number of state statutes governing access to medical records specifically address disclosure of a minor patient's records. A few states have statutes that permit the release of such records with the consent of either the patient's parent or the patient.[21]

The statutes of other states simply are not clear on the question of parental control of access to a minor's records. Most statutes permit access to records with the consent of "the patient"[22] or "the person."[23] In these states, hospitals should follow the generally accepted rule and obtain the authorization of the patient's parent before disclosing records to third parties. In some situations, state statutes authorize certain categories of minors (such as emancipated minors or those who are pregnant, parents, married, or suffering from drug abuse) to consent to their own medical care. It is a logical extension of these statutory rules to allow such minors to consent to disclosure of their medical records, but there is little clear authority for such a position. Hospitals should use caution when disclosing the medical records of these special types of minor patients.

Access to Medical Records by Others

There are exceptions to the general rule governing access to medical records. While certain types of medical records require a greater degree of confidentiality than others, in some circumstances medical records information may be disclosed to third parties without the patient's authorization. It is important for those involved with release of medical information to understand the exceptions.

Alcohol and Drug Abuse Patient Records

In the early 1970s, Congress enacted statutes that regulate the release of information from medical records relating to drug abuse patients[24] and alcohol abuse patients.[25] The regulations accompanying these amendments are found in 42 C.F.R. part 2 (1985) (the Rules). The general principle advocated by these rules is stated in section 2.18: "Any disclosure made under this part, whether with or without the patient's consent, shall be limited to information necessary in the light of the need or purpose for the disclosure."

The coverage of the prohibition is broad. It applies to records of the identity, diagnosis, prognosis, or treatment of any patient, which are maintained in connection with the performance of any alcohol abuse or drug abuse prevention functions.[26] The term "records" is defined to include *any* information relating to a patient that is acquired in connection with an alcohol or drug abuse program.[27]

The law and regulations are exceedingly complex. Any health care provider that receives federal funds and provides services to alcohol or drug abuse patients should have a patient records policy that complies with these rules. Moreover, hospitals must be wary of implicit disclosure of information. For example, if a drug or alcohol abuse patient is in a general care hospital, and the hospital fails to disclose information concerning him that it routinely discloses about other patients, the hospital could be liable for implicitly disclosing that the patient was being treated for drug or alcohol abuse. Hospitals should, therefore, be advised to delete such patients from their registers unless the patients consent to their presence being acknowledged. This practice presents a host of potential problems for hospitals that maintain patient registers at their switchboards and information desks. Institutions must devise methods of identifying drug or alcohol abuse patients so that their personnel do not inadvertently release information in violation of the law.

The courts have generally construed the statute and regulations in favor of protecting patients' confidentiality.[28] However, the courts have been reluctant to enforce the statute and rules where doing so would impede investigations under state child abuse statutes.[29] In August 1986, the Congress passed legislation permitting disclosures to be made from alcohol and drug abuse patient records without patient consent pursuant to state child abuse reporting statutes.[30]

Privacy Act Records

The Privacy Act of 1974[31] prohibits the disclosure of records maintained on individuals by federal government agencies (including those agencies that operate hospitals) and by government contractors, except under the conditions and subject to the exceptions specified in the Privacy Act. The records governed by the Privacy Act may be disclosed if requested by or with the prior written consent of the individual to whom the records pertain. The Privacy Act not only permits individuals to gain access to information pertaining to themselves in federal agency records but also to obtain copies of the records and to correct or amend the records.[32] Such records may also be disclosed without such individual's consent to the persons and agencies set forth in the act.

The Privacy Act requires federal agencies to collect, maintain, use, or disseminate any record of identifiable personal information in a manner that ensures that such actions are for a necessary and lawful purpose, that the information is current and accurate for its intended use, and that adequate safeguards are provided to prevent misuse.[33] Hospitals operated by the federal government are bound by the Privacy Act's requirements regarding the disclosure of their patients' medical records. Also, medical records maintained in a records system operated pursuant to a contract with a federal government agency are subject to the provisions of the Privacy Act.[34] For example, hospitals that maintain registers of cancer patients pursuant to a federal government contract or federally funded health maintenance organization are subject to the Privacy Act.[35]

Freedom of Information Act Records

The Freedom of Information Act (FOIA), enacted by Congress in 1966, requires agencies of the federal government to make certain information available for public inspection and copying.[36] Although the FOIA makes disclosure the general rule, it permits specifically exempted information to be withheld; one specifically exempt category includes "personnel and medical files and similar files the disclosure of which would constitute a clearly unwarranted invasion of personal privacy."[37]

There are three prerequisites for the application of this exception, commonly known as Exception 6: (1) the information must be contained in a personnel, medical, or similar file; (2) disclosure of the information must constitute an invasion of personal privacy; and (3) the severity of the invasion of personal privacy must outweigh the public's interest in the disclosure.[38] In determining whether information sought is within this exception, the relevant consideration is whether the privacy interests that arise from the information sought are similar to those arising from personnel or medical files and not whether the information is recorded in a manner similar to a personnel or medical record.[39]

In ruling on an Exception 6 claim, a court must determine *de novo* (1) whether the materials requested fall within the type of matter covered by the exemption, and if so, (2) whether the disclosure would constitute a clearly unwarranted invasion of personal privacy.[40] The courts have held that where there is an all-important public interest in obtaining the information, the private interest in preventing disclosure must give way to the superior public interest, particularly where the invasion of privacy is minimal.[41]

The language, "clearly unwarranted invasion of personal privacy," has been interpreted by the courts as an expression of a congressional policy that favors disclosure and an instruction to the courts to tilt the balance in favor of disclosure.[42] The United States Supreme Court has held that there is no blanket exemption for personnel files; nonconfidential information cannot be insulated from disclosure merely because it is stored by the agency in "personnel" files.[43] The exemption instead requires a balancing of the individual's right of privacy against the preservation of the public's right to governmental information.[44]

A file is considered "similar" to personnel and medical files if it contains intimate details of an individual's life, family relations, personal health, religious and philosophical beliefs, and other matters that, if revealed, would prove personally embarrassing to an individual of normal sensibilities.[45] Whether materials are "similar files" turns on whether the facts that would be revealed would infringe on some privacy interest as highly personal or as intimate in nature as that at stake in personnel and medical records; the court must then proceed to weigh this privacy interest against the public's interest in general disclosure.[46]

An agency is required to provide reasonably segregable nonexempt portions of an otherwise exempt record to any person requesting such a record.[47] Agencies that maintain medical records or have obtained medical records legitimately from a hospital are required by the Privacy Act[48] and by this exemption to the FOIA to withhold disclosure of such records unless a court, in balancing individual and public interests in the information, orders disclosure or unless such records are requested by Congress.

Although medical records maintained by an agency need not be disclosed, disclosure may be required of any information taken from a hospital's medical records by medical researchers in connection with government-funded medical investigation and incorporated into research reports to a sponsoring agency. The United States Supreme Court has held that a grantee's data will become subject to disclosure under the FOIA if it can be shown that the agency directly controlled the day-to-day activities of the grantee hospital.[49] Hospitals that receive federal funds for purposes of medical research, therefore, can minimize the risk of disclosure of research data by avoiding extensive agency supervision of studies conducted by hospital staff and by obtaining the agency's acknowledgment that the data are confidential and will not be disclosed except as required by law. Several states have adopted freedom of information acts. In construing these acts, state courts differ as to the extent of protection they will give records subject to the statutes.[50]

Peer Review Organizations

The Peer Review Organization (PRO) program, which replaced the Professional Standards Review Organization (PSRO) program in 1982, maintains many of the same recordkeeping requirements as those imposed on PSROs. The PRO law requires that PROs disclose, in accordance with procedures established by the federal Department of Health and Human Services (HHS), review information: (1) to state or federal fraud and abuse agencies; (2) to federal and state agencies responsible for identifying cases involving risks to the public health; and (3) to state licensure or certification agencies.[51]

One very significant provision in the PRO law expressly specifies that a PRO is not to be considered a federal agency.[52] The intent of this provision is to preclude litigation similar to that experienced under the PSRO law, where attempts to declare PSROs federal agencies for purposes of FOIA requests led to conflicting court decisions.

The PRO regulations require a PRO to hold patient-identifying information in confidence, unless such information is requested by the patient or the patient's authorized representative or unless disclosure of such information is otherwise permitted by statute or regulation.[53] If the PRO intends to disclose confidential information, it must notify the patient's treating physician and appropriate institution, except in cases involving possible violations of fraud and abuse prohibitions. The regulations provide for fines or imprisonment for unauthorized disclosure of such information.

A PRO is authorized to have access to and obtain the records pertinent to services furnished to Medicare patients and held by any institution in the PRO's area. The PRO may also gain access to non-Medicare patient records relating to a non-Medicare review by the PRO if such access is authorized by state law.[54]

Statutory Reporting and Other Disclosure Requirements

Many state statutes and regulations and a few federal regulations require hospitals to disclose confidential medical record information without the patient's authorization. Medical records, for example, may be released to the receiving facility when a patient is transferred to another health care facility,[55] when they are required by the state's board of medical examiners,[56] when state health department inspectors[57] or county medical examiners[58] request them, or when the hospital closes and must send its patient records to another institution.[59]

Disclosure of medical record information made pursuant to statutory or regulatory requirements does not subject a hospital or practitioner to liability, even if the disclosure is made against the patient's express wishes. As these statutory provisions authorizing release of medical records vary from state to state, hospitals should be aware of the special disclosure rules applicable in their jurisdictions.[60]

Child Abuse

The child abuse reporting laws of most jurisdictions require hospitals and practitioners to report cases of actual or suspected child abuse. The statutes also protect persons making such reports in good faith from liability for improper disclosure of confidential information, even if the report is erroneous.[61]

Drug Abuse

Some states require physicians and others to identify patients who obtain drugs that are subject to abuse so that patient names and addresses can be entered into a state registry.[62]

Poison and Industrial Accidents

A few states require physicians to report any illness or disease that they believe was contracted in connection with employment.[63] The purpose of these statutes is to enable public health officials to investigate occupational diseases and to recommend methods for eliminating or preventing them.

Abortion

Several states require hospitals and practitioners to report abortions they perform[64] and any complications that may develop.[65] Other states require hospitals to report fetal deaths, including those resulting from abortions.[66] Courts have held these requirements to be rationally related to a compelling state interest in maternal health and not to be an infringement upon the physician-patient relationship, the right to an abortion, or any personal right of privacy.[67]

Cancer

A few states require disclosure of information from the medical records of cancer patients to central state or regional tumor registries.[68] Usually operated by statewide tax-exempt organizations funded by federal grants, the registries rely to a large extent upon the cooperation of individual hospital registries. They obtain patient information directly from participating hospitals pursuant to agreements between the hospitals and the registry.

In the absence of a state reporting statute or other statutory or regulatory authority for reporting patient information to a registry, disclosure of such information without the patient's authorization may subject the hospital to liability for improper release of confidential data. Hospitals that have chosen to participate in a cancer or other registry should seek statutory or regulatory authority for release of medical record information to such registries. If legislative action is impractical, participating hospitals should exercise care in drafting agreements with registries. Such contracts should contain safeguards against improper disclosure of confidential information by the registry and an indemnification of the hospitals for claims against them that may result from their release of data to the registry or from improper disclosure by the registry.

Communicable Diseases

Communicable disease reporting laws requiring hospitals and practitioners to inform public health authorities of infectious disease cases are among the oldest compulsory reporting statutes in many states.[69] The laws attempt to balance a patient's right to confidentiality against the government's need for identifying information in order to protect the general welfare. Hospitals should disclose only the information required by the statute.

AIDS

The competing policy interests surrounding the issue of confidentiality are particularly acute in the context of the recent AIDS (acquired immune deficiency syndrome) crisis. While AIDS victims have a compelling interest in preserving confidentiality, government surveillance and research are imperative to protect the general public and eradicate this fatal disease.

In response to these conflicting policy considerations, several states have enacted legislation addressing the distribution and use of AIDS screening test results. Laws in California, Florida, and Wisconsin prohibit the disclosure of AIDS test results to third parties, except as provided by the statutes.[70] While the California and Florida statutes forbid the use of test results for insurance and employment purposes,[71] the Wisconsin law restricts insurance companies from considering test results unless the state authorities determine that the test is "reliable" for use in underwriting insurance policies. The Wisconsin law also imposes specific restrictions on use of test results by employers unless the state declares that a particular individual poses a significant risk of transmitting the infection through employment.

Reporting and notification requirements mandated at the local, state, and federal levels present a real threat to the confidentiality rights of AIDS victims. Florida law requires hospitals and physicians to notify individuals who have been in direct contact with patients subsequently diagnosed with AIDS, although specific names remain confidential.[72] In New York, the state health commissioner declared AIDS a reportable disease and provided that all such reports shall be confidential.[73]

Thus far, no specific federal regulations have been imposed instructing hospitals to follow special disclosure procedures regarding the medical records of AIDS patients.[74] Nonetheless, the Centers for Disease Control (CDC), which is authorized to assume the surveillance of communicable diseases, receives reports of AIDS cases from state and local health departments. The CDC's Field Activities Unit instituted an AIDS surveillance and monitoring program aimed at obtaining AIDS reports. While some hospitals, state health departments, and physicians voluntarily comply with the CDC's reporting requests, they are not legally required to do so.[75] Once the CDC acquires information pertaining to the AIDS victims, it must comply with the Privacy Act of 1974 and the regulations promulgated by the Department of Health and Human Services in its confidential maintenance of the medical records.[76] The Privacy Act's broad exceptions and permissive standards, however, may limit the confidentiality protection afforded to AIDS patients at the federal level.

Misadministration of Radioactive Materials and Blood Transfusion Reactions

Federal regulations require hospitals to report to the Nuclear Regulatory Commission any misadministration of radioactive materials. Misadministration is defined as the administration of a radiopharmaceutical or radiation other than the one intended, and of a radiopharmaceutical or radiation given to the wrong patient or administered to the right patient by a route other than that prescribed by the physician.[77] Regulations also require hospitals to report to the director of the Bureau of Biologics of the federal Food and Drug Administration all fatalities resulting from collection or transfusion of blood.[78]

Access by Hospital Staff

Hospital policy generally allows members of its medical and nursing staff access to patient records, without patient consent, for certain authorized purposes. It is the hospital's responsibility, however, to safeguard both the record and its content against loss, defacement, and tampering, and use by unauthorized individuals. These guidelines are generally set forth in hospital or medical staff bylaws, and less frequently in state statutes or regulations.

In the absence of state statutory law,[79] the majority of hospitals allow access to a patient's medical record to those persons directly involved in the care of that patient. Patients' medical records may also be examined for required clinical and financial auditing purposes, for utilization review and for other quality assurance activities. Records may also be available for research purposes provided that all patient identifying information is deleted when the research data are tabulated and reported. Nontreating physicians, therefore, will generally not have automatic access to patients' medical records unless the records are used for the purposes previously discussed.

Hospital policies should include the procedures that medical and hospital staff members should follow to obtain access to medical records. These procedures may be incorporated in hospital or medical staff bylaws and regulations as well as in appropriate hospital policy manuals.

Disclosures for Medical Research

Many medical research projects involve the use of patients' medical records. These records are typically used to determine response to specific types of therapy relative to population characteristics and incidence of illness, or to obtain statistical information important to the development of more efficient treatment protocols. Most states, therefore, have adopted the position that medical and nursing staff members may examine patient records for medical research purposes.[80] A minority of states also allow approved medical investigators access to patients' medical records.[81] Hospitals that permit their staffs to conduct medical research studies, however, should establish an institutional review board (IRB) or other medical review committee to evaluate the risk to the patient and the potential benefits of the research.

State statutes and regulations are not uniform in their regulation of access to records for research purposes. Some grant access to individuals who undertake studies with appropriate medical staff approval.[82] Others limit access to health care providers and insurers.[83]

In the absence of state regulations establishing stricter standards for the disclosure of patients' medical records for use in conducting biomedical or epidemiological research, without patient authorization, the IRB or research committee should require that the following safeguards are met before authorizing disclosure of these confidential records to medical investigators:

1. The information will be treated as confidential.
2. The information will be communicated only to qualified investigators pursuing an approved research program designed for the benefit of the health of the community.
3. Adequate safeguards to protect the record or information from unauthorized disclosure will be established.
4. The results of the investigation will be presented in a way that prevents identification of individual subjects.

Hospitals should prohibit access to medical records by investigators whose medical studies do not include at least these safeguards as determined by the IRB or other appropriate committee, barring statutory law to the contrary.

Government Agencies

Health care facilities have a strong privacy interest in their medical records, and as a general rule the hospital may refuse to release records to government officials. However, such government officials are entitled to search and seize medical records if they first obtain a judicially issued search warrant. Because a search warrant requires the approval of a neutral magistrate and must specifically state the place to be searched, the objects to be seized, and the reason for the search, it effectively denies general "fishing expeditions" by the government. Nevertheless, in some instances government officials are entitled to access to medical records even in the absence of a search warrant.

The Fourth Amendment to the United States Constitution is the source of the search warrant requirement. It protects persons and their houses, papers, and effects from unreasonable searches and seizures.[84] Although the amendment was intended to apply primarily to private residences, its proscription of warrantless searches as presumptively unreasonable applies to commercial premises as well.[85] Generally, therefore, government access to medical records without a search warrant is presumptively unreasonable and violates the Fourth Amendment.

Although the search warrant requirement has been almost exclusively associated with criminal investigations, the Supreme Court of the United States has specifically stated that administrative or regulatory searches also come within the Fourth Amendment's scope.[86] Whether a court will impose a warrant requirement on an administrative search, however, depends on whether the search is designed to enforce a general regulatory scheme or is aimed at specific licensed industries.[87] The Supreme Court has required a warrant when an administrative search is conducted pursuant to general regulatory legislation that applies to all residences, structures, or employers within a given jurisdiction. Recent state and lower federal court decisions also recognize these two basic types of administrative searches, concerning both general regulatory schemes and specific licensed industries, and have analyzed situations involving government access to health care facilities generally and medical records specifically.

State courts have upheld warrantless searches of nursing homes,[88] convalescent hospitals,[89] pharmacies,[90] and day care centers,[91] but have invalidated statutes that allowed warrantless searches of hospitals and clinics that perform abortions.[92]

If the government does obtain a search warrant, a medical facility could nevertheless be subject to a government "fishing expedition" if the warrant is not sufficiently detailed. The warrant must state with particularity the scope and place to be searched. A court cannot properly issue a warrant based on a government assertion of "valid public interest"; rather, the government must state specifically why it requires a search of specific medical records. The object of the warrant procedure is to take away from the government the unfettered discretion to inspect and seize any medical records. Thus, a hospital that believes a search warrant is insufficiently particular should affirmatively withhold consent to the search, for consent to an administrative search can be easily implied. On the other hand, a search warrant that states in detail the time and place of the search, and the specific records to be searched, must be obeyed.

Law Enforcement Agencies

As a general rule, hospitals should not release medical records or other patient information to law enforcement personnel without the patient's authorization. In the absence of statutory authority or legal process, a police agency has no authority to examine a medical record. If, however, a law enforcement official provides the facility with a valid court order or subpoena, the hospital with the advice of its attorney should provide the information requested.

Upon the advice of its attorney, the hospital may determine that it would be in the community's best interest to release specific medical record information to law enforcement personnel. To do so, the hospital may rely upon the doctrine of qualified privilege. This common law doctrine permits a party (i.e., the hospital) with a duty or a legitimate interest in conveying the information to make communications to a second party (i.e., the law enforcement agency) with a corresponding interest in receiving the particular information. The data must be transferred in good faith, given without malice, and based upon reasonable grounds.[93] Thus, the doctrine of qualified privilege protects the hospital only if the law enforcement officer who receives the medical record information acts under the authority of law. Before releasing such information, hospital personnel should determine that there is a basis for the request and that the officer requesting it is performing official duties. The information should be released only if appropriate to the purpose for which the particularized request is made; a hospital should not release a patient's entire record unless there are reasonable grounds for doing so. For example, if the law enforcement officer is requesting the results of a blood alcohol test, the hospital should not release information concerning the patient's unrelated prior hospitalization for a fractured leg.

In addition to the doctrine of qualified privilege and cases involving court subpoenas, there are statutory exceptions to the general rule requiring hospitals to refrain from releasing patient information to law enforcement agencies in the absence of patient consent. State law varies widely concerning the release of medical record information to government agencies without patient authorization.

Thus, some patient records, such as those concerning victims of crime or carriers of contagious disease not specifically designated by statute, may be revealed to government officials without the patient's consent in the course of routine police investigations or public health inquiries. Such a disclosure, however, should only be made pursuant to the state statute's confidentiality restrictions. In these situations, the hospital should demonstrate respect for the patient's privacy rights by seeking disclosure consent from the patient, preferably during the hospital admissions process.

State law also varies widely as to a hospital's duty to report certain kinds of information, such as cases involving gunshot or knife wounds,[94] child abuse,[95] and disorders impairing a motorist's ability to drive safely.[96] In states having these types of reporting statutes, a patient's consent is not required in order to release the record. In fact, under some statutes hospitals may be guilty of criminal misdemeanor if they do not report certain cases.[97]

NOTES

1. Joint Commission on Accreditation of Hospitals, Accreditation Manual for Hospitals 101 (1987).

2. See Miss. Code Ann. §41-9-65 (1972); Tenn. Code Ann. §68-11-304 (1983).

3. Pa. Regulations on General and Special Hospitals §115.28, 7 Pa. B. 3657 (1977); Kan. Hosp. Regulations, §28-34-9 (1974).

4. Rabens v. Jackson Park Hospital Foundation, 40 Ill. App. 3d 113, 351 N.E. 2d 276 (1976); ·Pyramid Life Insurance Co. v. Masonic Hospital Association of Payne County, 191 F. Supp. 51 (W.D. Okla. 1961).

5. Hampton Clinic v. District Court of Franklin County, 231 Iowa 65, 300 N.W. 646 (1941).

6. See generally, Killion, Patients' Rights to Their Medical Records, Health Span, Vol 2 No. 2 (Feb. 1985).

7. See, e.g., Iowa Code Ann. §22.7-2 (West Supp. 1986); Minn. Stat. Ann. §144.69 (West 1970); N.H. Rev. Stat. Ann. §126-A: 4-a (1977); N.M. Stat. Ann. §14-6-1 (1978); N.Y. Pub. Health Law §2805-g(3) (McKinney Supp. 1983–84); N.D. Cent. Code §23-16-09 (1978).

8. See, e.g., Cal. Civ. Code §§56.10–56.11 (West Supp. 1986); M.D. Health-Gen. Code Ann. §4-301 (1982).

9. See Parkson v. Central DuPage Hospital, 105 Ill. App. 3d 850, 435 N.E. 2d 140 (1982); Rabens v. Jackson Park Hospital Foundation, 40 Ill. App. 3d 113, 351 N.E. 2d 276 (1976); Cannell v. Medical and Surgical Clinic, 21 Ill. App. 3d 383, 315 N.E. 2d 278 (1974).

10. JCAH, Accreditation Manual for Hospitals 101–102 (1987).

11. Wallace v. University Hospitals of Cleveland, 164 N.E.2d 917 (Common Pleas Ct., Ohio, 1959), aff'd and modified, 170 N.E.2d 261 (Ohio Ct. App. 1960), motion to dismiss granted, 171 Ohio St. 487, 172 N.E.2d 459 (1961). See also Pyramid Life Ins. Co. v. Masonic Hosp. Assn, 191 F. Supp. 51 (W.D. Okla. 1961).

12. Hutchins v. Texas Rehabilitation Commission, 544 S.W.2d 802 (Tex. Civ. App. 1976).

13. 40 Ill. App. 3d 113, 351 N.E.2d 276 (1976); See also Thurman v. Crawford 652 S.W. 2d 240 (Mo. Ct. App. 1983).

14. Ill. Rev. Stat. ch. 110, §8-2001 (1985).

15. 396 F.2d 931 (D.C. Cir. 1967).

16. Several of the statutes that authorize the patient or the patient's representative to inspect records do not permit inspection of records until after the patient has been discharged from the hospital. See, e.g., Fla. Stat. Ann. §395.017 (West Supp. 1986); Ill. Rev. Stat. ch. 110 §8-2001 (1985).

17. See, e.g., Wisc. Stat. Ann. §51.30 (Supp. 1985).

18. See, e.g., Ill. Rev. Stat. ch. 91 1/2, §804 (1985).

19. See, e.g., Cynthia B. v. New Rochelle Hosp. Med. Center, 60 N.Y. 2d 452, 458 N.E. 2d 363, 470 N.Y. S. 2d 122 (1983) involving a hospital whose policy barred disclosure of sensitive psychiatric

records even when authorized by a former patient; Doe v. Comm'r of Mental Health, 372 Mass. 534, 362 N.E.2d 920 (1977); Sullivan v. State, 352 So.2d 1212 (Fla. Dist. Ct. App. 1977).

20. 144 N.J. Super. 579, 366 A.2d 733 (1976).

21. *See, e.g.*, MISS. CODE ANN. §41-41-11 (1972); MINN. STAT. ANN. §144.335 (West Supp. 1986).

22. *See, e.g.*, COLO REV. STAT. §25-1-801 (Supp. 1985); ILL. REV. STAT. ANN. ch. 110, ¶8-2001 (1985); S.D. CODIFIED LAWS §34-12-15 (Supp. 1983).

23. *See, e.g.*, MONT. REV. CODE ANN. §50-16-311 (1985); OKLA. STAT. ANN. tit. 76, §19 (Supp. 1986); WISC. STAT ANN. §804.10 (1977).

24. *See* current version at 42 U.S.C. §290ee-3 (Supp. 1986).

25. 42 U.S.C. §290dd-3 (Supp. 1986).

26. 42 C.F.R. §2.12(a) (1985).

27. *Id.* at §2.11(o).

28. *See, e.g.*, In the Matter of the Death of William Kennedy, No. SP-1724-80 (D.C. Super. Jan. 14, 1981); Raleigh Hills Hospital v. KUTV, No. C-81-0800 (D. Utah, Nov. 19, 1981); United States v. Banks, 520 F.2d 627 (7th Cir. 1975); Heartview Found. v. Glaser, 361 N.W.2d 232 (N.D. 1985) (holding that patients' failure to use pseudonyms to conceal their identities, while undergoing treatment at alcohol and drug abuse treatment center, was not a waiver of their privilege to confidentiality under North Dakota law); United States v. Smith, 789 F.2d 196 (3rd Cir. 1986) (holding that the public interest in confidentiality outweighs the defendant's need when disclosure of alcohol treatment records would only marginally impugn the witness-patient's credibility).

29. *See, e.g.*, State of Minnesota v. Anedring, 342 N.W. 2d 128 (Minn. 1984).

30. The Children's Justice and Assistance Act of 1986, Pub. L. No. 99-401, 100 Stat. 903 (1986).

31. 5 U.S.C. §552a (1977 & Supp. 1986).

32. *Id.* §552a(d) (1977).

33. *Id.* §552a(f) (1977).

34. *Id.* §552a(m) (1977).

35. *Id.* §552 (1977 & Supp. 1986).

36. 5 U.S.C. §552(a)(2) (1977).

37. 5 U.S.C. §552(b)(6) (1977).

38. Metropolitan Life Ins. Co. v. Usery, 426 F. Supp. 150 (D.D.C. 1976); De Planche v. Califano, 549 F. Supp. 685 (W.D. Mich. 1982); Ripskis v. Dept. of Housing and Urban Development, 746 F.2d 1, 241 U.S. App. D.C. 8 (1984).

39. Harbolt v. Dept. of State, 616 F.2d 772 (5th Cir.), *cert. denied*, 449 U.S. 856 (1980).

40. Plain Dealer Publishing Co. v. U.S. Dept. of Labor, 471 F. Supp. 1023 (D.D.C. 1979).

41. Campbell v. U.S. Civil Service Comm'n, 539 F.2d 58 (10th Cir. 1976). *See also* Florida Medical Ass'n, Inc. v. U.S. Dept. of Health Education and Welfare, 479 F. Supp. 1291 (M.D. Fla. 1979); Washington Post Co. v. U.S. Dept. of Health and Human Services, 690 F.2d 252 (D.D.C. 1982).

42. Dittow v. Shultz, 517 F.2d 166 (D.C. Cir. 1975); Celmins v. U.S. Dept. of Treasury, 457 F. Supp. 13 (D.D.C. 1977).

43. Dept. of the Air Force v. Rose, 425 U.S. 352 (1976).

44. *Id.* at 380. *See also* Jaffee v. C.I.A., 573 F. Supp. 377 (D.D.C. 1983); New England Apple Council v. Donovan, 725 F.2d 139 (1st Cir. 1984).

45. Pacific Molasses Co. v. N.L.R.B. Regional Office 15, 577 F.2d 1172 (5th Cir. 1978); Rural Housing Alliance v. U.S. Dept. of Agriculture, 498 F.2d 73 (D.C. Cir. 1974); Sims v. C.I.A., 642 F.2d 562 (D.C. Cir. 1980).

46. Board of Trade of City of Chicago v. Commodity Futures Trading Comm'n, 627 F.2d 392 (D.C. Cir. 1980); Shaw v. U.S. Dept. of State, 559 F. Supp. 1053 (D.D.C. 1983); Public Citizen Health Research Group v. F.D.A. 704 F.2d 1280 (D.D.C. 1983).

47. 5 U.S.C. §552(b) (1977).

48. Id. §552a (1977 & Supp. 1986).

49. Forsham v. Harris, 445 U.S. 169, 180 (1980). See also Ciba-Geigy Corp. v. Matthews, 428 F. Supp. 523 (S.D.N.Y. 1977).

50. See, e.g., Baxter County Newspapers, Inc. v. Medical Staff of Baxter General Hospital, 622 S.W. 2d 495 (Ark. 1981); Head v. Colloton, 131 N.W. 2d 870 (Iowa 1983); Short v. Board of Managers of The Nassau County Medical Center, 57 N.Y.S. 2d 399 (1982). In the absence of a state freedom of information act, the New Jersey Supreme Court applied a judicially created standard of disclosure for confidential investigative hospital records. McClain v. College Hospital, 99 N.J. 346, 492 A.2d 991 (1985). Referring to the federal FOIA as a model, the court held that

the standard is a showing of particularized need that outweighs the public interest in confidentiality of the investigative proceedings, taking into account: (1) the extent to which the information may be available from other sources, (2) the degree of harm that the litigant will suffer from its unavailability, and (3) the possible prejudice to the agency's investigation. Id.

51. 42 U.S.C. §1320c-9(b)(1) (1983).

52. Id. §1320c-9(a).

53. 42 C.F.R. §476.101-143 (1985).

54. 42 C.F.R. §476.111(b) (1985).

55. MD. HEALTH-GEN. CODE ANN. §4-301 (1982).

56. NEV. REV. STAT. 629.061 (1985).

57. N.Y. MENTAL HYGIENE LAW §31.09 (McKinney 1978).

58. Cook County Ordinance, ch. 5 §36 (1980).

59. MISS. CODE ANN. §41-9-79 (1972).

60. See generally Lehner, Disclosure of Patient-Health Care Records, WISC. BAR BULL. 16 (August 1984) for discussion of the challenge confronting health care professionals in attempting to interpret and apply complex confidentiality laws.

61. See, e.g., FLA. STAT. ANN. §827.07(g) (West 1976); MONT. CODE ANN. §41-3-203 (1985); Harris v. City of Montgomery, 435 So.2d 1207 (Ala. 1983); c.f., Hope v. Landau, 21 Mass. App. Ct. 240, 486 N.E.2d 89 (1985) (noting that correctness or good faith of psychologists' suspicions of child abuse were not material to issue of liability for improper disclosure) (emphasis added). For a thorough discussion of child abuse reporting, see Fraser, A Glance at the Past, a Glance at the Present, a Glimpse at the Future: A Critical Analysis of the Development of Child Abuse Reporting Statutes, CHICAGO-KENT L.R. 641 (1978).

62. See, e.g., ILL. ANN. STAT. ch. 56 1/2 §§1311, 1312(a); (Smith-Hurd 1985); CAL. HEALTH AND SAFETY CODE §11167 (West Supp. 1986); Whalen v. Roe, 429 U.S. 589 (1977). See also Volkman v. Miller, which held valid the maintenance of computerized cases on crisis center outpatients, 52 A.D. 2d 146, 383 N.Y.S. 2d 95 (1976). But see Commonwealth v. Donoghue, 4 Mass. App. Ct. 752, 358 N.E. 2d 465 (Mass. App. 1976), reporting statute was held to be unconstitutionally vague.

63. See, e.g., GA. CODE ANN. §34-9-209 (1982); MINN. STAT. ANN. §144.34 (West Supp. 1986).

64. MINN. STAT. ANN. §145.413 (West Supp. 1986).

65. See e.g., ILL. ANN. STAT. ch. 38, §81-30.1 (Smith-Hurd Supp. 1986).

66. See e.g., N.Y. PUBL. HEALTH LAW §4160 (McKinney 1985).

67. *See e.g.*, Schulman v. New York City Health and Hosp. Corp. 38 N.Y. 2d 234, 342, N.E. 2d 501, 379 N.Y.S. 2d 702 (1975).

68. *See, e.g.*, MINN. STAT. ANN. §144.68 (West. Supp. 1986).

69. *See, e.g.*, CONN. GEN. STAT. ANN. §19a-215 (West 1986); N.Y. PUB. HEALTH LAW §201 (McKinney 1971 & Supp. 1986).

70. 1985 CAL. STAT., ch. 23; FLA. STAT. ANN. §381.606; 1985 Wis. Laws, Act 73.

71. 1985 CAL. STAT., ch. 22; FLA. STAT. ANN. §381.606.

72. FLA. STAT. ANN. §395.0147; 1985 Proposed Rules, Fla. Dept. of Health and Rehabilitative Services, §§10D-28.129 through 10D-28.131.

73. 10 N.Y.C.R.R. §§24-1.1, 24-1.2 (1985).

74. In addition, the JCAH 1986 ACCREDITATION MANUAL FOR HOSPITALS fails to mention AIDS.

75. *See* Siegner, *AIDS Patients' Confidentiality is Medical Records Challenge*, MODERN HEALTHCARE, November 22, 1985, at 86; National Academy Press, CONFRONTING AIDS: DIRECTION FOR PUBLIC HEALTH CARE AND RESEARCH, at 64 (1986).

76. *See* LAMBA LEGAL DEFENSE AND EDUCATION FUND, INC., *AIDS LEGAL GUIDE: A PROFESSIONAL RESOURCE ON AIDS-RELATED LEGAL ISSUES AND DISCRIMINATION*, at 22 (1984).

77. 45 Fed. Reg. §31701 (1980).

78. 21 C.F.R. §606.170(b) (1986).

79. *See e.g.*, R.I. GEN. LAWS §5-37.3-4 (Supp. 1985); WYO. ANN. STAT. §35-2-601 (1977); ILL. ANN. STAT. ch. 110 §§8-2101-2105 (Smith-Hurd 1985 & Supp. 1986); (S.C. Health and Environmental Control Dept. R61-16 (1982)); JCAH, ACCREDITATION MANUAL FOR HOSPITALS 101-102 (1987).

80. R.I. GEN. LAWS §5-37.3-4 (Supp. 1985); WYO. ANN. STAT. §35-2-601 (1977); ILL. ANN. STAT. ch. 95-1/2 §11-501.3 (Smith-Hurd Supp. 1986) (authorizing the use of chemical testing results of patient-drivers' blood alcohol levels for medical and traffic safety research).

81. *See, e.g.*, Pa. Dept. of Pub. Health Rules and Regulations for Hospitals §115.27 (Purdon 1981). *See also* Kelsey, *Privacy and Confidentiality in Epidemiological Research Involving Patients*, IRB Rev. Hum. Subjects Research, Feb. 1981 at 1 (Publication by The Hastings Center, Hastings-on-Hudson, N.Y.).

82. *See* Hershey, *Using Patient Records for Research: The Response from Federal Agencies and the State of Pennsylvania*, IRB Rev. Hum. Subjects Research, Oct. 1981 at 8 (Publication by The Hastings Center, Hastings-on-Hudson, N.Y.).

83. OR. REV. STAT. §192.525 (Supp. 1981).

84. Camara v. Municipal Court, 387 U.S. 523 (1967).

85. *See* Marshall v. Barlow's, Inc., 436 U.S. 307, 312 (1978).

86. *See* See v. City of Seattle, 387 U.S. 541, 545 (1967). *See also* Camara, *supra* note 83, at 535.

87. *See, e.g.*, Colonnade Catering Corp. v. United States, 397 U.S. 72 (1970) (licensed liquor dealers); United States v. Biswell, 406 U.S. 311 (1972) (licensed firearms dealers).

88. People v. Firstenberg, 92 Cal. App. 3d 570, 155 Cal. Rptr. 80 (1979), *cert. denied*, 444 U.S. 1012 (1980); Uzzila v. Commissioner of Health, 47 A.D. 2d 492, 367 N.Y.S. 2d 795 (1975).

89. People v. White, 259 Cal. App. 2d Supp. 936, 65 Cal. Rptr. 923 (1968).

90. People v. Curco Drugs, Inc., 76 Misc. 2d 222, 350 N.Y.S. 2d 74 (1973).

91. Rush v. Obledo, 517 F. Supp. 905 (N.D. Cal. 1981).

92. Akron Center for Reproductive Health, Inc. v. City of Akron, 479 F. Supp. 1177 (N.D. Ohio 1979); Margaret S. v. Edwards, 488 F. Supp. 181 (E.D. La. 1980).

93. *See* Tarasoff v. Regents of the University of California, 17 Cal. 3d 425, 551 P.2d 334, 131 Cal. Rptr. 14 (1976) where the court held that the physician or the hospital had an affirmative duty to report a patient to law enforcement agencies because the patient's medical or psychological condition represented a foreseeable risk to third persons. The physician or hospital in this situation should have disclosed information that the patient had threatened to kill the eventual victim, since the physician and hospital are protected by the doctrine of qualified privilege. *See also* Hicks v. U.S., 357 F. Supp. 434 (D.D.C. 1973), *aff'd.* 511 F.2d 407 (D.C. Cir. 1975).

94. *See e.g.*, N.Y. PENAL LAW §265.25 (McKinney 1980 & Supp. 1986); CAL. PENAL CODE, §11160 (West 1982).

95. *See* Landeros v. Flood, 17 Cal. 3d 399, 551 P.2d 389, 131 Cal. Rptr. 69 (1976). *See generally* Paulsen, *Child Abuse Reporting Laws: The Shape of the Legislation*, 67 COLUM. L. REV. 1 (1967).

96. *See, e.g.*, CAL. HEALTH AND SAFETY CODE §410 (West 1982).

97. *See* CAL. PENAL CODE §11160-62 (West 1982).

Part V
Professional Management
Issues

Chapter 15

Institutional Ownership As an Ethical Issue

Kevin D. O'Rourke, OP

Does the type of institutional ownership present an ethical issue in health care? To put it another way, is it more fitting that health care be offered by a not-for-profit corporation rather than an investor-owned for-profit corporation? (The terms investor-owned and for-profit are often used synonymously. In this study, it is more accurate to use the term investor-owned.) The presence of for-profit or investor-owned corporations in health care is well established, and their activities have been evaluated frequently in relation to not-for-profit corporations. Most such evaluations have been made from an economic perspective.[1]

This evaluation of for-profit health care corporations will be from an ethical perspective. Ethics is the science and art of making beneficial human decisions; decisions that help individuals fulfill their innate and cultural needs. If one has a need, then fulfilling that need is a good or value for the person concerned; hence, ethics is concerned with needs, goods, and values. Values influence and determine human actions and human personality.[2] When a person has a need and capacity to pursue a value, we say that person has a right. If the need is innate or intrinsic to the person's well-being or goal in life, the need gives rise to a fundamental or inalienable right. Rights are fostered, protected, and attained through responsible actions. Hence, our consideration of values will necessarily bring into discussion the rights and responsibilities of those who need health care and those who provide this care. We shall therefore be concerned with the human values that are intrinsic to or intimately associated with striving for health and the provision of health care. After delineating and explaining these values, we shall consider whether or not investor-owned health care corporations promote or prevent the acquisition of such values.

Observers of the medical care scene in the United States may react to the consideration of values in health care with skepticism at best. After all, most American business executives and administrators are loathe to talk about or write about values.[3] Indeed, those who do pay lip service to values tend to treat them as gross abstractions, acceptable for discussion at conventions but too impractical to apply in planning or operations. Moreover, many will say that applying value considerations to the present health care situation in the United States is anachronistic. After all, investor-owned corporations are part of health care in the United States, so why call into question their right to exist?

While the quality of health care in the United States is defensible, the delivery system is flawed and thus many people do not have sufficient access to health care. The inequities of care, shortcomings in funding, monopolistic tendencies of suppliers, and lack of access for the poor have been too thoroughly documented to allow anyone to defend the present delivery system (or lack of system) as an ideal.[4] To those who react skeptically to this value analysis, I would offer two considerations. First, if change and renewal in the provision of health care are needed, then beneficial changes will not result if we merely tamper with the present delivery methods. Rather, let the changes in the system be dramatic, fundamental, and oriented to achieving the values inherent in health care. If we contend therefore that the breakdown in the health care system in the United States is due to a substitution of money for service as the goal of health care, it is not sufficient to say the service model of health care no longer exists in this country. Rather, if the service model responds to the needs and rights of the people seeking health care, then we must ask, "What changes are needed in the attitudes, ethics, and laws of people and corporations offering health care to restore the service model?" Second, in response to the view that a value-oriented analysis of health care is overly idealistic, especially in the face of present realities, we would affirm the fundamental worth and importance of value orientation. As Peters and Waterman state in their volume *In Search of Excellence*:

> Let us suppose that we were asked for one all-purpose bit of advice for management, one truth that we were able to distill from the excellent companies research. We might be tempted to reply, "Figure out your value system. Decide what your company stands for. What does your enterprise do that gives everyone the most pride? Put yourself out ten or twenty years in the future; what would you look back on with greatest satisfaction?"[5]

With these caveats in mind, let us proceed to consider the values inherent in health care and the rights and responsibilities associated with the attainment of those values.

THE MEANING OF HEALTH CARE

Health and health care are interdependent. Restoring health and preventing illness (a lack of health) are the goals of health care; hence, to understand the values associated with health care, one must possess a clear idea of human health. Ask the physician, nurse, or hospital administrator, "What is health?," and you are likely to receive a blank look in reply. Though there are thousands of people involved in health care in the United States, there is no consensus concerning the nature of health.

In an effort to formulate a health planning guide, Henrik Blum suggests the following definition:

> Health consists of the capacity of an organism (1) to maintain a balance appropriate to its age and social needs, in which it is reasonably free of gross dissatisfaction, discomfort, disease or disability; and (2) to behave in ways which promote the survival of the species as well as the self-fulfillment or enjoyment of the individual.[6]

Blum ends his discussion of human health with the brief formula, "Health is the state of being in which an individual does the best with the capacities he has, and acts in ways that maximize his capacities."[7] Because a human being is an organism, it is an open system. Hence, in maintaining balance or homeostasis, persons are continually relating to their environment. For our purposes, then, we shall conceive of health as optimal human functioning, which implies not only an internal harmony and consistency of function but also the capacity to maintain oneself in one's environment.

To understand this notion of health more fully, we must understand the needs and functions of the human person and how they are related. Otherwise, we may have a confused notion of human health. Briefly, human beings are born with the capacity to perform certain functions in response to felt needs. We have a capacity for knowledge; and because we feel a need for truth in order to understand and fulfill our purpose in life, we perform the function of learning. It is widely acknowledged that there are four categories of human needs and corresponding functions:

1. Biological or physiological functions, which correspond to needs human beings share with all living organisms: to maintain themselves homeostatically in a dynamic relation with their environment, to grow and mature to full biological development, and to continue the species through reproduction. Biologically, we need food, air, shelter, warmth, and so on.
2. Psychological functions, which correspond to the human needs to sense, imagine, and feel, and which enable humans to meet their needs for security, affirmation, and acceptance.
3. Social functions, which enable individuals to meet their needs for self-control and for peaceful and productive social relations within the context of their culture.
4. Spiritual or creative functions, which enable people to fulfill their need for commitment, integration, and transcendence. This function enables

persons not only to live within a culture but to criticize it, transcend it, and contribute to it.

The Limits of Medical Care

Given these basic needs and functions, it is extremely important to discern how they are related, for this will provide a blueprint for the quest for health and the limits of medical care. Is one function more important than another? If so, will it contribute more to health? Are the relationships among the various functions cooperative or competitive? Can one need or function be sacrificed for another without impairing the individual's health?

These four functions are not stories in a building, one on top of the other, but rather interrelated dimensions of human activity. Just as the length, height, and depth of a cube can be distinguished conceptually for sake of study, but not separated in reality, so the four functions of the human act are interconnected. Every truly human act involves all four functions. A human spiritual act, whether the creative act of a scientist or the loving act of a parent, at the same time involves a biological, psychological, and social function. True, one type of function will predominate in a human act, but all types will be present. The task of the creative function is to integrate the biological, psychological, and social functions. Thus, creative functions are the deepest, most central, and most complete.

At the same time, however, all these activities are rooted in and dependent upon the other functions in a network of interrelations. One cannot think unless one's brain is physiologically sound. Moreover, each function is to a certain extent autonomous, structurally and functionally differentiated, so that when help is needed to restore function, each function is served by a different discipline. To restore the physiological function, we call one trained in medicine; for the psychological function, one trained in psychology or psychiatry; for the social function, a social counselor or lawyer; for the creative-spiritual function, a teacher or spiritual director.

The Value of the Person

No matter which type of professional is called upon in an effort to integrate or improve human function—that is, to restore or maintain health—that individual does not assume the right to make decisions for the person being helped. The professional must always recognize the interrelatedness of all human functions, even if his or her effort is directed toward restoring only one function. Hence, the client must retain the creative function of making free, value-based decisions. This creative decision-making function is generally considered the essence of human worth and the primary activity by which one fulfills one's destiny or purpose in life. Through that type of creative action, basic decisions and commitments are made, leading to the integration of all human functions. By virtue of this function or power, people are of inestimable worth, and anyone who seeks to help another regain health must do so with reverence for this worth. The reverence and respect for the person and the creative function is the basis for requiring informed consent and other ethical norms such as confidentiality and truth telling that have been stressed in the practice of medicine in recent years.

The Meaning and Values of Medical Care

From the foregoing consideration of human health and human function, it is clear that physicians and all other medical care professionals must be concerned primarily with healing and physiological and psychological functions. However, their efforts at restoring these functions or preventing their failure must be performed with the awareness of the interrelatedness of all human functions. Thus, the term health care is more comprehensive than the term medical care because it refers to the restoration of the individual's capacity for integrative functioning. The term medical care refers more properly to what physicians and nurses do to help people regain or maintain health—that is, to restore physiological and psychological functioning. Confusion about the appropriate domain of medical care can lead to serious mistakes in the physician-patient relationship or in using the resources of society. Physicians who do not realize the interrelatedness of all human functions might think they have the right to make all decisions for the patient; health planning might be directed only to the amelioration of physiological problems without regard for their origin in psychological, social, or spiritual problems.

In keeping with this notion of human health, the patient is not passive in medical care. Rather, he or she retains the right of choosing medical means in accord with his or her value system. Even though patients present themselves in a wounded state of health, as a result of which they have lost some degree of self-determination, the patient's power to make his or her own decisions must be respected by the physician and all other persons in health care. Because of the good in question, and because there is a need to respect the spiritual integrity of the person who comes for help, a specific type of relationship arises between the physician and the patient, known familiarly as the professional relationship. The heart of this relationship is the avowal (profession) on the part of one person that he or she is willing to help another person attain a very important human good while at the same time respecting his or her personal worth and dignity. The professional promises to serve people in need; the ability of the person to pay for the help is a secondary consideration.

Today the term professional is applied casually to anyone who is adept at a job or trade and seeks to perform the work in a competent and honest manner. Thus, we might call an accountant or a plumber a professional. But in the proper meaning of the term, to be a professional implies something more than knowledge and skill. It implies as well a desire and ability to help a person with impaired function so that the person can become a better human being. Though an accountant or plumber may help a person with income tax or water supply, those services do not necessarily make the recipient a better human being. What makes a person a better human being is restoration of the capacity for fully integrated functioning, which in turn enables the person to strive for a meaningful life in an effective manner.

The professional, then, is concerned with a good that enables the person to become a better human being. Robert Merton explains the values of a professional as follows: "First, the value placed upon systematic knowledge and intellect: knowing. Second, the value placed upon mechanical skill and trained capacity: doing. And third, the value placed upon putting this conjoint knowledge and skill to work in the service of others: helping."[8] Kenneth Underwood further explains the service dimension of public responsibility: "These four concerns—concern for persons, trained skills, values and basic theory, and public responsibility—are the central themes of professional ideology always mentioned in the sociological literature on the professions and the professions' statement of purpose."[9]

Given the service value in the relationship between the professional and the person in need of help, it is evident that the relationship must be built upon trust. This is especially true in medicine, where the patient's vulnerability is multidimensional and the patient-physician relationship is intrinsically imbalanced. As Pellegrino and Thomasma state: "Medicine is . . . assistance and explanation, skill and commitment, all based on an ethic of trust which, in turn, is based on the ontological and sociological reality of an imbalanced relationship."[10]

To develop trust in the patient, the medical professional must do four things:

1. Develop knowledge and skill in medicine, good judgment, and facility at performing procedures. Personal warmth does not substitute for medical expertise.

2. Show concern for the patient's well-being. Trust will never exist if the patient believes that the physician is concerned only about the fee or is acting out of mere routine, like a machine or a functionary of a for-profit enterprise. Thus, the professional undertakes to help the client not because the client is worthy of help, nor because he or she is able to pay for the service, but primarily because of human need and the essential human rights based on need rather than on merit or ability to pay.

3. Communicate effectively with patients. A well-known study of hospital care showed that a high percentage of patients were incorrectly diagnosed because of the failure of physicians to listen carefully to patients' complaints and to recognize nonmedical factors in their condition.

4. Set or refuse an appropriate fee. Nothing destroys a trust relationship more quickly and more thoroughly than emphasis upon money as the basis for the relationship. Medical professionals, because of the good involved and the relationship to the patient, should not be paid according to laws of supply and demand. The good they are concerned with—health and life—is beyond price. At no time in the history of medicine has the profession operated totally in accordance with the market system, because there have always been people who needed help desperately but could not pay for it. Either the professional had to offer service free to the poor or a third party—for instance, a religious institution or the state—had to pay for it.

If our account of the values inherent in the medical relationship is accurate, then it is clear why profit cannot be the primary basis of any profession but must be considered a secondary and highly variable feature. Traditionally, a principle fundamental to all professions has been that the professional must be ready to give services free to those who are in need but cannot pay. The medical profession, like any true profession, must rest not upon bargaining or supply and demand but upon trust and service to those in need. No monetary value can be set on the spiritual guidance given by a minister, the defense of human rights provided by a lawyer, the search for truth shared by a teacher. Nor can any price be set upon the services of a physician in the battle to live. Thus, professional fees are not payments measured by the value of the service provided—which is truly priceless—but stipends that should be based solely on what professionals require to live in a manner that will free them to work without distraction, with liberty of mind and health of body, and adequately fulfill present and future family and social obligations. That some physicians still recognize this professional tenet is clear from a prominent physician's recent statement: "We must also be reasonable in our own demands for recompense. Doctors deserve a good living, but not an extravagant one. Greed and medical care are not compatible."[11]

Ultimately, the rewards in any profession are not to be found in extraneous gain. The rewards are intrinsic: the satisfaction of knowledge and of interesting and absorbing work and the joy that comes from helping people in their striving for a better life and in serving the individual and common good. Such an altruistic ideal is not easy to realize, nor is it often realized in its purest form; but even when imperfectly realized, it is the source of the medical profession's purpose and values. Whether this ideal is explicit or implicit in the physician's practice, for centuries medicine has brought out the best in people because of this ideal.

The specific responsibilities associated with professional trust apply as much to health care corporations such as clinics, hospitals, or surgicenters as to individual health care professionals. Corporations, after all, are recognized by law as entities (moral persons) pursuing the same goals as individuals, although ostensibly in a more effective manner. Thus the health care corporation is assessed and its responsibilities are determined not on the basis of its material constitution, since this differs from that of the individual person, but on the basis of its purpose. Corporations in medical care, then, must have the same primary goal as health care professionals: service to individuals in need of healing.

To build an atmosphere of trust, the corporation must maintain fiscal stability and make a surplus or profit. However, the ethical health corporation does not use its surplus to enrich investors, because this makes profit rather than service the purpose of the health care endeavor. Those who object that they can make a profit for investors and strive for service-oriented, compassionate medical care at the same time are confusing contradictory objectives. The situation in health care in our country illustrates this dichotomy. More and more, the poor are underserved as profit becomes the overriding goal of health care corporations. Unfortunately, even some nonprofit health care corporations misplace their priorities. Moreover, taking money out of the medical care system makes it more expensive than it should be and often results in more affluent individuals profiting from the suffering of the less affluent.

Conclusion

In view of the foregoing analysis of health care and the professional-patient relationship, the following value statements are normative for individuals and corporations involved in health care:

1. The primary and overriding purpose of medical care must be a desire to serve all whose physiological or psychological health is impaired, to enable them to lead a better life. Thus, assuring access to medical care for all persons is an important value to all health care professionals.
2. Those offering medical care must remember and respect the worth and autonomy of the individual.
3. The patient-physician relationship must be permeated by trust.
4. Medical care should not be considered a commodity, something to be bought or sold in a market system, because it is a precious and vital good to which no price can be attached, and because it is a prerequisite to the attainment of other human goods as well as to the pursuit of a meaningful life. Moreover, those who are most in need of medical care often have the least ability to pay for it.
5. Surplus funds over and above the money needed for expenses should not be taken out of the health care system by distribution to individual investors. Rather, the only appropriate disposition of any surplus is to continue and improve the quality of medical care and access to it.
6. Though persons and corporations offering medical care should receive an adequate stipend for service, they must fulfill their fundamental responsibility to care for those who cannot offer a stipend.

7. Because of their skill and their prominence in society, medical care professionals and corporations must assume leadership in the effort to establish
equity of access to medical care.

INVESTOR-OWNED MEDICAL CARE CORPORATIONS

The Nature of Investor-Owned Corporations

The term investor-owned medical care corporation refers to a for-profit corporation, usually a hospital or long-term care facility, that offers medical care
to patients and:

- involves a market system approach to health care, treating health care basically as a commodity;
- makes a profit for investors who are not personally involved in offering
  health care;
- in fact, and usually in self-description, considers "making a profit" to be
  the primary goal of the enterprise;
- renounces the personal responsibility of the corporation to care for the poor
  and to develop equitable access to health care for all persons.

Clearly, the goals and actions of the investor-owned medical care corporations
do not correspond to the value statements developed in the previous section.
Neither the goals nor the activities of these corporations coincide with service-
oriented, compassionate medical care. Moreover, these corporations consider
medical care not a profession, but a business—or, as the currently popular,
misguided phrase has it, "an industry." These corporations take money out of
the medical care system and refuse to assume the responsibility of offering care
for the poor and developing equal access to health care.

In order to substantiate our position that this description of investor-owned
medical care corporations is accurate and that these corporations are unethical,
because they do not serve the proper values of medical care, we shall consider
the arguments often put forth in support of investor-owned medical care corporations. The main defenses for the existence of investor-owned health care
corporations state that (1) treating medical care as a commodity will improve
the system of delivery by lowering costs and making the system more efficient
and more effective; (2) the investor-owned hospitals pay taxes and thus help care
for the poor; and (3) all medical care corporations must make a profit; therefore,
there is no difference between charitable and investor-owned hospitals.[12]

Medical Care As a Commodity

Proponents of investor-owned hospitals state that treating health care as a commodity is a logical step in creating a more effective and cost-efficient health care system. Competition is put forward as the solution to health care expense. But competition has led to higher prices in health care, especially given the well-documented realization that competition as we know it in United States health care is a word more than a reality.[13] While cost efficiency is a worthwhile goal, it must be subordinated to the more important and fundamental goal of assuring equitable access to medical care. Thus, to consider the assertion about effectiveness and efficiency from a value perspective, the type of good that health care offers must be considered carefully.

In its report entitled *Securing Access to Health Care*, the President's Commission for the Study of Ethical Problems in Medicine and Biomedical and Behavioral Research points out the nature of the human good involved in health care and the essential immorality of the market approach to health care:

> The private market does not adjust the financial burden of care to differences in income. Yet poverty and ill health are correlated—with the causal factors working in both directions. Therefore, the poor are in a double bind; they need more medical care but they have less money to purchase it or less insurance to secure it.[14]

Thus, the market approach deprives of health care those who need it most. Insofar as many cultural needs are concerned, it is appropriate to expect people to adjust their desires and wants (the fulfillment of their potential) to their ability to pay. The person who desires to see a movie or buy an automobile must pay for it. In this manner other people are enabled to earn income and to purchase goods and services.

But health care differs from most other goods and services because it is a good upon which the acquisition of income is based and upon which most other goods depend. It is an innate need. If one is ill or infirm, it is difficult to earn money to pay for the care that will enable one to regain health. Often the illness or infirmity is so severe that maintaining a limited health status is all that can be foreseen. Are people of such limited capacity to be declared ineligible for health care because they cannot pay for it? As the economist Eli Ginzberg points out, "To view the practice of medicine as just another business undertaking like retailing or banking is to blind to the role of agency in the work of a professional."[15] We should no more look upon medical care as a market commodity than we should police and fire protection. There is an element of public good and dire need in both of these services, as in health care, which makes it unethical to demand payment from those unable to pay. Thus, cost effectiveness is only one dimension of effectiveness—and a secondary one—in medical care. The primary measure is the service relationship and the access to care afforded to those who are most in need.

Taxes and Care for the Poor

Although we endorse a professional-patient relationship that involves a professional's personal responsibility to care for the poor, this does not signify that responsibility for improving the provision of health care rests solely with the health care professional or with health care corporations. Assuring access to health care is an obligation that must be borne by all the people and institutions of society.[16] Though state and federal governments are elements in society, they do not remove the personal responsibility from individuals or institutions. Therefore, it is invalid for doctors, nurses, hospitals, or other health care corporations to say, "Let the federal government take care of the poor." Nor is it valid to say, "We pay taxes, and care for the poor should come out of our taxes." Medical professionals, whether individuals or corporations, must realize their personal ethical responsibility to help those who cannot help themselves. They will fulfill this responsibility through personal care and through political activity designed to help those in need. The President's Commission expressed the complex balance of personal and social responsibilities in the following manner:

> Society has a moral obligation to ensure that everyone has access to adequate care without being subject to excessive burdens. . . . But the recognition of a collective or societal obligation does not imply that government should be the only or even the primary institution involved in the complex enterprise of making health care available. It is the Commission's view that the societal obligation to ensure equitable access for everyone may best be fulfilled in this country by a pluralistic approach that relies upon the coordinated contributions of actions by both the private and public sectors. . . . There is a strong tradition of private charity in the United States, including free services by health professionals, and charitable organizations continue to play an important role in health care delivery.[17]

Every person and corporation involved in health care has an ethical obligation to care for the poor, individually and collectively, and to work for equitable access to the system. The government should move in as required to fill the gaps and assure equity of access. Do investor-owned health care corporations accept a personal responsibility? Paul Starr notes:

> The profit-making hospitals clearly benefit from the structure of private health insurance and can be counted on to oppose any national health program that might threaten to end private reimbursement. The cor-

porate health services industry will also represent a powerful new force resisting public accountability and participation. A corporate sector in health care is also likely to aggravate inequalities in access to health care. Profit-making enterprises are not interested in treating those who cannot pay. The voluntary hospital may not treat the poor the same as the rich, but they do treat them and often treat them well.[18]

The de facto behavior of investor-owned health care corporations seems to confirm our evaluation. Leaders of the investor-owned hospitals have been heard to deny a personal responsibility to care for the poor. Michael Bromberg of the Federation of American Hospitals stated that investor-owned hospitals pay taxes "which in turn are used to support public hospitals."[19] One doubts that the accountants preparing the tax returns for investor-owned hospitals are told, "Don't cut any corners or claim any borderline exemptions; remember, our taxes will mean better health care for the poor." It seems far more likely that efforts would be made to pay as little tax as possible so there will be more profits to enrich investors. To put it another way, one seeks evidence to substantiate Bromberg's inference that investor-owned hospitals are committed to their responsibility to support society's efforts to provide adequate access to health care. For health care professionals and corporations, care for the poor is both a personal and a social responsibility. Is there evidence that either responsibility is fulfilled in investor-owned medical care? The pertinent literature does not justify an affirmative response.[20]

Profit and Medical Care

Could it not be argued that making a surplus or a profit is incumbent upon all health care corporations if they are to continue in existence and that therefore investor-owned corporations have a place in health care? Here we must be careful in our understanding of terms. A profit simply means that a corporate entity takes in more than it spends. In this sense, every health care corporation must make a profit in order to care for the future as well as the present. If there is no profit, the corporation will cease to exist. The denominations "for-profit" and "not-for-profit," then, are not clear enough for this discussion. Rather, the concern is what happens to the profits. Returning them to the health care system by using the surplus to improve quality of care, improve access, or provide needed equipment or buildings is an ethical use of profits; distributing them to investors who have no direct interest in supplying medical care is not.[21]

To distribute profits to investors has two results, both of which are unethical: (1) money is removed from the health care system, thus making health care cost more than it should; and (2) the trust that should characterize medicine is weakened and eventually destroyed. Paul Starr points out the inevitability of these results in discussing the consequences of the "coming of the corporation" into medical care:

> The organizational culture of medicine used to be dominated by the ideals of professionalism and voluntarism, which softened the underlying acquisitive activity. The restraint exercised by those ideals now grows weaker. The "health center" of one era is the "profit center" of the next.[22]

Not only do investor-owned medical corporations take money out of the system, but the manner in which they obtain their profits is open to ethical questions. "Creaming" the lucrative services and patients and avoiding unprofitable activities, which are part of a complete medical care service, are not uncommon for investor-owned corporations.[23] "Dumping" is another common practice today.[24] In the process of "creaming and dumping," the goal of compassionate service to ailing humanity is supplanted by the goal of profit. Is it possible to take surplus funds out of the system and still have service as the primary goal of medical care? Long ago a wise man said, "No one can serve two masters." Today the de facto goal of the investor-owned hospital is clear in the following vignette:

> To stimulate admissions, Humana offers physicians office space at a discount in building next to its hospitals and even guarantees first-year incomes of $60,000. It then keeps track of the revenues each doctor generates. "They let you know if you're not keeping up to expectations," says one young physician. Humana's president is frank about what happens if they fail to produce: "I'm damn sure I'm not going to renegotiate their office leases. They can practice elsewhere."[25]

CONCLUSION

Because of the values inherent in health care and because of the values, dispositions, and attitudes which should typify the individuals and corporations that offer health care in the United States, investor-owned health care corporations seem to be unethical. They neither strive for nor reflect the values proper to health care. In fact, the conditions and attitudes that allow investor-owned health care corporations to survive in our society lead us to ask some far more serious questions: What type of society are we creating for ourselves? What type of society are we creating for future generations? What values do we wish to dominate society in the present and in the future? Are we espousing values that promote service, trust, and compassion for the weak, or values that promote competition, exploitation, and profits for the strong at the expense of the weak? There are some goods so important and so intrinsic to human development that we cannot expose them to the vagaries and manipulations and inequities of the free market.

NOTES

1. J. Michael Watt et al., "The Comparative Economic Performance of Investor-Owned Chain and Not-for-Profit Hospitals," *New England Journal of Medicine* 314, no. 2 (Jan. 9, 1986):89–96; Stephen Remm et al., "The Effects of Ownership and System Affiliation on the Economic Performance of Hospitals," *Inquiry* 22 (Fall 1985):219–236; A.S. Relman, "Investor-Owned Hospitals and Health Care Costs," *New England Journal of Medicine* 309 (1983):54, 370–372; D. Ermar and J. Gabel, "Multi Hospital Systems, Issues and Empirical Findings," *Health Affairs*, Spring 1984, 50–64; R. Pattison and H. Katz, "Investor-Owned and Not-For-Profit Hospitals: A Comparison Based on California Data," *New England Journal of Medicine* 309 (1983), 53 (347); B. Gordon, "For Profit Hospital Care, Who Profits, Who Cares?" National Council of Senior Citizens (1986).

2. As the text indicates, values are discerned through an analysis of objective reality, not from feelings or emotions, which are rationally indefensible. Cf. Robert Belloh et al., *Habits of the Heart* (Berkeley: University of California Press, 1985), 80.

3. Thomas Peters and Robert Waterman, *In Search of Excellence* (New York: Warner Books, 1983), 279.

4. President's Commission for the Study of Ethical Problems in Medicine and Biomedical and Behavioral Research, *Securing Access to Health Care* (Washington, D.C.: Government Printing Office, 1983), especially vol. II and III.

5. Peters and Waterman, "Excellence."

6. Henrik Blum, *Planning for Health: Development and Application of Social Change* (New York: Behavioral Publishers, 1974), 93.

7. Ibid.

8. Robert Merton, "Some Thoughts on Professions in American Society" (unpublished paper presented at Brown University, 1960).

9. Kenneth Underwood, *The Church, the University and Social Policy*, vol. 1 (Middleton, Ct.: Wesleyan University Press, 1972), 422.

10. Edmund Pellegrino and David Thomasma, *A Philosophical Basis of Medical Practice* (New York: Oxford University Press, 1981), 23.

11. Charles Davidson, "Are We Physicians Helpless?" *New England Journal of Medicine* 310 (April 26, 1984):1118.

12. For a detailed study in accord with this chapter, cf. B. Gordon, "For Profit Hospital Care." For opinions contrary to ours, cf. Richard Rosett, "Doing Well by Doing Good: Investor-Owned Hospitals," *Frontiers of Health Service Management* 1 (Sept. 1984):1–9; Frank Sloan and Robert Vraciu, "Investor-Owned and Not-For-Profit Hospitals: Addressing Some Issues," *Health Affairs* 2, no. 1 (1983):25–37.

13. Eli Ginzberg, "The Grand Illusion of Competition in Health Care," *Journal of the American Medical Association* 249, no. 14 (April 8, 1983); Council on Medical Services, American Medical Association, "Effects of Competition in Medicine," *Journal of the American Medical Association* 249, no. 14 (April 8, 1983).

14. President's Commission, *Securing Access*, 20.

15. Eli Ginzberg, "The Monetarization of Medical Care," *New England Journal of Medicine* 310 (May 3, 1984):1163.

16. Unfortunately, some not-for-profit institutions are indistinguishable from investor-owned. Cf. "Transfers to a Public Hospital," *New England Journal of Medicine* 314, no. 9 (Feb. 27, 1986): 552–557.

17. President's Commission, *Securing Access*, 22–23.

18. Paul Starr, *The Social Transformation of American Medicine* (New York: Basic Books, 1982), 448.

19. Michael Bromberg, quoted in "Conference on For-Profits," *AHA Washington Memo* no. 494 (March 16, 1984), 6.

20. Cf. footnotes 1, 12, 13.

21. Though the issue will not be debated here, there is a significant difference between the interest on bonds paid by a not-for-profit corporation and the dividends paid to investors; cf. K. O'Rourke, "Investor-owned Catholic Teaching Hospitals," *New England Journal of Medicine* 313, no. 20 (Nov. 14, 1985):1297.

22. Starr, *Social Transformation*, 448.

23. Arnold Relman, "The Commercialization of Medicine" (unpublished paper presented to the Hospital Superintendents of New England, September 1983).

24. Cf. footnote 16.

25. Starr, *Social Transformation*, 446.

Chapter 16

Ethics and Health Care: The Importance of the Profit Motive

Michael D. Bromberg, LLB, and Thomas G. Goodwin, BA

Rarely are issues of ethics debated more hotly than in medicine and health care; and in recent years the temperature of the debates has been rising. This is due almost entirely to revolutionary upheaval in the financing of medical care, a commodity whose true costs have been hidden from patients and health care payers until only just recently. A national revolt in the private and public sectors against the high costs of health care has brought about a new competition in a new health care "marketplace."

The changing patterns of medical practice away from the traditional fee-for-service system and toward a more market-oriented scenario are inexorable and inevitable. Equally inevitably, these changing patterns have elicited a host of worries from those who fear change and who insist on presupposing a lack of ethical behavior on those others who are pioneering new territory to meet the realities of changing public policy.

Raising institutional ownership in the hospital field as an ethical issue indicates the extent to which the ills of revolutionary change occurring in medical care are laid on the doorstep of the for-profit sector. This attempt most frequently is manifest in efforts to draw a meaningful distinction between for-profit and not-for-profit hospitals, and to assume as a basic premise that a free enterprise health care system is inherently more concerned with the bottom line than care of patients.

The answer to the question, "Does institutional ownership of health care facilities present an ethical issue?" is no. There is virtually no difference whatsoever between not-for-profit and for-profit hospitals in their admissions practices, in their staff/patient ratios, in the quality of care offered, in their social contributions, and probably most importantly, in their need to earn a profit.

It is around that last point that the debate seems to revolve. The so-called health care revolution has brought to light the beliefs of some that it is unseemly for hospitals to be concerned about "profits." In health care, this concern is peculiar to hospitals, a function no doubt of their historic role as institutions that were either publicly supported or charitably endowed refuges for the sick, rich and poor alike.

The focus on hospitals in the debate over profit in health care is demonstrably misplaced, and increasingly irrelevant—particularly in a society founded on the capitalistic approach.

The health care system in the United States has always been oriented toward, and dominated by, the private sector reflecting the tenets of a free enterprise system as established by our Founding Fathers.

Physicians, who serve as the "gatekeepers" of health care, are among the most entrepreneurial of all professional groups. The profit-making abilities of these guardians of our health are well documented; yet ethical concerns are for the most part left undiscussed (except with regard to the susceptibility of physicians to succumb to the lure of financial incentive arrangements with hospitals).

Likewise, the companies who produce important pharmaceuticals that often make a life-or-death difference pursue profits unfettered by ethical questions.

There are interesting distinctions between health care and some other commodities that are basic to human existence. We cannot live without food, yet we do not find it inherently unethical for supermarkets to earn a profit on their operations. Neither do we find it inherently unethical for landlords or real estate developers to offer shelter for more than the construction or operating cost of a property.

In a dynamic environment, the issues of ethics in health care must inevitably be viewed, as Princeton Professor Uwe Reinhardt puts it, as a "state of nature." In many nations of the world, health care is regarded as a community service to be distributed equally according to need. Although there are those in our society who would imbue our system with this premise, there is in fact little widespread public support for it. Indeed, in recent years it has become quite clear that the American people have decided to regard health care as more a commodity than a service.

There is no dispute that American public policy toward health care in the past few years has been, and will continue to be, oriented toward cost containment. The government has determined to pursue this objective by cutting back its commitment to national health care programs, thus increasing the role of private investment as a means of protecting quality and services.

Likewise, the private sector has forced a new competition among health care providers by demanding discounted health care for employee groups.

The impact of the health care revolution cuts across hospitals of all stripes. It adversely affects the ability of both not-for-profit and for-profit institutions to raise capital, to add new services, to offer care to those who cannot afford it or are uninsured.

A recent report issued by the Institute of Medicine following a three-year study about the profit motive in health care noted that:

Historically, charitable donations and governmental grants were the major sources of capital and important sources of revenue. . . . However, the revenues of not-for-profit hospitals have increasingly come from billing for the services they provide and now, with the rising capital intensity of health care, the relative decline of charity, the rapid inflation in the 1960s and 1970s, and the end of the government's Hill-Burton program, leave capital requirements to be met mostly from retained earnings and debt. . . .

Economic pressure is not peculiar to the for-profit sector. Thus, it is not surprising that many observers see similarities in the behavior of for-profit and not-for-profit hospitals. . . .

Not-for-profit organizations can and do make profits (usually termed a "surplus") in the customary accounting sense of the term. . . . The ability of any organization to survive requires that it generate revenues beyond those necessary to cover operating expenses, not only because of the need for working capital but also because the equipment and renovations needed to keep an institution up-to-date and acceptable to doctors and patients require new infusions of capital.[1]

In fact, then, there are really only two meaningful distinctions between for-profit and not-for-profit institutions: for-profit hospitals pay taxes, while not-for-profit hospitals are tax-exempt; and not-for-profit hospitals return their "surplus" to the institution itself, while for-profit hospitals offer a return on investment to their stockholders, who in turn reinvest new capital into the facility.

Those who question the ethics of profit in health care ignore several realities—the new facts of life in a changing environment. They also misdirect their wrath at health care providers, who can, after all, only react to shifts in public health policy.

Better we should question the ethical implications of governmental policies that view societal spending for health care in terms of reducing a federal budget deficit rather than maintaining quality care, and access to it. Better we should question the ethical implications of deep budget cuts in Medicare and Medicaid—programs that together provide funds that total more than one-half of the nation's hospital bill. Better we should question the ethical implications of a national health policy that spends not one dime to extend health care to those who are ineligible for Medicaid or uninsured.

What happens when ethical considerations collide with the facts of life? In health care, the ethical considerations appear to be that it is wrong for hospitals to earn a profit from caring for the sick. The facts of life are that without a profit, hospitals would be unable to offer that care.

Profit, in health care or in any other business, is not an end. Rather, as Humana chairman David Jones pointed out, "Profit is always a requirement."

Any institution, be it private not-for-profit, public or for-profit, must be able to retain some funds over and above its expenses. Whether one calls it "profit" or "surplus," it is a must. Without it, salary increases cannot be met, new equipment cannot be acquired, renovations or additions cannot be realized, the quality of care might not be maintained.

Hospital care has become a service that must make a profit to remain in business. Simply stated, profit is a cost: the cost of being able to stay open. For a hospital, there is no ethical consideration more compelling than that it must stay open.

NOTE

1. National Academy of Sciences, Institute of Medicine, "For-Profit Enterprise in Health Care" (Washington D.C. 1986, unpublished), 9–11.

Chapter 17

Conflict of Interest in Health Care

K. Bruce Stickler, JD, and Mark D. Nelson, JD

CONFLICT OF INTEREST

The primary purpose of a health care institution is to provide competent health care to the sick and aged within the community it serves. Ideally, the hospital's mission to provide quality care is coextensive with the interests and needs of its employees and other individuals, such as physicians, who are integral components of the hospital's ability to fulfill its responsibility. However, conflicts of interests can develop between a health care provider and its employees and agents where their interests or goals are not coextensive; indeed, such interests often are mutually exclusive of one another.

The phrase "conflict of interest" is used most often with respect to public officials and their involvement in matters of private interest or personal gain to them. In the public sector, an individual usually takes an oath to uphold the responsibilities of his or her position. Moreover, the responsibilities and obligations are frequently established and clearly set forth by statutory law. The competing and conflicting interests are the individual's ethical or fiduciary responsibilities associated with the position occupied versus the personal or private gain or benefit that flows to the individual either through or as a result of his or her position. Resolving a conflict of interest is relatively straightforward; the duties are defined and the standard of conduct is established. The individual's actions or interests either violate the standard of conduct or not; if the standard is violated, either the position or the private interests must be discontinued.

Conflicts of interest outside public office are more difficult to resolve. For example, hospitals themselves face conflicts between competing internal interests. Hospitals are providers of health care and, in the purest sense, offer their services to those who need them without regard to the individual's ability to pay or economic status. Simultaneously, hospitals must function with a consistent and realistic view of the economic realities of operation, the "bottom line." The advent of diagnosis-related groups (DRGs) and the substantial increase in alternative health care delivery systems have created new dramatic financial

254

pressures on hospitals. They are experiencing unprecedented competition for patients. Thus, in order to survive as a health care provider a hospital must effectively meet this competition and operate with a view toward the bottom line by increasing revenues and/or reducing costs.

A conflict can arise because these costs include uncompensated care for patients unable to pay for their care. At the same time, however, a hospital's responsibility to serve these people continues. Before a conflict of interest can be resolved, however, the various interests must be identified and whether they are, in fact, in conflict must be determined. Many institutions have resolved this conflict by accommodating both interests; the hospital continues indigent care while addressing the associated financial impact by increasing revenues or reducing costs elsewhere. Other health care providers have resolved the conflict by encouraging indigent and welfare patients to seek care at another hospital, usually a public facility. While the latter approach may be unethical, it represents a conscious resolution of a conflict of competing interests. If, however, the hospital has a legal obligation to care for these patients, or these patients have a legal right of access to care at this hospital, the conflict would be resolved before administrative or judicial bodies.

The physician-hospital relationship presents unique conflict of interest concerns. The relationship is one of necessary symbiosis; a physician needs a hospital as a place to treat patients and hospitals need physicians to admit patients for whom the hospital provides inpatient and outpatient services. Both physicians and hospitals derive significant revenues from this relationship. However, substantial conflicts of interest can and do result. Moreover, as physicians and hospitals separately and jointly explore service ventures and investment opportunities, conflicts can arise between the physicians, the hospital, and members of the administrative team who may have a financial interest or stake in a particular venture.

For example, some physicians at some hospitals enjoy advantageous bargaining positions by virtue of their specialty, their political or community stature or their ability to generate revenue or patients for the hospital. In joint ventures or other relationships with these physicians, a hospital can face a conflict between its interest in maintaining a positive relationship with the physician and entering into an agreement that may not be in the best interests of the hospital.

Similarly, the individuals involved in the decision-making process could have personal interests that interfere with their impartiality and perspective in evaluating the venture in terms of the hospital's interests. For example, an administrator may enter into an agreement on behalf of the hospital, motivated in part by personal gain from the venture, such as through personal investment in the deal or long-term security arrangements. Not only does this situation raise the appearance of impropriety but it may commit the hospital to an obligation that is not in its interest whatsoever.

Mergers and acquisitions present conflict of interest concerns due to the potential varied interests of the individuals involved, particularly the principals representing the hospital that is to be acquired. Consider this situation: a not-for-profit hospital is approached by a for-profit hospital system seeking to acquire the not-for-profit entity. The present administrator is very concerned with his employment status after the acquisition. The hospital board of directors is concerned with the acquisition's impact on their community hospital's status, as well as its impact on the hospital employees and the community. Because of the potential conflict and its fiduciary responsibility, board involvement in the acquisition discussions is critical; the possibility and the opportunity exist for the administrator and others to "cut a deal" to guarantee employment on favorable terms at the expense of the hospital in the contract terms.

Acquisitions or mergers involving municipal or religious institutions warrant consideration of continuing their special obligations and value after the change is effected. A municipal hospital is responsible to the community it serves, and the hospital decision makers must consider whether the public interest is protected in the change; will the for-profit hospital provide the same level of indigent and low-income care as the municipal hospital? A religious hospital should evaluate whether a merger acquisition will further the purposes, mission, and values of the institution, for example, will the "new" hospital now begin performing abortions?

Antinepotism policies, which prohibit or limit the employment of related individuals, involve conflicting interests for hospitals. Where a close relative of a current excellent employee applies for employment with the hospital, a natural inclination is to presume that the relative too is a good worker and would be an asset to the institution. Conversely, a bad experience with an employee may lead to disqualification of relatives. Also, particularly in smaller communities, it may be difficult to hire qualified employees without hiring an individual who is related to a current employee. On the other hand, related individuals working in a hospital can create problems where familial disputes are brought to the workplace or when an employee becomes upset or objects to the treatment of a relative.

Courts have held that an employer's policy that uses family relationship as a hiring criterion may inherently "select out" certain applicants and, as a result, may violate Title VII of the Civil Rights Act of 1964 and similar state laws if it has an adverse impact on a protected class. On the other hand, an antinepotism policy designed to limit employment of relatives is valid if it is applied even-handedly and does not have an adverse effect on males or females. In evaluating nepotism policies or situations, a hospital can generally balance the competing interests. A blanket prohibition against employment of related individuals may well prove unduly restrictive of the hospital's need to hire qualified employees. Indeed, a hospital may recruit an employee who, as a condition of accepting the offer, requires hospital employment for the employee's spouse. An overly broad nepotism policy would interfere with the hospital's interest in recruiting. A policy prohibiting related individuals from working in a supervisor-subordinate position is advisable because the situation is fraught with potential conflicts and allegations of favoritism. In many cases, conflicts of interest arising from employment of related individuals can be resolved by evaluating the various interests.

THE ANALYTICAL FRAMEWORK

In order to resolve conflict of interest situations, one must determine whether an actual or potential conflict of interest exists. This process requires the identification of the interests of the parties involved—generally the hospital and the employee. The next phase is critical evaluation of the nature and extent of the conflict of the interests involved. Then the conflict, if one exists, can be resolved using the proposed analytical framework.

Many conflict of interest issues that confront hospital administrators and managers escape legal definition, classification, or resolution. Nevertheless, decisions made by management should be based on solid legal principles whenever possible. Indeed, failure to do so may result in an inappropriate or unlawful decision and subject a hospital to liability for its actions. For example, a hospital might discipline or discharge employees for writing a letter to the local newspaper critical of hospital administration or operations. It could be liable for such action if the purpose underlying the employees' interest in writing the letter has a legal foundation. In a situation involving a public hospital, discipline for such conduct could violate the employees' rights to freedom of speech guaranteed by the Fourteenth Amendment. A private hospital could be liable for an unfair labor practice for infringing on the employees' right to engage in protected concerted activity under the National Labor Relations Act by seeking to publish concerns over working conditions.

A difficult situation is presented when both the hospital's interest and the employee's interest appear to have legal support. First, the apparent legal foundation must be scrutinized for validity and relevancy; does the law actually support the interest claimed? For instance, consider a situation where a pregnant employee refuses to care for a patient who shares a room with a chemotherapy patient. The employee may claim that exposure to the chemotherapy patient may harm her fetus, and that she and the fetus have a right to a safe and healthful workplace. The hospital's interest is the fundamental management right to assign employees as it deems appropriate, so long as the assignment is not unlawful. The assignment to care for the nonchemotherapy patient would not, in most circumstances, violate the employee's interest in safe working conditions. The employee's fear of risk in this situation would probably be deemed unreasonable. Thus, the employee's concern is unjustified, and the employer's interest would take precedence, requiring her to perform the service.

Second, the legal foundation should be evaluated. In a conflict between federal law and state law, the federal mandate generally governs except where the state law provides greater protection or rights to individuals. Similarly, state regulations usually precede local or municipal ordinances. Administrative regulations represent an agency's interpretation of a specific law it is charged with enforcing, and while such regulations are entitled to deference by the courts, they are not laws in and of themselves. Thus, in a conflict between a law and a regulation, the law will generally control.

Third, the analysis should weigh the respective public policies advanced or articulated in each legal foundation. For example, where the hospital's interest is based on a public policy to control contagious diseases and the competing employee interest is supported by a personal right of privacy, the public interest may be paramount. Thus with the fear of spreading AIDS a health care institution may arguably require testing for the AIDS virus even though an employee may wish to avoid any test.

Fourth, the penalties or sanctions associated with an interest, or the violation of the legal basis for the interest, should be determined. In some cases, the resolution of a conflict may be based upon selecting the lesser of two penalties.

Fifth, the importance of the hospital's interest to its essential responsibilities and mission should be considered. A valid hospital interest and a competing employee interest must be balanced.

Where neither competing interest is founded on a law or regulation, each interest should be analyzed to determine which is more compelling and, consequently, should control. The likely impact of the conflict resolution should also be considered. If the hospital's interest is more compelling in the immediate conflict but would be destructive of employee morale, the situation should be reevaluated. Generally, the hospital's interest will be the more compelling where its interest is integral to the hospital's role and philosophy. For example, a hospital's interest in not having employees who abuse alcohol or drugs is more closely tied to the hospital's role and philosophy than a hospital's interest in seeing that its employees do not work part-time for another employer.

Figure 17-1 sets forth this analytical framework.

SPECIFIC CONFLICTS OF INTEREST

Conflicts of interest occur in a wide variety of situations. These conflicts can be divided into two general categories: disputes over outside employment and conflicts regarding outside activities unrelated to employment. Application of the foregoing analytical framework to conflicts in these categories should provide a useful tool for approaching these frequently emotion-charged situations from a reasoned perspective.

Figure 17-1 Conflict of Interest—An Analytical Framework

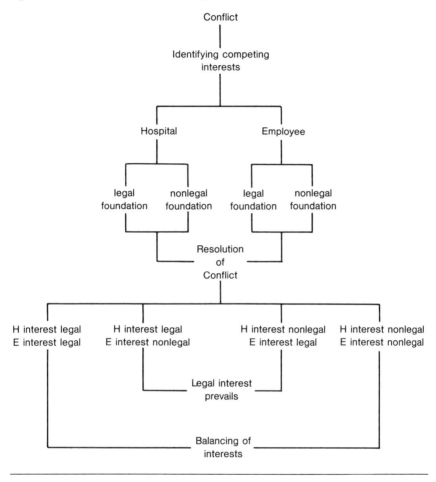

A Case Study: Outside Employment

When a hospital offers employment to an individual, it expects that if the individual accepts the offer he or she will perform to the best of his or her ability and will be loyal and dedicated to the hospital. Indeed, many hospitals expect, or at least hope, that the job and the hospital will be a very important facet of the employee's life. Conversely, many employees expect that they will work hard during work hours but that their activities when they are away from the hospital are strictly their own business, beyond the hospital's legitimate interests or concern. So long as an employee's outside activity such as working a second job does not cause the employee to perform unsatisfactorily, an employee would contend that moonlighting is of no legitimate concern to the employer. The hospital is concerned with actual and potential problems; the employee believes such concern is valid only when actual, significant problems such as inadequate performance develop.

The hospital's interest in limiting the outside employment of its employees does not have a statutory or regulatory foundation; it is grounded in the traditional notion that management has the right (absent specific legal prohibitions) to establish the terms and conditions of employment for its workers. Similarly, an employee's interest in having a second job is not guaranteed by law. The right to privacy arising from amendments to the U.S. constitution extends only to certain personal interests such as family and marriage, and even then not to all matters that can be characterized as personal.

A hospital can create a legal foundation for restricting or prohibiting outside employment through an employment contract. A specific prohibition contained in a written employment contract would resolve a potential conflict of interest where in agreeing to the contract, the employee waives his or her right to assert any interest in outside employment. Similarly, if an employee can negotiate a right to outside employment, that interest would have a legal foundation and the hospital would have waived its competing interest.

The primary conflict created by an employee's interest in outside employment is interference with the individual's job performance at the hospital. Such interference can manifest itself in several ways: decreased employee productivity due to exhaustion from working the second job, absenteeism or tardiness, and scheduling inflexibility including unavailability to work overtime due to a conflict with the second job. An employer can and should discipline employees for job performance deficiencies caused by outside employment. Indeed, failure to do so could be viewed by other employees as approval of otherwise unacceptable work standards. Clearly, such a situation must be avoided. In disciplining employees, the effects of the outside employment should be the focus and basis for the discipline. The reasons for the performance deficiencies are not material. Absenteeism problems due to outside employment or other reasons such as health problems have the same impact on the hospital: the employee is not at work performing his or her duties.

In limiting an employee's ability to work outside the hospital, each situation should be evaluated individually based upon the specific circumstances in that case. Several important factors should be considered: the employee's status, the employee's level of responsibility in the hospital, and the nature of the requested outside employment. Outside employment undertaken by a full-time employee has greater potential to interfere with hospital interests and operations. Moreover, the hospital's commitment to full-time employees is usually greater, as full-time employees generally receive greater benefits than part-time employees.

Employees who work on a part-time basis do so for a variety of reasons, including the desire to work another job. A policy prohibiting moonlighting by part-time employees could have an adverse effect on the hospital's ability to recruit qualified personnel, and recruitment of capable employees is a significant interest of hospitals. Thus, limiting outside employment can advance the employer's interest in avoiding potential conflicts of interest while conflicting with the employer's interest in recruiting personnel.

An employee's level of responsibility should be a criterion in reviewing outside employment situations. Generally, the higher the employee is in the organization, the less appropriate it is for that individual to have outside employment. An integral part of the responsibilities of hospital managers and administrators, and a basis for their compensation, is that they have 24-hour responsibility and commitment to the institution. In addition, such employment would reflect adversely on the institution; hospital managers working for two employers would raise questions regarding their loyalty and the hospital's pay practices (i.e., management is underpaid and needs to work a second job to "get by"). Management involvement in community activities and philanthropic ventures is frequently encouraged, on the other hand, because it creates good will for the hospital and fosters the image of the hospital as an active participant in the community.

The specific nature of an employee's outside employment should be evaluated in determining whether a conflict of interest actually or potentially exists. Outside employment that could harm the institution's reputation or image in the community can be prohibited. However, caution should be exercised in this area. For example, a hospital could determine that an employee's work with, and advocacy of, a gay rights group is harmful to the hospital's reputation in the community. However, prohibiting the employee from such work could be unlawful discrimination, particularly in jurisdictions that prohibit discrimination on the basis of sexual orientation or preference. In this case, the employee's interest would supersede the hospital's interest because the employee's interest has an articulated legal foundation.

Where an employee provides services to an entity that does business with the hospital, it creates the appearance of, and the potential for, a conflict of interest between the employee's loyalty and responsibility to the hospital and the employee's personal gain in doing business with the hospital. For example, a computer services supervisor at a hospital also operates a computer hardware and software sales business. As the computer services supervisor for the hospital, the employee has input into the design and selection of the hospital's computer system. The potential exists for the employee, with either innocent or self-serving motives, to plan a system that uses the products he or she sells. Even if the hospital does not purchase its system from the employee and the employee does not receive a commission or other credit for the sale, an appearance of impropriety or a conflict of interest would exist. If the hospital actually purchased the computer equipment from the employee, the situation would be fraught with significant problems. In this regard, the conflict of interest should be resolved in favor of the hospital's interest in having employees not associate with an entity that does business with the hospital.

An employee's outside employment can create special problems where the employee has special skills or expertise that is not readily available in the marketplace, or the employee is not easily replaced. Particular difficulties can arise when the employee has an opportunity to work outside of hospital work hours and earn additional income performing duties similar to the employee's duties at the hospital. Suppose a nonmetropolitan hospital offers physical therapy services on both an inpatient and outpatient basis and has three physical therapists on staff, a department head who treats patients and two staff therapists. For this hospital, and many others across the country, recruiting and retaining physical therapists, as well as other specialty employees, is difficult at a time when the demand for their services is increasing substantially. The hospital learns that the department head has, or is intending to, begin providing private physical therapy services after hours at the therapist's home. The hospital must decide how it will address the situation; initially, the hospital must determine whether a conflict of interest exists. If the employee's access to these patients results from hospital employment, a conflict of interest may well exist because the employee is using the hospital employment for personal financial gain and patients are being diverted from the hospital. If the patients are otherwise generated by the employee, a conflict of interest may exist because of the potential to compete with the hospital for patients. The employee should be informed that the outside venture is impermissible and that continuing it could result in discipline including discharge.

The employee may respond that, if forced to quit treating patients outside the hospital on his free time, he or she will resign. The hospital's position can be firm unless it cannot readily replace the employee. If the employee leaves, the hospital's ability to provide physical therapy would be compromised. However, allowing the employee to continue to work outside would establish a precedent; at the very least, other employees would see that a difficult-to-replace employee has a very strong bargaining position with the hospital. Other similarly situated employees may follow the lead, while replaceable employees may perceive the hospital's policies and practices as inequitable. If a resolution cannot be achieved, the hospital's commitment to providing patient care may dictate retaining the employee, at the cost of establishing a significant precedent.

Conflicts Arising from Off-Duty Activities

An employer's interest in limiting the outside employment of its employees is clear, but it faces significant conflict of interest issues when it attempts to monitor or limit an employee's off-duty, nonemployment activities. However, when an employee's off-duty activities interfere with performance, employers may be required to consider the reasons for the inadequate performance in order to address the issue effectively and legally. The critical inquiry is: To what extent can and should an employer delve into the off-duty activities of its employees? Perhaps the most controversial outside activity is employee recreational use of alcohol or drugs. A hospital employer is not a law enforcement agency and the fact that an employee may use or abuse illicit drugs, prescription drugs, or alcohol is not, standing alone, of concern to the hospital. Indeed, hospital inquiries into such conduct may constitute an invasion of privacy or defamation of the employee. However, when off-duty activity affects the employee's job performance, it becomes a legitimate and compelling concern to the hospital. An employee impaired by alcohol or drugs not only performs at a less efficient level but also presents a threat to the health and safety of the hospital's patients and employees. In addition, these employees use health insurance benefits more and are more likely to be involved in workplace accidents or injuries.

The respective interests are significant: the hospital has a legal duty to protect its patients and to provide a safe and healthful workplace for its employees, a right to receive satisfactory job performance and productivity from its employees, and a right to maintain the integrity of the workplace. The employee has a legal right to privacy, an interest (or a right if a public employee) in being free from unreasonable searches, a right in some jurisdictions to be treated fairly and in good faith by the employer, and an expectation that the terms and conditions of employment will not be changed without, at least, prior notice to the employee.

Physical testing for alcohol or drugs is a volatile issue articulating a classic conflict of interest: the employer's right to police the workplace and monitor employee performance versus the employee's right to be free from unreasonable intrusion, particularly intrusion into the employee's body. Random testing for drugs and alcohol is probably the most effective means of discouraging employee substance abuse.

Random testing is particularly effective when it is combined with a tough disciplinary policy on substance abuse. Random testing is strongly opposed by many labor unions and civil rights groups. They claim it can be used by supervisors to harass employees by subjecting them to frequent testing. In addition, where testing is not based upon employee job performance or conduct, a positive result indicates no more than that a substance was present in the employee's system at the time the sample was taken. Urine and blood testing do not indicate impairment or precisely when the substance was ingested. In addition, it has been argued that random testing violates a public employee's Fourteenth Amendment guarantee against unreasonable searches.

Physical testing, such as urine, blood, or saliva tests, is an important ingredient in an effective substance abuse program. While current testing cannot identify whether an employee is impaired by alcohol or drugs, testing can be useful as a confirmatory tool to support other evidence of substance use. A substance abuse policy that provides for physical testing based upon a supervisor's reasonable suspicion that the employee may be under the influence of alcohol or drugs can be a reasonable resolution of the hospital/employee conflict of interest in this area. Reasonable suspicion testing protects employee personal privacy and freedom interests consistent with the hospital's right to test employees for substances to protect patients, employees, and the hospital itself. Under this approach, testing would be initiated only when the employee's performance or conduct gives rise to a supervisor's belief that the employee may be under the influence of a substance.

CONCLUSION

Resolution of conflicts of interest requires identification of the competing interests and evaluation of the foundation for the interest. In addition, the short-term consequences and the long-range impact of a particular resolution of a specific conflict must be considered. The analytical framework set forth in this chapter offers guidelines for health care professionals to address conflicts of interest.

While conflicts of interest cannot be avoided altogether, they can be minimized by developing and implementing a personnel policy on conflicts of interest. Such a policy dealing with outside employment should address the following matters:

1. whether employees are permitted to work outside the hospital and, if so, the parameters of the outside employment;
2. whether a distinction is made between full-time and part-time employees in working outside the hospital;
3. whether prior approval of outside employment is necessary and, if so, the standard that will be applied (i.e., a case-by-case determination);
4. whether outside nonemployment activities will be restricted, including activities that may injure the reputation or image of the hospital; and
5. what disciplinary action will be taken if the policy is violated.

An analytical approach to conflicts of interest, combined with written personnel policies, gives notice to employees of the hospital's expectations and will assist supervisors and managers in resolving conflicts in an appropriate, consistent, and legally supportable fashion.

Chapter 18

Discharging Patients: Limiting Length of Stay in a Cost-Conscious and Resource-Limited Environment

Valerie A. Glesnes-Anderson, MHSA, and Ruth L. Garvey, MSW

Health care institutions have three primary service concerns: accommodating, treating, and discharging patients. Each major task involves the skills and services of a variety of health care professionals guided by institutional policies.

Discharge planning is accomplished by assessing individual patient needs, formulating an adequate and acceptable plan of posthospitalization placement, and implementing this plan.[1] The goal for such planning is to ensure the safety, well-being and, to the degree necessary, continuing care of the former patient. However, the process and the resulting plan are created by professionals who might face conflicting definitions of what is in the best interests of the patient, difficulty with respecting the patient's right of self-determination, and broader issues related to the interests of the health care professional or institutions involved. In fact, if this process and plan are inadequate, unacceptable, or poorly implemented, serious harm to the patient may result.

ETHICAL ISSUES IN DISCHARGE PLANNING

Although service challenges and ethical dilemmas abound in discharge planning, there are some areas of relative clarity and agreement. Most would agree that an institution is obligated to treat an emergency patient in spite of financial loss if the patient is uninsured. Most would agree that it is wrong and inappropriate to discharge an acutely ill patient to a setting unprepared to provide minimally necessary care. It would also be inappropriate to discharge an acutely ill patient in a manner that would endanger his or her well-being (such as transporting an acutely ill patient a great distance to a public hospital). Such actions, sometimes called "dumping," have received dramatic media attention and resulted in public and legislative clamor.

Financially motivated decisions that clearly harm patients are difficult to justify. However, self-enriching motivation may be difficult to determine. Posing more complicated ethical dilemmas, issues of quality of care, professional values, and the role of patient autonomy may also be difficult to clarify.

Quality Issues Versus Cost Containment

A primary ethical concern with regard to discharge planning has centered on the issue of time. For several decades this concern for time was evidenced by fears that patients were being maintained in hospitals longer than their illnesses might require. Extended hospitalization was viewed as harmful to the patient and family, causing disruption and delay in reestablishing private life and undue dependency on the institution. This length of stay was attributed to payment schemes that financially rewarded institutions for long patient stays.

In recent years, time concerns have been at the opposite extreme—the fear that patients are being discharged from hospitals too quickly. The identified motivational culprit is financial incentives that reward short hospital stays. Both extremes affect the patient's quality of life. The current incentive for speed may also affect the quality of placement and the resulting level of care after hospitalization.

Issues related to discharge planning have always attracted attention as hospitals tried to care effectively for patients who no longer needed acute care and who would no longer be the direct responsibility of the hospital. With today's economic realities, this commitment to patient care is joined by the hospital's fiscal pressures. The regulatory pressure of diagnosis-related group (DRG) reimbursement has resulted in the need for rapid discharge for the financial viability of the institution. DRG reimbursement has introduced a specific dollar amount assigned to treating each illness. This shift in financial incentives from a charge-based method of payment to a prospective method has meant that a patient admission can result in a financial loss to the hospital if discharge is delayed. The rationale for prospective payment is cost containment: if a hospital is paid a set amount for an illness regardless of the resources used in treating a patient, the natural incentive would be to provide care in a cost-efficient manner, encouraging patients to leave the hospital as soon as possible. This incentive could result in a conflict of interest between the hospital's need to contain costs and the potential level of care and extent of treatment that an individual patient might require.

While hospitals are responding to these new payment schemes and resulting incentives, government agencies are also using peer review mechanisms to encourage decreased length of stay by denying reimbursement for hospital days and services regarded as inappropriate. These heightened pressures on hospital administrators have positively resulted in higher awareness, interest, and attention to the components of discharge planning. Less positively, some of this pressure has thwarted the discharge planning process as responsible professionals are encouraged to move patients out of the institution as quickly as possible.

Consequently, there is increased pressure on discharge planners that may introduce further conflicts of interest involving loyalty to one's professional standards (such as social work or nursing) and loyalty to one's institution and employer. A professional commitment to patient self-determination and to quality care may be taxed by the interests of the institution that, in turn, is attempting to balance a service function and its financial "bottom line."

Regulations and reimbursement policies have underscored that hospitals are *acute* care facilities and are not intended to provide long-term care for the chronically ill or recovering patient. This has resulted in a social process similar to the deinstitutionalization of psychiatric patients in the 1970s. Similarly, it has assumed a network of intermediate care and alternate care settings outside of the hospital to meet the discharged patient's continuing need for some degree of service or supervision. However, that network does not yet exist. Noting increased pressure on aftercare facilities and programs, Congressman Waxman (D-Cal.), chair of the House's health subcommittee, observed, "The cracks in the patchwork of programs and services are staggering."[2]

In response to anecdotal reports and "horror stories" about the discharge of patients and the allegation that peer review organizations (PROs) are concerned with cost containment to the neglect of quality issues, Congress has begun to act. Senator Heinz (R-Penn.) and Congressman Stark (D-Cal.) concluded that "quality of care has deteriorated under the PPS (prospective payment system) and that the PROs are doing an inadequate job monitoring quality."[3] Consequently, the Medicare Quality Protection Act of 1986 was introduced in Congress. This extensive bill required:

- refinement of the prospective payment system;
- distribution to patients of a written statement of rights with regard to hospital and posthospital care;
- a modified appeals process for "continued stay" denials;
- prohibitions against hospital incentive programs for physicians meeting specific length of stay targets;
- further study of quality assurance and reimbursement strategies;
- improved review of quality by peer review organizations.[4]

Critics have noted that congressional concern has been based primarily on anecdotal stories as opposed to sound, scientifically based methodology. Others have testified that a "premature discharge" problem is not evident in their states. For example, in testimony before the New Jersey Senate Committee on Aging, the president elect of the PRO of New Jersey stated that a review of 74,183 Medicare records identified eleven cases (0.014%) where patients might have been discharged too early. He added that in these eleven cases there was no evidence of intent to discharge for financial gain and in fact, professional judgment deemed that patients were stable at the time of discharge.[5] However, the high number of patient stories, nationally, and the basic agreement of organizations such as the American Hospital Association have given credibility and impetus to regulatory reform.

An institution's need for financial solvency in order to provide its service to patients and communities is obvious. The scarcity of health care dollars and the access issues raised by the allocation of limited resources makes cost containment imperative. The dilemma is posed when balancing institutional interests and the well-being of patients.

Professional Values

Further conflict might be introduced by the differing individual value systems of professions, patients, and family members. For example, a discharge planner or physician who is biased against the frail elderly may fail to formulate a plan that will consider the rehabilitation potential of the older patient. Or the discharge planner who believes that health care is a "right" will expend greater effort to establish a discharge plan and will often include continued hospitalization as an option when community services are unavailable, particularly to the patient who cannot pay for needed community services.

A more serious dilemma arises when the physician treating a patient believes a patient should receive only what he or she can pay for and refuses to order the services that are not covered by insurance. Will a poor patient needing a respirator and a nonexistent Medicaid bed in a nursing home be given the same consideration as a patient who will pay privately for services after discharge? A physician operating from this belief may also respond to utilization review denials by discharging the patient before all plans are in place. Conversely, a physician who believes that health care is a right may overutilize hospital resources and ignore guidance of DRG coordinators and utilization review.

Paternalism Versus Patient Autonomy

Involving the patient, and the patient's family, in planning and decision making related to discharge requires time and resources that may be very difficult to invest in this process. In addition, health care provider attitudes may influence this planning process: Do patients receive all the information available to make decisions or are they given only the information they need to make the "right" decision (as defined by the discharge planner)? Are patients and families involved in the planning stages and exploration of alternative plans or are they presented a final package that they must either accept or reject?

Autonomy issues might also include professional autonomy—the right of professionals to make independent decisions consistent with their training and values. Interdisciplinary teamwork in discharge planning ideally illustrates the contributions and expertise of a number of professionals. However, accountability measures and review of one's decisions could potentially threaten the decision makers' assessments, judgments, and choices.

Discharge planning pressures have challenged not only social workers and nurses (typical discharge planners), patients and their families, and administrators and physicians, but also the network of agencies, institutions, and informal networks that support patients after they leave the hospital. At one time patients who were no longer in need of acute care but still required medical supervision and intervention might have remained in the hospital. This is no longer fiscally possible, resulting in increased need to discharge patients to settings capable of providing nursing and health-related care.

The deemphasis of expensive institutional care has assumed outpatient support services that often do not exist or do not have the capacity to meet this increased demand for their services. In fact, under prospective pricing, discharges to skilled nursing home care are up almost 40 percent, and discharges to home health care have similarly risen by 37 percent.[6]

Discharge planning requires several innate ethical considerations:

1. Is the discharge of an acutely ill patient premature?
2. Is a nonacutely ill patient being discharged to a setting that is appropriate?
3. Does the planning process consider the desires and choices of the patient or the patient's family?
4. Does the discharge planning process allow financial considerations to supersede the professional judgments of physicians and discharge planners?
5. Are professionals involved in discharge planning sensitive to their own values in establishing and implementing patient discharge plans?

In summary, discharge planning must address professional and patient autonomy, result in a placement that is in the best interests of the patient, and not result in social, financial, psychological, and physical harm to the patient and the patient's family. Poor discharge planning has always had the potential for harm to patients. The lack of careful planning poses no ethical dilemma—it is wrong and should be corrected. However, the conflicting and often unidentified values of the professionals who are involved in patient discharge may pose confusing or contradictory options.

CASE EXAMPLE

The pressures to effect early discharges bring greater emphasis to the need for coordinated discharge planning, professional and patient education, and continual reaffirmation of the importance of appropriate discharges. The circumstances in the following case are not extraordinary, but they illustrate the interaction of role, values, and behavior that extends beyond a described process.

A frail, elderly woman was admitted to Memorial Hospital with a diagnosis of septicemia. The patient was incontinent, dependent on others for personal hygiene, and somewhat confused. Early in the admission, a social worker picked up the case because the patient was elderly. Further information about home care needs were hard to obtain—the patient had difficulty speaking because of a stroke many years before. Her admission slip showed her next of kin residing at the same address. Upon contacting the next of kin, the social worker discovered that patient's "home" to be boarding home and the next of kin to be the owner.

The results of the social worker's investigation and reports from the physician and nurses led the discharge planning team to propose nursing home placement as the optimal discharge plan. The boarding home operator initially opposed this plan, stating that she had taken care of the patient successfully for two years and could continue to do so. The patient agreed with the operator, but the social worker did not believe the patient fully understood the type of care she would receive at a nursing home. Furthermore, the social worker believed the patient had strong ties with the boarding home and suspected the boarding home operator did not want to lose the revenue she received from the patient.

The social worker could not pursue nursing home placement in opposition to the patient unless a competency petition was made. The patient's occasional confusion did not warrant a competency hearing. Eventually the boarding home operator decided that she could not care for the patient. She stated that the patient's sister, who lived in the next state and had managed the patient's finances through a local bank, would assist with nursing home and Medicaid applications. The patient accepted this decision.

The physician, born and educated in the Far East, had been practicing at Memorial for eight years. He was one of the hospital's top admitters and had a growing practice. He believed he was responsible for initiating all aspects of patient care and consequently rebuffed suggestions from hospital personnel. He did not believe the patient's personal life or social problems were to be addressed during the course of hospitalization. The physician operated under increasing stress as his practice grew. On many occasions he had reported employees to the hospital administrator for incompetence or interference in his cases. However, he was intimidated by the utilization review process and viewed a denial of benefits as a serious criticism of his skill.

The social worker had a bachelor's degree in social work and five years experience including three years at Memorial as a discharge planner. She averaged a monthly caseload of fifty patients, which was considered appropriate for the intensity of services required. Performance appraisals showed her to be a consistent, competent professional. On two prior occasions the physician on this case had accused her of incompetence when she failed to obtain Medicaid beds in nursing homes. These charges were unsubstantiated.

Memorial's chief executive officer had been at the hospital for less than one year. His priority of increasing admissions had met with success because he aligned himself strongly with physicians. In prior discharge planning cases brought to his attention for mediation the administrator supported the physician.

The boarding home operator lived in her boarding home. Although uneducated, she had shrewdly turned her ability to take care of frail elderly people into a means for survival in a poor urban community. This small income came into jeopardy when the state passed the Rooming and Boarding Home Act. All such facilities were to be licensed and regularly inspected by the Department of Community Affairs. Violations could result in removing the license or closing the home. Many of the boarding home operators regarded their residents as family and had difficulty meeting standards requiring eviction of residents who needed skilled care.

An interdisciplinary discharge planning committee chaired by the social work director reviewed policy and procedures and coordinated interdepartmental efforts. However, no single person or department was formally designated as having responsibility to oversee the process. A nurse hired to make visiting nurse referrals reported to the director of nursing and all other discharge planning activities were carried out by social workers.

During the lengthy wait for a nursing home bed the patient began to improve. At the same time the utilization review committee began to question the physician about discharge plans. The physician reevaluated the patient and found her to be independent in ambulation, continent, and self-feeding. The physician wrote an order to contact the boarding home and arrange to discharge the patient ''home.''

The social worker contacted the sister and the boarding home operator to relay the physician's wishes. Despite their earlier decision, the sister and operator decided the patient could go home as long as it was in accordance with the physician's wishes. The patient agreed and nursing home plans were dropped.

Approximately two months after discharge the boarding home was inspected by the Department of Community Affairs (DCA). The operator was cited for having a resident who needed a higher level of care. Because the patient had been placed there by the hospital, the DCA referred the case to the Department of Health (DOH) as an inappropriate discharge.

The DOH investigated and cited the hospital for making an inappropriate discharge. The penalty was a fine of $15,000 calculated at $250 per day for every day that the patient was in the ''inappropriate setting.'' No charges were filed against the boarding home operator or the physician. Neither the patient nor her sister had initiated any complaint.

When cited, the hospital administrator and the social work director reviewed the medical record, interviewed the social worker, and reviewed existing policies and procedures. The medical record showed documentation inconsistencies. The physician notes indicated the patient was ambulatory without assistance, fed herself, and was continent. The nurses' notes for the same date showed the patient being assisted from bed to chair, incontinent of urine, and restrained at night to prevent her from wandering. Social work notes documented the initial assessment and the progress of the nursing home placement efforts. The notes did not reflect a reassessment at the time the plan changed from nursing home to boarding home.

The social worker was familiar with all aspects of the case but had retreated from her convictions when she was the only person questioning the plan that was in keeping with patient and family wishes. At the time, the social worker had eight other patients awaiting Medicaid beds and was aware that the patient could feasibly await a nursing home bed for several months at great cost to the hospital and restraint to the patient. She also admitted a reluctance to have another confrontation with the physician in light of past difficulties.

The attending physician was not interviewed by the state or the hospital administrator. In fact the physician was not told of the incident until all appeals had been filed. The issue of shared responsibility between physician and hospital was never addressed. Revised policies and procedures reflected the position of the state that hospitals are accountable for the actions of physicians who practice in the institution.

Analysis

In this case existing discharge policies and procedures were followed appropriately but four areas of improvement needed to be implemented:

1. The hospital needed in-service education and a tool to assist physicians in determining appropriate post-discharge levels of care.
2. A mechanism for mediation of disputes between discharge planners and physicians needed to be established.
3. The discharge planning function needed to be recognized and responsibility for coordination centralized under a single authority formalized on the table of organization.
4. A monitoring system needed to be established to review the appropriateness of discharge plans.

These recommendations for revision of the existing policies and procedures provide an ideal mechanism for ensuring appropriate discharge planning. Realistically, the duplication of supervisory review of 100 percent of all discharge placements would not be feasible within the staffing limits of most hospitals. The regular review and evaluation of discharge placements would have to monitor a sufficient number of placements to assure compliance with procedures.

This case illustrates the complexity of decision making viewed from the perspective of conflicting belief systems and overlapping authority. The state clearly placed the responsibility for discharge planning on the hospital, yet the administrator deferred to the "process." In that "process" neither the social worker nor the physician perceived their own authority. The physician was intimidated by utilization review and the social worker by the physician.

The question of who is responsible for a discharge plan and action is further highlighted by a 1986 California case that held the physician the sole determinant of discharge decisions.[7] In this case a patient received necessary vascular surgery and ten days of hospitalization, authorized by Medi-Cal. Because of a stormy recovery after surgery and the risk of infections or blood clots, the patient's physicians requested an additional eight days of acute care hospitalization. This request was reviewed by a Medi-Cal nurse, who spoke with a consultant physician. After this telephone conversation the physician consultant authorized only an additional four-day extension. Within a few days after discharge, the patient began to suffer severe pain in her right leg, and nine days later she was readmitted to the hospital. Her physicians concluded she had developed clotting in the right leg along with an infection at the site of surgery. The leg had to be amputated.

The patient filed a complaint against Medi-Cal, arguing that the original eight-day requested hospitalization would have allowed for early intervention, thus saving her leg. Her primary physician testified that, "to a reasonable medical certainty," the patient would not have lost her leg if she had remained in the hospital for the requested period.[8] A jury's verdict in favor of the patient was overturned by the Court of Appeals, thus accepting the state's argument that the discharge decision was made by the patient's physicians based upon her condition at the time of discharge and that Medi-Cal was not liable for her injuries as it played no part in the discharge.

The court stated that the principal issue was "who bears responsibility for allowing a patient to be discharged from the hospital, her treating physicians or the health care payor." With regard to physicians, the court said: "a physician who complies without protest with the limitations imposed by a third party payor, when his judgment dictates otherwise, cannot avoid his ultimate responsibility for his patient's care."[9] The court noted that the physician was intimidated by the Medi-Cal plan but not paralyzed or rendered powerless. It added that the physician should have advocated for the patient's best interests.

Although the Medi-Cal plan was not held liable, the court stated:

> Third party payors of health care services can be held legally accountable when medically inappropriate decisions result from defects in the design or implementation of cost containment mechanisms as, for example, when appeals made on a patient's behalf for medical or hospital care are arbitrarily ignored or unreasonably disregarded or overridden.[10]

In summary, the physicians should have protested or requested a reconsideration of Medi-Cal's authorized four-day extension, at least requesting an additional four-day extension when the first expired. The court reaffirmed the "fundamental principle" that physicians, and not other actors in the discharge process, are ultimately responsible for the medical care of their patients. This case represents the first time that a state appellate court has clearly discussed cost containment pressures and their effect on discharge decision making. This case may have implications for hospital responsibility for discharge decisions made by physicians. It also illustrates the cost of inappropriate discharge for both the patient and physician, and potentially the health care institution.[11]

EFFECTIVE DISCHARGE PLANNING

As the above-described cases indicate, discharge planning must be accomplished with care and vigilance for each hospital admission, as misdirections and errors can easily translate into harm for the patient. Appropriate mechanisms to meet patients' needs after hospitalization require programs, personnel, and a process for assessment, decision making, action, and follow-up. These component parts of discharge planning cut across a broad range of activities. (See Figure 18-1.)

Discharge Program

An effective discharge planning program is a coordinated multidisciplinary approach to patient care. This program maintains written, mutually agreed upon procedures outlining responsibilities for each discipline interfacing with the patient during treatment. The components of this program should include, but not be limited to: (a) written criteria for identifying patients in need of special attention, (b) documentation of assessment and plan, (c) clearly defined roles and responsibilities for team conferences, and (d) a mechanism for ongoing evaluation of the quality and appropriateness of discharge planning activities.

Discharge Personnel

Personnel responsible for discharge planning compose an interdisciplinary team within the hospital and ideally function as a team consistent with program guidelines. This team includes all individuals who interface with the patient and have information (medical, psychological, or social) that will facilitate a smooth transition from hospital to home or extended care facility. Each team member should be identified by the role he or she plays; the titles will vary from hospital to hospital.

The team consists of, but is not limited to: patient, physician, primary care nurse, social worker, home health intake coordinator, utilization review coordinator, patient educator, and discharge planning coordinator (if not already named). Other persons such as dietician, physical therapist, pastoral care counselor, or pediatric play therapist may be available for specific case conferences. Although the attending physician has ultimate responsibility for total patient

Figure 18-1 Discharge Planning Process Flow Chart

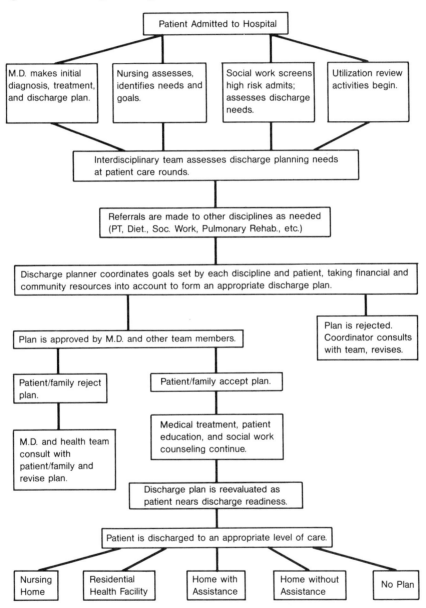

care, each team member has a responsibility to assess the patient's needs and establish a care plan whenever appropriate.

Discharge Process

Ideally the discharge planning process is an interdisciplinary team approach coordinated by a central authority accountable to the hospital's chief executive officer. An effective discharge process prevents any delays in discharge and—in many cases—eliminates the need for continued care referrals after discharge. The process begins with the patient's entrance into the health care system and ends with the implementation of the aftercare plan.

A. Admission Screening

At admission the physician assesses the patient for possible discharge planning needs and makes appropriate referrals to other services. The primary nurse completes a nursing assessment and establishes a treatment plan that includes goals and anticipated discharge needs. Social workers are responsible for screening all admission slips for potential discharge planning needs. Those patients in the high risk categories must be assessed by the assigned social worker within a specified number of days (usually three working days). The utilization review coordinator reviews each patient record for potential discharge planning needs and makes appropriate referrals to other services.

B. Referrals

Not all discharge planning needs are identified during the screening phase, and subsequent referrals are responded to within the guidelines of that department. Discharge planning referrals should be responded to within one working day.

C. Assessment

The patient's and the patient's family's capabilities in relation to the patient's anticipated needs are identified through assessments. Assessments should address activities of daily living, environmental obstacles, social, emotional, and financial needs as well as the patient's and family's reliability and expectations. The assessment is a fluid process that must be kept current as patient needs change and other risk factors are identified.

D. Patient Care Conferences

One means for structuring time to ensure collaborative review of patient needs and evolving plans is the patient care conference. The team members meet on a regularly scheduled basis to evaluate each patient's physical, intellectual, medical, and psychosocial functioning to make treatment recommendations. This conference is attended by key team members and encourages a holistic approach to discussing patient needs and progress. Referrals to other disciplines can be initiated through these meetings.

E. The Plan

Strategies for obtaining necessary posthospital services are established in collaboration with the patient and team members. The discharge planner coordinates goals set by each discipline and, taking financial and community resources into account, forms an appropriate discharge plan. Once the plan is approved by both the physician and the patient it is put into action. Medical treatment, patient education, and social work counseling continue as the patient progresses toward discharge readiness. As the discharge date draws near the plan is reevaluated and implemented.

F. Follow-Up

The hospital is responsible for follow-up and/or follow through on care plans for patients discharged to home care or transferred to other institutions. This follow-up shall include determinations that planned services were received and that initial contact was made with the referral agency.

Exhibit 18-1 can be used to help professionals, particularly physicians, understand the decision making that must occur. It also provides a chart that is effective documentation for the discharge plan.

CONCLUSION

In reality, the discharge planning process may be fraught with obstacles such as turf battles between professionals, conflicting values, poor coordination, failure to include the patient or key family member in the planning process, competency questions, and lack of appropriate community resources. These obstacles can be reduced with clear policies and procedures that identify roles and responsibilities of team members, provide a mechanism for educating the medical, nursing, social work, and utilization review staffs and the patient, and formally recognize the discharge planning function, whether the function lies within a department or stands alone. The two cited cases illustrate that the body of law, whether regulatory or judicial, is still evolving in relation to discharge planning. While familiarity with specific state law is essential, the only real "guarantee" against charges of wrongful discharge is an effective process that strives to make discharges appropriate.

Communication is the key to an effective and efficient process. Communication between members of the health care team and the patient and family

Exhibit 18-1 Guidelines for Assessing Postdischarge Level of Care

Instructions:
1. Review levels of care provided by each type of facility.
2. Check the box in each of the areas (I–IV) that best describes the care your patient will need.

	Skilled Nursing Facility (S.N.F.) Intense, Skilled Nursing Level	Intermediate Care Facility		Residential Health Care Facility Nonmedical Facility	Boarding Home Nonhealth Facility
		Level A Upper Level Medical Care	Level B Lower Level Nonmedical Care		
I. *Nursing Services* required for assessment and management, changing conditions, patient instruction	24 hour care by R.N. under physician supervision. □	24 hour R.N. supervision on premises. □	24 hour R.N. or L.P.N. supervision on premises. □	No nursing supervision required. □	No supervision required. □

II. Treatments (i.e., decubitus care, catheter care, tube feedings, I.V., I.M. injections)	Given or supervised by R.N. Treatments necessary on a daily basis. ☐	Given by L.P.N. or R.N., but supervised by R.N. on a daily basis. ☐	Provided by L.P.N. or aide under supervision of R.N. or L.P.N. ☐	No nursing care required. Medication distribution supervised by *nonprofessional*. ☐	Maintenance and medications not requiring assistance or supervision. ☐
III. Physical/Medical Functioning	Requires intense observation and treatments. ☐	Requires substantial assistance with personal care. ☐	May be partially ambulatory with physical and/or mental dysfunction. ☐	Must be ambulatory (with minimal assistance device). Must be alert and oriented. May require assistance with financial affairs. Must be continent. ☐	Must be ambulatory, alert, and oriented. Must not require health care. ☐
IV. Personal Care Needs	2.7 hours direct personal care in every 24 hours. ☐	2.5 hours direct personal care in every 24 hours. ☐	1.25 hours direct personal care in every 24 hours. ☐	May require minimal personal care with dressing and bathing. 1 hour direct personal care in every 24 hours. ☐	No personal or financial services offered (except at Level "C" home). ☐

requires time. In today's health care environment there may be many demands on limited professional time plus additional pressures to discharge quickly. The discharge planning process should clearly identify points where communication takes place and provide a structure to ensure time is set aside for this communication. This preparation for and prioritization of discharge planning is necessary to prevent harm and complete the health care professionals' service to the patient.

NOTES

1. K.W. Davidson, "Evolving Social Work Roles in Health Care: The Case of Discharge Planning," *Social Work in Health Care* 4, no. 1 (Fall 1978):43–53.

2. "Premature-Discharge Allegations Intensify," *Hospitals* 59, no. 22 (November 16, 1985):31.

3. Ibid.

4. "The Medicare Quality Protection Act of 1986," *New Jersey Hospital Association* (NJHA), *Government Relations*, July 18, 1986, 1–8.

5. Ibid., 1.

6. "Premature-Discharge," 31.

7. *Wickline v. State of California*, No. B010156, Slip opinion, Cal. Ct. App. 2nd Dist., July 30, 1986.

8. S.M. Mitchell, "Discharge Decision Is Physician's Responsibility," *Health Law Vigil* 9, no. 17 (August 29, 1986):5.

9. Ibid., 5.

10. Ibid., 5.

11. Ibid., 6.

Chapter 19

Whistle-Blowing: A Problem of Values in the Workplace

Leah L. Curtin, MS, MA, RN, FAAN

At 35, with ten years of grade school teaching behind her, Sister M. Angelique* was an exceptionally mature and sensitive nursing student: an ideal person to assign to care for Muriel Feldstein, the 52-year-old wife of one of the hospital's benefactors. Admitted for gall bladder surgery, Mrs. Feldstein had a history of emphysema and congestive heart failure—a challenging nursing care study for Sister Angelique. All in all, it seemed a perfect match, which indeed it was. Sister Angelique's intelligence and gentle ways quickly won Mrs. Feldstein's trust; so much so that she formally asked that Sister be present during her surgery. Sister Angelique promised that she would be there, and arrangements were made for Sister to observe the surgery (a not uncommon practice for nursing students even today).

Following the surgery, Mrs. Feldstein spent several hours in the surgical intensive care unit before she was returned to her room. As she became more alert, she asked Sister Angelique many questions about her surgery. Sister assured her that everything had gone beautifully, textbook-perfect, and that Dr. X's technique was exquisite.

"Dr. X?!" Mrs. Feldstein exclaimed. "Who is Dr. X? Dr. Y, the chief of surgery, is my doctor?"

"Oh yes," Sister Angelique replied, "I am very sure it was Dr. X. He is a surgical resident here. I know Dr. Y quite well. I taught all of his children in grade school, and Dr. Y wasn't even in the room."

At this, Mrs. Feldstein simply said "Thank you, Sister," and settled down for a rest. A short time later, Dr. Y entered her room and cheerily informed her that her surgery had gone very well indeed. Mrs. Feldstein said, "How would you know? You weren't even there."

"What ever gave you that idea, Mrs. Feldstein? I am your surgeon."

---

*All names are fictitious, although the situation is reported accurately in all its essentials.

"That's what I *thought*," she said, "but Sister Angelique said you weren't there, and Sister Angelique doesn't tell lies. If you think for one minute that I'm going to pay your bill, you've got another thing coming."

Mrs. Feldstein closed her eyes, and Dr. Y stalked out of the room and headed for the closest telephone. Within minutes he was in the vice president for nursing's office demanding Sister Angelique's immediate dismissal for breach of professional confidentiality.

Several hours later, Sister Angelique was in the same office trying to explain what happened. She asked this hospital's chief nurse, "Have I done something wrong?"

"No, Sister, you have not. You've done something very right. It's just a little difficult to handle. Mrs. Feldstein is very angry with Dr. Y and has refused to pay him." And despite the problems, the chief nurse laughed.

"I know," said Sister in a woebegone voice, "Her husband handed me this check for $5,000 just before I came down here. He said it was the doctor's fee, but I was the only one who earned it."

As a result of Sister Angelique's naivete, "phantom surgery," long a problem in this institution, was placed squarely before the medical and administrative staff. Eventually, stringent measures were taken to lay this ghost to rest. However, one wonders whether the situation would have been handled differently if Mrs. Feldstein had not been powerful, and Sister Angelique had not been a member of the religious order that owned the hospital.

THE CASE FOR "BLOWING THE WHISTLE"

Few things challenge traditional work values as clearly as what has come to be called "whistle-blowing." In American society we associate the *right* and *duty* to "blow the whistle" with the authorities in our lives. We expect our teachers, referees, managers, and bosses to be the ones who say, "Wait a minute," "That's enough," "Something's wrong," "Let's start over," "Foul!" Students, players, and workers often are admired if they can "get away with something." Group loyalty demands silence or even collusion. We are puzzled, suspicious, or even outraged when someone in the ranks yells "Stop!" What right does that voice in the crowd have to halt our pleasure in the game, to disrupt our routines, to prick our consciences, or to challenge our authority?

There probably never were any "good old days" when people knew what they ought to do and did it—and were respected for doing it. Nonetheless, life today is more complex than it once was, and one aspect of that complexity is that it has become even more difficult to determine what to do and when to do it. Bhopal, Challenger, Chernobyl: it seems a long way from Sister Angelique to these screaming headlines; yet each disaster could have been prevented if a Sister Angelique had been there—if someone had reported warning signs or if managers had listened when that person did.

Much has been written about the impact of technology on our value systems: how it has increased options, blurred traditional principles, and posed unprecedented questions. However, a great deal more needs to be said about the ways in which technology heightens the moral responsibility of the worker. Technological advances compress time and decrease the tolerable margin for error. Moreover, division of labor has placed many in positions of power with little knowledge about producing a good or service and even less about the complex technological trade-offs involved in their production.*

Today, when practical, even prosaic, everyday decisions may have awesome consequences, it has become imperative for each person to be *vested* in his or her job—in the ultimate outcome of the work. Each has a special responsibility and accountability that must become part of an employee's identity, commitment to life, and place in society. Ignoring the importance of that investment—however misguided or imperfect it may be—risks the integrity of the worker and the whole institution.

To put the matter succinctly, advanced technology and its complex systems demand what Nicholas Rescher calls "value restandardization." Contemporary developments stretch traditional lines of authority and loyalty beyond their limits. For example, while loyalty, authority, honesty, and integrity still are found in the workers' hierarchy of values, their relative positions and what *constitutes* each of them have been (or need to be) revised.

PROBLEMS AND EVASIONS

Few things illustrate the importance of rethinking and restandardizing work values as clearly as "whistle-blowing" or, more properly, its absence. Despite popular notions to the contrary, "whistle-blowers" pose many problems for someone in a position of authority:

- How much weight should one give to the complaint and to the complainer?
- Does this report make the institution look bad?
- Can it be covered up?
- Should it be covered up?
- How can the damage be contained?
- Who, in the end, will pay the damages?
- Is it safer (psychologically, socially, economically, politically) for me *not* to know?

---

*It is equally appalling that a Morton-Thiokol executive could override his engineers' decision about the safety of Challenger's rockets and that a hospital purchasing agent could override clinicians' decisions about the safety of oxygen equipment.

Knowing and not knowing are *choices* in mature persons of reasonable capacity. Ignorance (used here in its precise, technical sense, i.e., deliberate, self-chosen lack of knowledge) distances the decision maker in time and space from painful and threatening information. The manifestations of ethical ignorance include: (1) refusing to place credence in evidence, (2) failing to ask pertinent questions, (3) blindly following established routines, (4) burying data that contradict prevailing norms or political trends, (5) depositing information "in the files" (without analysis) for one's successor(s) to handle, and (6) segmenting information so that no one can understand the implications (outcomes, possibilities) of the whole.

We are not talking here about mere abstractions. What is involved is real and demonstrable—and dangerous precisely because ignorance precludes resolve. If knowledge is a prerequisite for judgment, then ignorance enables one to avoid (at least temporarily) the duty to decide. By intellectually distancing oneself, one escapes both conscience and accountability—and shirks personal and social liabilities.

The problems of conscience encompass both ethics and integrity. While I'm not at all sure that I can defend this distinction philosophically, practically speaking it is enormously helpful to separate the two. In any case, ethical problems arise when one is not sure—or even reasonably confident—that one knows what is the right thing to do in a given situation. For example, loyalties to a friend, coworker, leader, or team may conflict with one another or with ideals like justice and honesty. Problems of personal integrity arise when one has figured out the right thing to do—or at least thinks one has—and yet does not want to do it or is prevented from doing it.

LOYALTY AND COERCION

As short a time ago as 1908 Royce, in his book *The Philosophy of Loyalty*, held that one could center one's entire moral world around a rational concept of loyalty provided that loyalty is defined as the willing and practical devotion of a person to a cause. While this approach helps to clarify conflicting claims on one's loyalty, it seems a bit too simple. For example, China's Cultural Revolution, which certainly operated on devotion to the "cause," not only decimated the intelligentsia but also undermined any pretense of trust in human interactions. It seems to me that any approach that places ideology above persons is perilous at best. However, if one measures the *safety* of others (many or only one) against the convenience, comfort, status, or profit of a friend, coworker, leader, or institution, even the professional *ethos*, which focuses almost exclusively on the covenant between professional and *individual*, recognizes the superior claim of those endangered by the decision, action, or omission of the one to whom one owes loyalty.

Even when the "right" thing seems clear, a prospective whistle-blower faces difficult value choices. Consider the questions this person must grapple with *before* taking action:

- Have I got my facts straight?
- If so, is it my problem?
- Why should I do anything about it?
- Is is my fault?
- Who am I to judge?
- Should I ignore the situation? tolerate it?
- Is anything to be gained?
- What do I get out of this?
- What might it cost me?
- Must I do something about it?
- Is it worth the trouble?

Moreover, when the consequences seem out of all proportion to the problem (error, offense), yet another dimension is added. For example, it has been noted that nurses frequently will not report colleagues for suspected substance abuse because the consequences are draconian: in most instances, dismissal, loss of livelihood and health insurance, suspension of license to practice, personal and professional ostracism, and perhaps criminal charges as well. Few people want to be "responsible" for such personal devastation and so they "look the other way." The situation is all the more easily ignored because the dangers usually are potential rather than actual. At any rate, effective and appropriate reporting will not occur until less punitive or, preferably, genuinely helpful approaches are developed. At those institutions (such as Crawford W. Long Hospital in Atlanta) where a humane program has been established to help impaired nurses, reporting is much more frequent *and* timely.

Problems regarding judgment and safety are far more immediate than problems of honesty and, thus, more likely to be reported. For example, in one case a surgical nurse was appalled when a urological surgeon bragged about doing the bare minimum possible to restore micturation for patients with BPH (benign prostatic hypertrophy): that way he could collect another fee next year, and the next, and year after year. This surgeon's indiscretion implicated the nurse. If she remained silent she became a moral accomplice to his malfeasance. However, she faced severe problems if she chose to report the situation: (1) the near impossibility of obtaining corroborating information, (2) the likelihood that he would deny that he ever made such a statement, and (3) the probability of personal reprisals. Sensibly skeptical of her own authority and influence, this nurse faced not only problems of personal integrity (how much was she willing to risk to do what she thought right?) but also the pragmatic problem of whether the risk could produce any positive results at all. It is good to be a martyr for a just cause; it's quite another thing altogether to suffer in vain. Other than expressing her disapproval (primarily by avoiding him), this nurse did nothing.

We ignore at our own peril the power of informal, often invisible coercion. Because we traditionally think of force in physical terms, we may forget that the stuff of psychological coercion is ridicule, social ostracism, and economic loss—in that order of importance. To a social and cerebral animal like man, the need for approval and acceptance is associated with survival. To belong to the group is psychologically comparable to being worthy, safe, and secure. Behaviors that threaten group norms are punished with rejection and even abandonment, temporary or permanent. If we really do want people to "blow the whistle" appropriately, we must devise a way to affect group norms without destroying personal trust.

RESTANDARDIZING VALUES IN THE WORKPLACE

An effective approach to restandardizing group norms demands pragmatic, not merely philosophical activity. To begin, we must:

1. develop clearly defined parallel lines of technical and administrative authority,
2. promulgate clearly understandable procedures for reporting errors or problems and challenging decisions,
3. design appropriate rewards and protections for those who are instrumental in reporting and solving problems,
4. devise measures that will inhibit vindictive use of the system, and
5. compose a program of values clarification and ethical responsibility for each of the interconnected, interdependent layers of administrators, professionals, technicians, and workers.

These reflections become particularly significant when one considers the great social phenomena that are shaping society today. Professionals, moving rapidly from entrepreneurial to employee status, live and work in a society in transition— culturally, morally, and technologically. A pervasive sense of transition breeds skepticism. As institutions, customs, and mores are challenged and change, stability is undermined, and people lose faith in the constancy of the values, norms, and authorities that shaped the past. The result is a general tendency to distrust and debunk those in positions of authority, past and present. Moreover, the high rate of mobility in the population inhibits familiarity with persons, places, and traditions that are basic to acknowledging professionals, institutions, and symbols; it also leads to personal withdrawal and alienation. Fear of large scale institutions adumbrates those who represent them (business and labor leaders, lawyers, doctors, nurses, and so on). Thus, individuals in these positions are required to prove themselves constantly because the institutions they represent no longer are deemed trustworthy.

The one constant guaranteeing status and representing success is money. The monetization of status—the equation of worth or value with income—further inhibits recognition of those aspects of professional life and status that are not amenable to such quantitative analysis: commitment, ethical standards, presence, judgment, and concern for the social good inspire trust or confidence. To illustrate, the word "professional" today is generally used as the antonym for "amateur." A professional is paid, an amateur is not. The more a professional is paid, the better professional he or she is. Thus, the entertainer who earns two million dollars a year is more valuable to society than the physician who earns one hundred thousand dollars a year. In this manner, social utility becomes secondary to financial gain, which in turn sparks fears that professionals exploit the public to augment their own incomes (witness the malpractice crisis). These changes in social values, exacerbated by technologically induced pressures in the workplace, further complicate attempts to actualize such professional values as altruism and accountability in the agencies that employ professionals. Given both the public's expectations of success *and* distrust of the system, it is little wonder that physicians and institutions feel pressure to practice protective medicine and may seek to cover up more than to correct errors and problems. Nonetheless, despite public skepticism—or perhaps because of it—public institutions and the personnel they employ must demonstrate increased accountability and must stop errors before more damage is done both to their credibility and to the public's well-being.

Restandardizing values in work settings that contain a mix of professional and management personnel is challenging because the groups usually have (and ought to have) considerable differences in work values. For the professionals, work is an instrument to effect human well-being directly. For the managers, work is an instrument to effect organizational goals and indirectly to add to the social good. To put matters in different language, professionals view their work from a deontological perspective: my duty to this individual, one on one. Managers view their work from a teleological perspective: our commitment to produce the best outcome most efficiently.

Negotiating these differences demands a reconceptualization of employer-employee relationships—a move from hierarchical to interactive models. The whole notion of "superior/subordinate" breaks down when the expert power of the professional confronts the position power of the manager. An effective model recognizes parallel areas of clearly defined authority, with space at the interface continually negotiated to achieve mutually acceptable goals. (See Figure 19-1.)

When critical incidents occur (as they undoubtedly will), immediate intervention and negotiation must be initiated by whoever discovers the problem—

Figure 19-1 Critical Incidents: Range of Negotiated Outcomes

Value Orientation		Value Orientation
Deontological		Teleological

		CRITICAL INCIDENT		
	+4	Commitment to Changed Accountability Standards	+4	
• Expert Power	+3	Correction of Standards, Reconciliation of Accountable Persons	+3	• Position Power
• Access to Informal Network	+2	Correction of Situation, Mutual Tolerance of Accountable Persons	+2	• Access to Administrative Network
• Efficient Use of Resources	+1	Mitigation of Situation, Reconciliation of Persons	+1	• Distribution of Resources
EMPLOYEE'S RESOURCES		**CRITICAL INCIDENT**		MANAGER'S RESOURCES
	−1	Moratorium for a Short, Definite Period	−1	
				• Coercive Power
• Passive-Aggressive Resistance	−2	Toleration of Situation, Distancing of Persons, Prolonged "Study" of Problem	−2	
• Subversive Power	−3	Deterioration of Situation. Reassignment or Firing of Personnel	−3	• "Divide and Conquer"
	−4	Reinforcement of Negative Situation, Punishment	−4	

without prejudice. One simple way of beginning to create an environment that encourages accountability is to establish a "critical incident hotline" that would connect any employee directly to the risk management department. Each complaint should be received respectfully and investigated quickly. Whenever possible, the employee who has reported the problem should be involved in its resolution—and, in any case, should be apprised of what action was taken, or why action was not taken.

If this small beginning is augmented by ongoing in-service programs that stress the importance of the work each person or department contributes to the whole, a sense of personal responsibility may replace the alienation so common among today's workers. The more people *understand* how their work relates to the ultimate outcome, the more likely they are to become *vested* in that outcome. And the less likely they are to tolerate substandard or dangerous practices and situations. That is, the more likely it will become that they will report problems, i.e., "blow the whistle."

However, technicians, housekeepers, maintenance personnel, and the like are most unlikely to adopt such upscale professional values when or if the professionals themselves disown them.

Paid professionals are a difficult and volatile lot to manage—for those who fail to understand their work values. The professional ethos, combined with professional socialization patterns, tends to foster noncompliance with hierarchical patterns and policies, rejection of organizational authority (especially in regard to the particulars of their practice and the evaluation of their performance by nonexpert managers), and disinclination to engage in peer review. This latter tendency results from a deeply ingrained belief that true professionals self-evaluate and self-discipline. Rigid hierarchical and authoritarian management styles inevitably lead to conflict with professional staff. Insecure or dissatisfied professionals are bright enough to exploit any given system to their own advantage, sabotage the system, or transfer their education and skills to other, better paid fields. On the other hand, paid professionals may conform to organizational imperatives to such a degree that they (1) develop highly rationalized routines that look good but do not deliver the service, (2) sacrifice professional judgment to procedure ("follow the book" even when it is inappropriate to do so), (3) engage in absenteeism and vagabondage (drift from job to job), and (4) sell out (forfeit personal integrity to organizational goals) or burn out (give up).

If employers are to achieve organizational goals while at the same time accommodating the professional ethos, they must structure the environment according to professionally acceptable criteria. All employees need a standard of living that supports personal decency and physical security, continuing education, and the community respect that guards against corruption of professional values (education, commitment, achievement, dedication, and honor cost money, too). Otherwise the professional, rejecting "professionalism," will abdicate personal accountability for the quality and outcomes of his or her work. Decentralized management, participatory decision making, and peer involvement in selection and evaluation of personnel are prerequisites. The workplace should support professionally defined standards of practice, accord respect to the individual dignity of the practitioner, allow space for the integrity of professional judgment, and encourage personal commitment to professional goals. In such an environment, whistle-blowing is transformed into responsible reporting and the whistle-blower into a valued partner in the achievement of professional and organizational goals.

BIBLIOGRAPHY

Annas, George J. "Who to Call When the Doctor is Sick." *The Hastings Center Report* 8 (6):18–20.

Cassirer, Ernst. *Rousseau, Kant and Goethe.* New York: Harper and Row, 1944.

Curtin, Leah, and Zurlage, Carolina, eds. *DRGs: The Reorganization of Health.* Chicago: S-N Publications, 1984.

Curtin, Leah, and Flaherty, M. Josephine. *Nursing Ethics: Theories and Pragmatics.* Bowie, Md: Robert J. Brady Co., 1982.

Graner, John L. "Osler's 'A Way of Life'." *Humane Medicine* 2 (1):33–38.

Hunt, Robert, and Arras, John. *Ethical Issues in Modern Medicine.* Palo Alto, Cal.: Mayfield Publishing Company, 1977.

Jameton, Andrew. "The Nurse: When Roles and Rules Conflict." *The Hastings Center Report* 7 (4):22.

Levenstein, Aaron. *The Nurse as Manager.* Chicago: S-N Publications, 1981.

Levine, Carol, and Bermel, Joyce. "Revising the United States Senate Code of Ethics." *Hastings Center Report Special Supplement*, February 1981, pp. 1–28.

Mill, John Stuart. *On Bentham and Coleridge.* New York: Harper and Row, 1950.

Rescher, Nicholas. "What is a Value Change? A Framework for Research," in K. Baier and N. Rescher, eds. *Values and the Future.* New York: The Free Press, 1969.

Shannon, Thomas. *Bioethics.* New York: Paulist Press, 1976.

Singer, Peter. "Do Consequences Count? Rethinking the Doctrine of Double Effect." *The Hastings Center Report* 10 (1):42–44.

Walton, Clarence C. "Business Ethics: The Present and the Future." *The Hastings Center Report* 10 (5):16–20.

Part VI
Structure for Action

Chapter 20

The Role and Structure of Hospital Ethics Committees

George A. Kanoti, MA, STD, and Janicemarie K. Vinicky, MA

INTRODUCTION

The concept of an institutional ethics committee (IEC) attracts the attention of many health care administrators. Although committees for decision making are not novel to medicine (committees such as credentials, morbidity and mortality, institutional review, quality assurance, utilization review, and others do exist), the idea of organizing a standing committee to address ethical concerns in the clinical setting is new.[1] Many health care administrators and decision makers wonder whether they should establish an IEC in their institution. The answer to that question depends upon many factors.

The purpose of this chapter is to illustrate these factors, i.e., the need for institutional ethics committees; the investments of time, energy, and finances; the benefits, costs, and pitfalls in establishing an IEC; the mandates given to IECs; their place in organizational tables; and the structures they have taken. At the conclusion of this chapter readers will be able to understand the processes by which IECs are established, function, and grow.

An IEC can be defined as an interdisciplinary group of health care professionals, community representatives, and nonmedical professionals who address ethical questions in the health care institution, especially on the care of patients.

Since the court recommended in the *Karen Ann Quinlan* case (1979) the establishment of ethics committees to assist in clinical decisions,[2] the number of IECs has grown. The literature reports several years of IEC experience from which an understanding of the nature and functions of IECs can be gained.

NEED FOR IECs

Are IECs merely fads that have been precipitated by the federal government and by consumer rights and other advocacy groups? Although the growth of IECs has been influenced by these groups, they reflect a need in medicine rather than a reaction to political, governmental, advocacy, or legal pressures. The moral choices produced by economic factors and the medical, surgical, and technological options at the beginning, middle, and end of life have created the need for IECs. The allocation of resources, withdrawal of nutritional support for terminally ill patients, decisions concerning reproductive technologies (abortion, in vitro fertilization, and so forth), and other choices illustrate some of these moral choices.

In the past, in most health care institutions, moral choices were not addressed in any systematic ethical fashion. The moral choices usually were made by individuals (physicians, hospital administrators, patients) who reflected their personal moral convictions, rather than by a group that systematically discussed the ethics of alternatives and guidelines for policy and behavior in the health care institution. Further, not infrequently the choice raised disagreements about the correctness of the option, either among the staff, or between staff and allied health persons, between the staff and patients, between the patients and families, or among family members. A moral question that frequently raises very different and conflicting opinions is whether one should withdraw nutritional life support systems. An IEC provides a forum for systematic ethical discussion of these moral choices.

There is an extensive history of medical moral questions that have taken hospitals and staff into the courtroom. The *Karen Ann Quinlan* case in New Jersey is the classic example. Exhibit 20-1 lists the most significant legal/moral cases.

ORGANIZATIONAL STRUCTURE

The birth and growth of IECs have raised practical administrative questions such as the place of an IEC within the organizational and reporting structure of health care facilities. Four reporting models have evolved. (See Figure 20-1.) Each has its advantages and disadvantages. We believe the fourth model is the simplest and most appropriate—the IEC reports directly to the governing board, is mandated and supported by the board and the administration, and is peopled by medical, allied health, and other nonmedical professionals.

In some institutions the relationship of the IEC to other committees like the IRB committee (human research committee) is important. Although the mandates of the two committees are similar, a distinction does exist. The IRB is mandated by federal law to review the ethics of human research protocols funded by the federal government. IECs are mandated more broadly, i.e., to review the ethics of clinical cases and other ethical issues that affect the health care institution. Frequently the distinction is blurred because much medical research is clinical (patients are subjects of the research). In cases that have both clinical and research implications, or instances where proposals on the cutting edge of medical tech-

Exhibit 20-1 Landmark Cases on Life Support Decisions*

1976, *Matter of Quinlan*. New Jersey Supreme Court authorized discontinuance of respiratory support for the 21-year-old woman in a permanent vegetative state.

1977, *Superintendent of Belchertown State Schools vs. Saikewicz*. Massachusetts Supreme Court approved a decision not to provide chemotherapy for a 67-year-old retarded and institutionalized man with acute leukemia.

1978, *Matter of Dinnerstein*. Massachusetts Appeals Court upheld the validity of a ''No Code'' order for a 67-year-old woman with Alzheimer's disease.

1979, *Matter of Spring*. Massachusetts Supreme Court approved a decision to stop dialysis for a 77-year-old man with dementia.

1980, *Application of Eichner*. New York Appeals Court authorized discontinuance of respiratory support for an 83-year-old man in a persistent vegetative state.

1980, *Matter of Storer*. New York Court of Appeals refused to approve discontinuance of transfusion for a 52-year-old retarded man with bladder cancer.

1983, *Matter of Colyer*. Washington Supreme Court upheld removal of respiratory support for a 69-year-old woman in a chronic vegetative state.

1983, *Barber and Nejdl v. Superior Court*. California Appeals Court refused to reinstate homicide charges against physicians who discontinued respiratory and nutritional support from a 55-year-old man in persistent coma.

1985, *Claire Conroy*. Single 84-year-old woman in a nursing home, had severe organic brain syndrome, chronic decubitus ulcer, urinary tract infections, heart disease, hypertension, and diabetes; unaware of her surroundings, no cognitive ability, and no expectations for her condition to improve. In 1979, nephew was appointed guardian; doctors wanted to amputate her gangrenous leg but he refused; no surgery was performed. Nasogastric tube was inserted to improve feeding; removed Oct. 18, reinserted Nov. 3. Nov. 17, patient was transferred back to nursing home; physician refused to remove tube at nephew's request. Appellate court ruled that termination of feeding would be homicide. Conroy died February 15, 1983. In 1985, New Jersey Supreme Court permitted termination of *any* medical treatment for incompetent patients, including artificial feeding, so long as certain procedures were followed.

1986, *Helen Corbett*. Husband requested the feeding tube be removed from 75-year-old comatose woman. Trial court in Florida ruled that it could not be removed, since such removal would violate a Florida state statute. Corbett died during trial court proceedings. Appellate court reversed the decision and ruled that the right of privacy protected by the U.S. Constitution demands that such life-sustaining procedures may, at the request of the patient, be removed.

1986, *Paul E. Brophy*. During surgery for a cerebral aneurysm a 48-year-old patient lapsed into a persistent vegetative state. After 40 months, the family requested to have a feeding tube removed. The lower (probate) court in Massachusetts ruled that since Brophy was not being subjected to ''considerable pain and suffering'' and was not terminally ill or dying, it was in the state's interest to prevent a cessation of treatment. (Concern for Dying newsletter, Fall 1985.) State Supreme Court of Massachusetts had not yet decided the issue in 1986.

*Cases from 1976–1983 are taken from *Western Journal of Medicine*, pp. 358–363, California Medical Association, © September 1984.

nology raise questions of institutional policy, a working relationship between the IRB and the IEC is essential. A subcommittee, composed of membership from both, can review specific questions that might otherwise fall between the cracks. The subcommittee's charge is to recommend whether the issue should be directed to the IRB or IEC for judgment or whether a special joint ad hoc committee should be established to review the particular issue.

MANDATE

The IEC is mandated to address the ethical questions in the institution, especially those involved in the care of patients. Specifically, this general task has

Figure 20-1 Four Hospital Ethics Committee Structures

Model 1 (Governing Board)

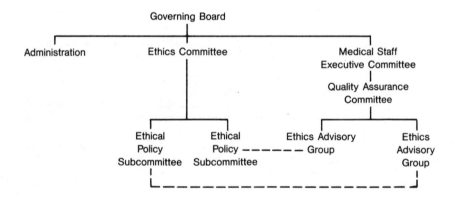

Model 2 (Administration)

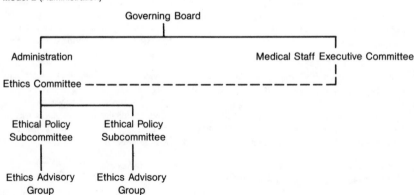

Figure 20-1 (continued)

Model 3 (Medical Staff)

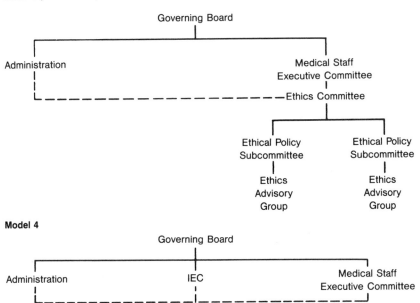

Model 4

Note: Solid lines are formal lines of authority. Broken lines are formal lines of communication.

Source: The first three models are reprinted from *Insight*, Vol. 8, No. 20, p. 3, with permission of California Hospital Association, © June 26, 1984.

been interpreted to mean the IEC has four roles, education, consultation, development of ethical policy guidelines, and retrospective review of decisions. The experience of most IECs indicates that the first three roles are essential.[3]

Consultation is the role most identified with IECs. Most IECs understand their consultative role to be not making decisions but rendering opinions on the ethics of clinical options.

The most persistent role is education, first of the IEC members and second of the health care staff. Education requires constant review and discussion of scientific, ethical, and legal literature and self-education.

Policy formation is becoming one of the most important roles of an IEC. Since behavior within an institution is directed by the mission, goals, and policies of the institution, clarity about the ethical dimensions of the institution's goals and mission is important. Clarity is attained by establishing policies that guide the choices of the members of the institution and provide criteria by which such behaviors can be assessed. However, policies are effective as long as the circumstances remain constant. The development of medical technology and new surgical techniques and changes in the economic climate create new possibilities that will require reassessment of policies.

The question of the power of the IEC is important. Should the IEC function merely as an optional consultative service or should consultation be obligatory? Several models have been proposed: an optional/optional model, an optional/ mandatory model, a mandatory/optional and a mandatory/mandatory model. The distinctions describe first the obligation to use the committee and second the force of the committee's judgment.[4] Most committees are optional/optional. However, in some institutions, specific cases must be referred to the IEC, e.g., care of severely defective newborns, removal of life support systems, and so forth.

BENEFITS

Institutional ethics committees do benefit the institution. They facilitate decision making on ethical aspects of clinical care; provide a forum for ethical discussions; and educate its members and staff on ethical issues and concerns. Moreover, IECs can assist in establishing clinical ethical guidelines and policies for the institutions, e.g., allocation of scarce medical resources, do-not-resuscitate orders, care of the terminally ill, and brain death. IECs assist the institution in presenting clear statements of the institution's policies and practices concerning ethical questions to its staff, its patients, and the public. Clear policies engender confidence and trust. A coherent set of policies provides standards to assess personnel's behavior and personal credentials. The lack of a coherent policy produces a splintered institution and the possibility of very diverse and even conflicting practices. Trust in the institution's ability to treat patients totally, not only medically but also ethically, is enhanced by a well thought out set of policies.

The institution's public ethical commitment to an IEC also gives assurances that there is a mechanism and a forum to which ethical dilemmas can be referred for advice and judgment. Further, if litigation is started, the institution can demonstrate that a decision in a contested case received detailed professional review not only for medical reasons but also for ethical and legal reasons through the IEC. This is admittedly protectionistic but a warranted protection because the interests of all parties (the patient, the institution, the physician, and society) are protected by ethical review.

In summary, IECs provide substantial benefits: a linkage between society and the institution; a systematic approach to moral analysis and judgment; a forum where discussion of moral issues can take place; an interdisciplinary mix of talents to develop functional guidelines and policies for the institution; and finally, the establishment and deepening of confidence in the institution's ability to decide ethical dilemmas in a systematic, professional way that involves consultation rather than independent decision making.

COST/RISK

Nothing is without cost and risk. Administrators must weigh the costs and risks against the benefits of any institutional change. An IEC's presence creates some costs and exposes the institution to some risks. They can be accepted when the change is important to the institution's life and future.

The costs and risks of an IEC include: (1) becoming merely a rubber stamp with no force and no respect, (2) directing some of the hospital's limited funds and energies to an endeavor that many believe has no patient care results, (3) creating suspicion and negative feelings among health care professionals, (4) raising suspicion that professional responsibilities will be taken away from physicians and given to a committee, (5) invading the privacy of the patient and intruding into the privileged therapeutic relationship between the patient and physician, (6) threatening to judge professional behavior by inapplicable criteria, (7) prolonging decisions because of the time necessary for review, (8) increasing costs within the institution by requiring liability insurance for the committee members.

Summation of Costs/Risks/Benefits

The experience has shown that well formulated, educated, and institutionally supported IECs are worth the acceptance of the costs and risks.[5] The IEC can stimulate ethical thinking and raise the consciousness of health care persons to the ethical dimensions of care. This enhances the quality of patient care. Members of ethics committees can grow in their knowledge of ethics and their ability to apply ethical principles to human choices.

The costs of an IEC are minuscule in comparison with costs of other committees and departments within a health care institution. Financially the costs involve secretarial support for the committee, a library budget, and scheduling part of the health care professional's time to devote to IEC deliberations and education. Probably the greatest challenge in a community hospital or a free-standing institution is to motivate physicians to give of their time to IECs' formulation, education, and operation.

A well-functioning IEC can reduce costs. Energy, time, and money spent in trying to put out brush fires of discontent or to ward off litigation or to develop public positions to preserve the reputation of the institution can be directed elsewhere. The presence of an IEC allows the administrator to direct controverted questions to the IEC to be processed in an organized fashion. It allows an administrator to buy time in a legitimate way when he or she is pressured to take action or make a decision. The IEC gives health care professionals a consultative service that will support their efforts to render ethically sound patient care. It also prevents scurrilous and arbitrary legal action because most persons will hesitate if they know the institution handles ethical questions in a professional manner.

MEMBERSHIP

IECs are multidisciplinary, usually composed of combinations of the following disciplines: medicine, surgery (including house officers in teaching institutions), nursing, chaplaincy, law, ethics, and social work. Community representatives are also included in many IECs. Professions with an interest in patient care as well as experience in patient care issues should be represented on the committee. Since the IEC's deliberations concern clinical matters, clinicians must be represented. Medical expertise (a member expert or a consultant) on specific issues is important. A surgeon, intensivist, oncologist, neurologist, or psychiatrist should be considered for membership or consultation. A nurse's perspective on patient care concerns is essential.

Many IECs include lawyers as members; others merely use lawyers on a consultative basis. The argument for lawyers being members of the IEC is that they will provide the legal perspective and give opinions about the legal implications of the case or policy question being deliberated by the IEC. However, some argue that the lawyer would be more concerned with the interests of the institution than the care of the patient and should be used only on a consultative basis. We feel the input of law is important in the IEC and the interchange between the members does provide opportunities for education, new perspectives, and growth for committee members.

ORGANIZATION/ACCESS

Most committees are accessed through the committee chairman or any committee member (at the Cleveland Clinic Foundation, entry is also through the Department of Bioethics). Ethical issues and problems affect individuals at all levels of the institution. Therefore it is important that all personnel, from trustees to maintenance personnel, are aware of the existence of the IEC and are encouraged to present their ethical concerns to the committee. Access to the committee must be publicized via a medium that has the widest exposure to the hospital and patient population. Further, other committees within the institution, whether trustee, administrative, or medical committees, should be given access to the IEC for ethical analysis and opinion.

The IEC's chair can have an executive committee serve as a screening group to decide whether a specific question is within the purview of the IEC or should be referred elsewhere.

Planning Phase

Careful preparation for an institutional ethics committee is imperative. Institutions find it useful to create an ad hoc planning committee that is charged to make recommendations concerning the establishment of the IEC. Most of these ad hoc committees operate for six months to a year and use consultants. The health care administrator should make certain that the planning committee's chair is respected by physicians and the committee has representation from staff, administration, nursing, chaplaincy, law, and even trustees.

The first task of the study committee is to decide whether an IEC is appropriate for its institution. This requires assessment of the need, the climate of acceptance, the institution's sociopolitical structure, the ethical preparedness of its staff, and the placement of an IEC within the mission and structure of the institution. It is useful to employ consultants to assist the committee.

Once the committee has accepted the desirability of an IEC, its next task is to define the structure and placement of the IEC within the table of organization. Some institutional ethics committees are subcommittees of the Board of Trustees, others are committees of the CEO's office, or subcommittees of the Department of Medicine or Surgery. Some institutions use a subcommittee of a standing committee such as quality assurance, whose minutes and proceedings are privileged information, in order to try to gain some protection for its committee's minutes and recommendations. (See Figure 20-1.) The study committees must select or create a place in the organization table that best reflects the institution's mission and sociopolitical reality.

Usually the study committee gives a general mandate: to address the ethical aspects of care. This allows the future IEC members to establish their own structure and to specify their mandate more completely.

Selection of Members

Selection of committee members must be done carefully. Besides the mix of professions, personal characteristics of members are very important. Professionalism, curiosity, open-mindedness, intelligence, and team consciousness are important to the success of the institutional ethics committee. Persons who are willing to participate in a decision instead of feeling compelled to direct decisions and analyses usually serve well on IECs.

Members also should be individuals who express interest in ethical questions and, ideally, have ethical skills and knowledge. Physicians and health care workers are becoming aware of the ethical aspects of clinical medicine and the methodology of ethics through reading, seminars, lectures, and so forth. Since ethical training in medical and nursing schools is increasing, more health care professionals are prepared to participate in IECs.

Start-Up Phase

The start-up phase in the IEC's development is crucial to its effectiveness. The members must have confidence in each other, respect their strengths and weaknesses, and develop a systematic method of addressing questions in order to reach closure. We recommend that the IEC keep a low profile for six months to a year until it educates itself and establishes its role within the institution.

Committees should meet monthly. The first six months to a year should be focused on organization, group dynamics, and education. As the committee begins to feel comfortable in its role it should accept cases and begin to study the policies of the institution concerning major questions such as do-not-resuscitate orders, care of the terminally ill, brain death, allocation of resources, and so on. It can apportion the work by creating subcommittees to study the policies of the institution and to make policy recommendations for the staff and administration's consideration.

During the start-up period the committee should use consultants skilled in group processes and in ethics. Ideally the chair of the committee should have these skills. Ethical issues do raise high emotions, and skills in directing group processes when these emotions surface are very important. The challenge is to bring the committee to focus on the ethical question without endangering the confidence and motivation of committee members. This requires adroit handling.

An ethicist, a philosopher, or a theologian who is aware of ethical theory and how to apply theory in medical circumstances can educate members. Ethical education cannot be overstressed. Most mistakes are made by IECs because of imprecise language, lack of understanding the ethical questions, and use of arbitrary means of analysis on a clinical case.

The education should include ethical language, the meaning and definition of terms, distinctions between law, ethics, and morality, knowledge of specific ethical dilemmas faced by medicine today (for example, withdrawal of life support systems), and knowledge of the logic of ethical thought that involves both utilitarian and deontological theories.

It is useful for committees to work with mock cases during this time. This allows committee members to address the ethical questions and test their moral reactions in a nonthreatening setting. Video cassettes and case books are available. The Hastings Institute, the Kennedy Institute for Ethics, the Department of Bioethics at the Cleveland Foundation, and others can provide bibliographies or materials for IECs to test their ethical knowledge and skills. It is important that committees do not consider active cases within the first six months to a year, until they are prepared to address the questions in a systematic way.

EDUCATIONAL ROLE

The educational role of the committee extends beyond the initial start-up period of self-instruction in ethics. Its first objective is to be proactive concerning issues in medicine that have ethical implications, whether they concern clinical practice directly, the impact of economic factors upon distribution and allocation of limited resources, or some developing medical technology such as gene therapy or in vitro technology. The second objective is to educate members of the institution in ethics by rounds or special lectures on ethical issues that are pertinent to the institution. This objective also can be achieved by contributing to the continuing medical education of the staff and other health care professionals by incorporating ethical topics into the regular CME programs.

CONSULTATIVE ROLE

When a clinical case is presented to the committee, it should meet within a given period of time. A good rule of thumb is to meet within 24 hours and to render an opinion in no more than 72 hours. The committee should address clinical cases in an organized fashion. A suggested model is: (1) Obtain as much medical information as possible by pulling the patient's chart and inviting the attending physician or representative, along with consultants, to present the medical data to the committee. (2) Invite all other health care persons who are intimately involved in the care of the patient to present their perspectives on the case. (3) If it is appropriate, invite the patient, patient's family, and/or patient representative to present the issue to the committee. (4) Analyze the facts by asking three basic questions: Who should make the decision? What are the options? And on what ethical basis should the decision be made? That is, what ethical principles and values apply to the decision? The IEC should indicate which of the options are ethically justifiable and present the arguments to support the justification to the attending physician and family for their decision. If the committee is not unanimous, the minority opinion should also be expressed along with the justification for this minority status.

In retrospective case review, the same methodology should be followed. However, the IEC's goal is to analyze the justification and the appropriateness of a decision rather than to give an opinion.

PITFALLS

Some of the pitfalls in establishing IECs are: noninvolvement of medical staff in planning, precipitous organization of a committee, arbitrary appointment of committee membership, ambiguity in mandate, lack of adequate support services, and lack of adequate time to educate the IEC.

The IEC should know the extent of its turf. The issue that causes most fear and resistance to IECs is interposing the IEC between the patient and the physician. The IEC should make every effort to reinforce the idea that its role is to be an advisor, or if it is within its mandate, to be an arbitrator, when the two parties are in disagreement. The IEC also should know its legal limitations and not intervene in areas outside its jurisdiction.

LAW AND IECs

The futile attempts to establish infant care review committees, the famous "Baby Doe committees," indicate the interest of the federal government to involve itself in ethical decisions, but at this time there is no legal requirement for IECs. Currently, the legal questions that surround IECs are issues such as liability of members, privileged nature of minutes, subpoena of IEC minutes and records, and impact of IEC deliberations on court decisions. There have been instances where ethics committees' deliberations have been incorporated in legal suits.[6]

Although the law has not directly addressed the question of IECs and their role in legal considerations, many health care institutions are anticipating that IECs or ethics consultation may become part of customary and usual medical practice. This raises a speculative question about the legal position of a physician who does not use an available IEC for consultation on a case that eventually goes to court. Lack of IEC consultation could be construed as a sign of inadequate professional practice. Further, if the IEC was consulted and its opinion disregarded by the physician, the physician's burden of justification would be greater.

RESOURCES

National as well as regional resources are available to help in both the establishment and education of an IEC. The Society of Law & Medicine, the Society for Health & Human Values, and the Society for Bioethics Consultation are major resources for qualified consultants and/or persons to serve on IECs.[7]

The institutional ethics committee also needs bibliographic and consultative resources for its ongoing work. Bibliographic services are available through the Kennedy Institute, the Hastings Center, the Cleveland Clinic Foundation's Department of Bioethics, and other local bioethical institutes.[8]

The IEC itself should serve as a resource to the institution. It should be a repository of information concerning the ethics of medicine that will be readily drawn upon by administrators, staff, and other persons when they address questions of an ethical nature or prepare educational programs. Hence the need to provide a library budget and support personnel.

ETHICS OF IECs

The creation of an IEC presents ethical responsibilities and challenges to its members. The major ethical responsibility of the IEC is patient and health care provider confidentiality. Since its discussions can reveal intimate information about professional practice and personal morality, all discussions, opinions, and names should be regarded as confidential. Not only moral constraints but also legal constraints and protections should be instituted to protect confidentiality.

Second, the protection of the anonymity of persons who access the IEC is a major responsibility. Since ethical questions can concern the practice of a superior, the person who presents the case must be protected from the fear of retaliation.

There is a danger that the IEC will use narrow criteria in making its judgments. For example, it may exclude any economic considerations or use only economic factors to guide its judgment. The responsibility of the IEC is to explore all ethical criteria and to educate itself constantly so that new or refined ethical criteria are not excluded from judgment.

Another danger is that the IEC may become effectively either a physician's or a nonphysician's committee where the judgment of the other members is not respected. The ethical challenge is to create the atmosphere of free exchange of perspectives and opinions from all members.

Finally, IECs must be aware of the responsibility to keep within their limits, i.e., to render an opinion when consulted and to avoid any impression that they are assuming an active role in the patient/physician relationship.

FUTURE

Every health care institution will have an IEC or share the services of a central IEC for several hospitals.[9] Further, as more IECs come into existence the opportunity for the organization of statewide networks of committees will present itself. These networks will pool resources, share experiences, and unite efforts to produce legislative or professional guidelines that will assist hospitals and physicians in the care of their patients.[10] Consultation with an IEC will become accepted as standard professional practice in patient care dilemmas.

Both profit and nonprofit health care corporations will have IECs at least at the corporate level in order to address policy questions for the corporate members.

Finally, IECs will become resources for legal cases and provide forums where social morality will be formulated, honed, and proposed for political action. The rise of required request legislation for transplantable organs was at least partially stimulated by IEC action.

The most significant role that hospital administrators play in the establishment and successful functioning of an IEC is to publicly support the committee's formation, education, and operation. Leadership is critical because it validates the enterprise and can bring support from physicians and others who are skeptical about the need for such committees.

NOTES

1. J.A. Robertson, "Ethics Committees in Hospitals: Alternative Structures and Responsibilities," *Connecticut Medicine* 48, no. 7 (July 1984):441.

2. "The court assigned the ethics committee the task of agreeing or disagreeing with the responsible attending physician's determination that there was no reasonable possibility of Quinlan ever emerging from her comatose condition to a cognitive, sapient state. However, this essentially medical function caused considerable confusion in subsequent development of ethics committees in American medicine since there was little (if anything) distinctly 'ethical' about the judgment which the court asked the committee to make." C.G. Ferguson, "Medical Ethics Committees, The Decision is Yours," *Dimensions*, Sept. 1984, 36.

3. D. Avard et al, "Hospital Ethics Committees: Survey Reveals Characteristics," *Dimensions in Health Services* 62, no. 2 (Feb. 1985):24–25; R.E. Cranford and A.E. Doudera, "The Emergence of Institutional Ethics Committees," *Law, Medicine & Health Care* 12, no. 1 (Feb. 1984):16–17.

4. Robertson, "Ethics Committees," 442–444.

5. R.M. Kliegman et al, "In Our Best Interests: Experience and Workings of an Ethics Review Committee," *Journal of Pediatrics* 108, no. 2 (Feb. 1986):178.

6. R.E. Cranford and E.J. VanAllen, "The Implications and Applications of Institutional Ethics Committees," *American College of Surgeons Bulletin* 70, no. 6 (June 1985):24.

7. The American Society of Law & Medicine, 765 Commonwealth Ave., Boston, Massachusetts, 02215. The Society for Health & Human Values, Suite 3A, 1311A Dolley Madison Boulevard, McLean, Virginia, 22101. The Society for Bioethics Consultation, % John C. Fletcher, Ph.D., Chief, Bioethics Program, CC National Institutes of Health, Building 10, Room 2C-202, Bethesda, Maryland, 20892.

8. The Joseph and Rose Kennedy Institute of Ethics, Georgetown University, Washington, D.C., 20057. The Hastings Center, 360 Broadway, Hastings-on-Hudson, New York, 10706. The Department of Bioethics, The Cleveland Clinic Foundation, 9500 Euclid Ave., Cleveland, Ohio, 44106.

9. C. Keenan, "Ethics Committees: Trend for Troubling Times," *The Hospital Medical Staff*, June 1983, 3.

10. See, e.g., "The Minnesota Network for Institutional Ethics Committees," *American College of Surgeons Bulletin* 70, no. 6 (June 1985):22–23.

BIBLIOGRAPHY

Avard, D., Frimer, G., and Longstaff, J. "Hospital Ethics Committees: Survey Reveals Characteristics." *Dimensions* (February 1985):24–26.

Brodeur, Dennis. "Toward a Clear Definition of Ethics Committees." *Linacre Quarterly* (August 1984):233–247.

Capron, Alexander M. "Twenty Questions About Ethics Committees." *Ethics Committee Newsletter* 1(4) (June 1984):2–10.

Committee on Ethics & Medical-Legal Affairs. "Institutional Ethics Committees, Roles, Responsibilities and Benefits for Physicians." *Minnesota Medicine* 68 (August 1985).

Cranford, R.E., and Doudera, A.E. *Institutional Ethics Committees and Health Care Decision-Making.* Ann Arbor, Mich.: Health Administration Press, 1984.

Cranford, R.E., and VanAllen, E.J. "The Implications and Applications of Institutional Ethics Committees." *American College of Surgeons Bulletin* 70(6) (June 1985):19–24.

"Ethics Committees Double Since '83 Survey." *Hospitals* (November 1985):60, 64.

Ferguson, Cherry G. "Medical Ethics Committees, The Decision is Yours." *Dimensions* (September 1984):36–41.

Fleischman, Alan R., and Murray, Thomas H. "Ethics Committees for Infant Doe?" *The Hastings Center Report* (December 1983):5–9.

Fost, Norman, and Cranford, R.E. "Hospital Ethics Committees: Administrative Aspects." *Journal of the American Medical Association* 253(18) (May 1985):2687–2692.

Gallo, Anthony E., Jr. "Hospital Ethics Committees: A Pediatric Neurosurgical Perspective." *Child's Nervous System* 1(3) (1985):132–136.

"Guidelines on the Establishment of Hospital Committees to Consider Biomedical Ethical Issues." American Hospital Association, 1984.

Hosford, Bower. *Bioethics Committees: The Health Care Provider's Guide.* Rockville, Md.: Aspen Publishers, Inc., 1986.

Infant Bioethics Committee. "Guidelines for Infant Bioethics Committees." *Pediatrics* 74(2) (August 1984):306–310.

Kalchbrenner, J., et al. "Ethics Committees and Ethicists in Catholic Hospitals." *Hospital Progress* 64(9) (September 1983):47–51.

Keenan, Carol. "Ethics Committees: Trend for Troubling Times." *The Hospital Medical Staff*:2–11.

Kliegman, Robert M., Mahowald, Mary B., and Younger, Stuart J. "In Our Best Interests: Experience and Working of an Ethics Review Committee." *Journal of Pediatrics* 108(2) (February 1986):178–188.

Levine, C. "Questions and Answers About Hospital Ethics Committees." *The Hastings Center Report*, June 1984.

McCormick, Richard A. "Ethics Committees: Promise or Peril?" *Law, Medicine & Health Care* (September 1984):150–155.

Monagle, John F. "Blueprints for Hospital Ethics Committees." *CHA Insight* (20) (June 1984):1–4.

Presidential Commission for the Study of Ethical Problems in Medicine and Biomedical and Behavioral Research. *Deciding to Forego Life Sustaining Treatment: Ethical, Medical and Legal Issues in Treatment Decisions.* Washington, D.C.: U.S. Government Printing Office, 1983.

Randal, Judith. "Are Ethics Committees Alive and Well?" *The Hastings Center Report* (December 1983):10–12.

Riga, Peter J. "The Care of Defective Neonates, Ethics Committees and Federal Intervention." *Linacre Quarterly* (August 1984):255–276.

Robertson, J.A. "Ethics Committees in Hospitals: Alternative Structures and Responsibilities." *Connecticut Medicine* (48)7 (July 1984):441–444.

Rosner, Fred. "Hospital Medical Ethics Committees: A Review of Their Development." *Journal of the American Medical Association* 253(18) (May 1985):2693–2697.

Thomasma, David C. "Hospital Ethics Committees and Hospital Policy." *Q.R.B.* (July 1985): 204–209.

Youngner, Stuart J., et al. "A National Survey of Hospital Ethics Committees." *Critical Care Medicine* 11(11) (November 1984):902–905.

Youngner, Stuart J., et al. "Patient's Attitudes Toward Hospital Ethics Committees." *Law, Medicine & Health Care* (February 1984):21–25.

Chapter 21

The Role of an Ethicist in Health Care

Terrence F. Ackerman, PhD

Every day, health care administrators and clinical care providers confront decisions that underscore the increasing moral complexities associated with the provision of medical care. These complexities can be traced to technological, economic, and social factors operating within the practice of medicine.

In recent decades, there has been a remarkable expansion of medicine's technological capacities. While these technologies create new opportunities for extending human life, they may also affect the quality of patients' lives in unacceptable ways. Major changes in the health care delivery system and mechanisms of reimbursement have also been implemented to control costs. As a result, decisions must be made about which services should be available to patients and how limited services shall be allocated among persons who need them. These changes have occurred against the backdrop of widespread social concern about the moral and legal interests of individuals, especially disadvantaged persons.

Faced with the intricate moral issues thus generated, health care administrators and clinical care providers might prefer to call upon specialists in ethics. Handling new complexities in medical care through increased specialization of personnel and services is a familiar strategy.

However, the prospect of specialists in ethics raises some unique doubts. First, moral philosophers themselves are quick to point out that we are not even close to the systematic knowledge of right and wrong to which the great moral systems have aspired. By contrast, a specialist in clinical pharmacology or clinical nutrition possesses a complex body of knowledge that can be effectively applied in resolving problems in patient care. If an ethics consultant lacks a similar information base, what elements of knowledge and skill can he or she offer in solving moral problems?[1]

Second, there is resistance to the idea of relegating to a "moral expert" the task of formulating solutions to ethical issues in clinical care. Moral issues arise from differences in values and interests, and the process of resolving them requires full airing of the viewpoints of different members of the moral community.[2] By contrast, clinical pharmacologists and nutritionists can appeal to

308

widely accepted bodies of facts and principles about drugs and diet in developing clinical recommendations.

Third, there is an ingrained belief that men or women of conscience who thoughtfully apply themselves to the moral problems faced in professional practice can arrive at morally correct decisions. Conscience is connected with conscientiousness in addressing moral concerns, and good people generally produce good results.[3] This belief sharply contrasts with our attitude about the scientific aspects of medical care, where we have given up the idea that the conscientious physician can know everything necessary to provide optimal clinical care—hence the need for clinical pharmacologists and nutritionists.

These are serious doubts, and if there is a legitimate use for specialists in ethics, we shall have to formulate their role in a way that satisfies the objections.

MORAL PROBLEMS AND MORAL REFLECTION

In daily life there are two varieties of moral problems. It is important to distinguish them, since only one variety is the unique concern of the ethicist.

Types of Moral Problems

One type of moral problem occurs when appropriate norms of conduct are commonly acknowledged, but persons are not treated in accordance with these norms. A frequent cause of this failure is immoral conduct. For example, an obstetrician decides to turn off his page unit while attending a baseball game, even though he knows that one of his patients, who may have a complicated delivery, will soon enter labor. The labor begins, complications ensue, and the inability of the nursing staff to locate the physician delays the performance of a cesarean section, resulting in the birth of a neurologically impaired child. The physician's behavior violates a clear obligation, inspiring moral outrage. Control of unprofessional conduct of this sort represents a serious moral problem.

Another cause of failure to treat persons in accord with acknowledged moral norms is the absence of essential social resources. For example, the same patient's husband must drive her nearly seventy miles to the nearest city hospital once her labor begins, because cost constraints have recently forced the closing of a small community hospital. Complications in her labor occur en route, and again a neurologically impaired child is born. Society's obligation to provide minimally satisfactory health care services is unfulfilled, and we feel a sense of moral tragedy. This moral problem requires a revision in current social services.

Another type of moral problem has significantly different properties. It involves situations in which different human values or norms suggest conflicting courses of action, and there is an initial lack of social consensus about which values should be endorsed and acted upon. Consider the following example:

A 76-year-old widow had been diagnosed several months previously with severe essential hypertension. She was a cantankerous patient who went to the physician only at her daughter's urging. She consistently failed to take her medications or restrict her diet. When the doctor warned that grave consequences might ensue, she said that she had little use for physicians and, no matter what happened, she never wanted to be "hooked up to any machines." The physician noted her wishes in the chart.

One morning several months later she called to tell her daughter that she had a severe headache and had vomited. Her daughter said that she would leave work to take her to the doctor. However, when she arrived three hours later, she found her mother unconscious and breathing shallowly. In the emergency room, it was determined that her mother had suffered a severe cerebral hemorrhage. As her condition deteriorated, she became deeply comatose and ventilatory support became necessary. Her physician explained to the daughter that there was little chance of her surviving more than a few days, and he related his earlier conversation with her mother. But the daughter was completely opposed to anything but fully aggressive therapy, saying that the Lord would decide matters. She also had to be constantly reassured that her delay in getting to her mother's house had not affected the seriousness of her mother's condition.

The physician was deeply troubled about how to proceed.[4]

This case clearly illustrates the second type of moral problem. First, there are different moral values suggesting divergent courses of action. Concern for the well-being of the daughter suggests that discontinuation of aggressive therapy should at least be delayed until she can be adequately reassured that she was not responsible for her mother's stroke. The delay would also forestall any future anxieties about whether "everything possible" had been done for her mother. By contrast, respect for the choices of patients suggests that treatment should be discontinued in accord with the previously stated wishes of the patient. Since the patient will survive only a brief period of time, discontinuation of aggressive treatment also seems consistent with a concern for the patient's well-being. Finally, if resources in the intensive care unit are scarce (beds, ventilators, nurses, and so on), fair treatment may require allocation of the resources in question to patients who have a better chance of surviving their current illnesses. Thus, different human values suggest conflicting courses of action.

Second, there is likely to be an initial lack of consensus among members of the moral community about how the physician should proceed. Persons placing highest priority upon respect for the wishes of patients will favor withholding aggressive treatment. However, other persons may believe that the daughter's well-being should take priority, provided that her mother's suffering is not exacerbated by continuation of aggressive therapy. They will point to the fact that how the situation is handled may seriously affect the daughter's emotional adjustment to her mother's death in the coming months.

Methods for resolving these distinct types of moral problems differ significantly from one another. On one hand, moral problems involving the failure to treat persons in accord with acknowledged norms of conduct are resolved through various mechanisms of social control and reform. Criminal and civil law, professional peer review, and social disapprobation control immoral conduct. Agencies of social welfare provide needed social resources such as health care. On the other hand, moral problems involving conflicting human values are treated through the social process of moral reflection. Since this second type of moral problem is the special focus of the ethicist's professional activities, we must now take a closer look at the purpose and process of moral reflection.

Moral Reflection

The purpose of moral reflection is determined by the social and practical character of moral problems that arise when there is a lack of social consensus about norms of conduct to be observed in our interactions with one another in specific kinds of circumstances. The purpose of moral reflection is to identify solutions to moral problems that effectively respect shared value priorities established by members of the moral community through careful study of each problem.[5]

This statement suggests several important features of moral reflection:

- It involves the attempt to establish an initially lacking social consensus. Norms of conduct are sought that are capable of evoking a shared social commitment.

- Achieving this objective requires social agreement about how we will jointly prioritize competing human values, such as respect for choices of patients and concern for the welfare of family members.

- We seek problem solutions and moral priorities that recommend themselves to persons who have thoroughly studied each problem.

- Moral reflection is not the process of taking an opinion poll, but involves careful social examination of the relevant values, alternative solutions, and the comparative consequences of their implementation.

- Moral reflection seeks to identify solutions to moral problems which are actually effective in achieving our moral priorities when implemented in practice.[6]

Thus, successful resolution of a moral problem involves broadening our shared interests or common moral bonds.

The process of moral reflection consists of analytic procedures useful in identifying plans of action that effectively respect shared moral priorities. One component is careful identification of the cherished values that members of the moral community consider relevant to the choice of a plan of action. For example, in the case presented, numerous human values might be considered: respect for the stated wishes of the patient, concern for the daughter's welfare, concern for the patient's well-being, and fair allocation of resources among patients. This set of values forms the framework from which development of a solution must proceed; it must be carefully and completely articulated.

Another feature of moral reflection involves understanding relevant data. In the case considered, these facts include the patient's previous statements about the use of artificial life supports, her current prognosis, the source of the daughter's anxiety, the chances of causing harm to the patient through further aggressive therapy, and others. Since conduct in accord with selected plans of action must interact with existing circumstances in producing consequences that we may value or disvalue, moral assessment of alternative solutions to a moral problem must include thorough familiarity with the facts.

A third aspect of moral reflection is the identification of alternative ways in which the moral problem might be resolved. In the stated case, the physician might: (a) pursue aggressive therapy until the daughter's emotional adjustment is secured; (b) surreptitiously reduce the level of support to guarantee the quick demise of the patient; or (c) straightforwardly refuse to initiate therapy contrary to the patient's previously stated wishes. Although many writers in medical ethics take an "either-or" approach to moral problems (either respect the patient's wishes or relieve the daughter's mental anguish), this may be an extremely creative phase of moral reflection. Frequently, plans of action can be fashioned to respect various relevant human values. This way identifies a solution that can evoke a broadly shared commitment among different members of the moral community.

A fourth component of moral reflection involves the comparative assessment of how alternative plans of action will achieve or fail to achieve the states of affairs represented by the relevant moral values. For example, while failure to initiate aggressive life support will respect the previously stated wishes of the patient, it will probably not constitute an effective strategy for dealing with the emotional needs of her daughter. By contrast, briefly delaying discontinuation of aggressive treatment while providing intensive counseling to the daughter may allow both moral concerns to be addressed. This phase of moral inquiry involves a moral cost-benefit assessment of the various options available. We project how alternative plans will interact with existing circumstances to produce various valued or disvalued outcomes. This is clearly the most crucial phase of moral reflection, since it is from this stage that a shared commitment to a particular plan of action must emerge.

This view about the purpose and procedures of moral reflection does not assume that we will achieve closure on all moral issues. However, lack of complete success in resolving moral problems does not undermine the usefulness of the methodology. Rather, the crucial question concerns which conceptualization of the process of moral reflection permits the *most effective* resolution of these problems, and no alternative conceptualization offers better results.[7]

Moreover, as a moral community, we are not confronted by the stark alternatives of either having a method that resolves all our moral problems or accepting intellectual chaos in our social affairs. Where reasonable people differ, political, legal, and administrative procedures can be created to assure orderly resolution of issues about how we will interact with one another. Properly devised, these procedures may themselves be the justified outcome of moral reflection.

THE ROLE OF THE ETHICIST

This preliminary description of the nature of moral problems and the process of moral reflection permits us to delineate the role of the ethicist in health care.

The analysis must begin by rehearsing the circumstances in which the assistance of the ethicist may be sought. The request will occur when a moral problem of the second type (moral reflection) arises, and health care administrators or clinical care providers are not able to readily employ the conceptual tools (e.g., moral principles and their constituent concepts), factual data, or analytic steps of moral reflection useful in resolving the problem. Thus, the basic function of the specialist in ethics is to *facilitate* the process by which reflective resolution of moral problems can be achieved.

The Ethicist As Facilitator

The previous description of moral inquiry suggests several ways in which the ethicist may facilitate the reflective process. First, the ethicist can contribute to the classification and diagnosis of the moral problem.[8] The conceptual framework of a moral problem is set by the diverse human values relevant to the situation. Moral principles categorize and summarize the types of human values that possible solutions must protect or promote. Familiarity with the content of key moral principles enables the ethicist to identify important human values at stake and to explain their meaning. For example, in the case presented, the ethicist can identify key principles such as respect for the choices of persons and concern for their welfare, and explain their meaning as applied to the situation under review. Since reflection on a moral problem proceeds from the framework of competing values, proper classification of the problem is an essential step in developing a satisfactory solution.

Second, the specialist in ethics can provide assistance in identifying alternative plans of action. The ability to catalogue the diverse human values forming the conceptual framework of the moral problem may allow the ethicist to suggest creative plans of action sensitive to these different moral concerns. Similarly, knowledge of important moral concepts and distinctions aids in assessing the moral impact of particular plans of action and in suggesting alternatives that may better satisfy the relevant human values. The ethicist should be familiar with recent professional guidelines, government regulations, legal cases, and other policy statements that recommend or restrict solutions to particular moral problems.

Third, the ethics consultant who is familiar with the results of relevant psychosocial research may promote a clearer understanding of the factual components of a morally problematic situation. In the illustrative case, an understanding of the grieving process may be useful in estimating whether it is possible to secure an agreement with the daughter about further care that does not substantially violate her mother's wishes and does not compromise her own emotional adjustment. Since plans of actions must interact with existing circumstances in producing valued or disvalued outcomes, the analysis of factual components may contribute to the resolution of the moral problem.

Fourth, the ethicist has an important role in assessing how alternative plans of action will promote or impede the realization of various valued states of affairs. This is a crucial aspect of moral reflection, since it is from this assessment that shared commitments must emerge. In this phase of the reflective process, the ethicist can introduce moral concepts and distinctions that allow the parties consulted to trace out the differential impact of alternative plans of action upon the human values identified.

For example, aggressive treatment of the patient seems to violate her wishes. However, an important issue is whether she made an informed choice to refuse artificial life supports. The consulting ethicist can identify the elements of informed decision making, explore the evidence that the patient made an informed choice, and explain how the absence of an informed choice might affect our obligation to respect the patient's decision. If the patient did not consider the prospect of emotional trauma to her daughter but had generally shown concern for her daughter's welfare, brief prolongation of her life to relieve the daughter's emotional distress might not violate the patient's considered wishes. Thus, the introduction of moral concepts and distinctions enables the ethicist to assist in the moral cost-benefit assessment of alternative plans.

Finally, the ethicist can make recommendations regarding the proper resolution of moral problems. This role must, however, be carefully circumscribed. The specialist in ethics cannot deliver "right answers" to the moral quandaries faced by health care administrators and clinical care providers. Moral reflection is a process for establishing *shared* moral commitments. Appropriate plans of action and moral priorities cannot be determined apart from the confirmatory reflection of other members of the moral community. Thus, an ethicist's recommendation constitutes a proposal requiring thorough assessment by the parties consulted. However, the ethics specialist may be well situated to make sound recommendations. The social process of moral reflection is represented in myriad academic journals, books, newsletters, government publications, and public discussions devoted to moral issues in medicine. From this reflective social dialogue, there often emerge tentative solutions to moral problems (e.g., recognition of the right of competent adult patients to refuse treatment that merely prolongs the dying process). The reputable ethicist is presumably current in his or her knowledge of these social developments, and recommendations that reflect the tentative results of the social process of moral reflection merit special consideration. Thus, the specialist in ethics cannot deliver "right answers" to moral problems, but may provide informed recommendations.

The ethicist's role as a facilitator of moral reflection can be implemented in various activities, differing in the directness of their relationship to patient care decision making. There are three basic activities: staff education, policy formation, and clinical case consultation.[9] In providing staff education, the ethicist might present seminars on such topics as refusal of treatment, withholding life-prolonging therapies, and allocation of scarce resources. The ethicist might also assist in hospital policy formation regarding such matters as do-not-resuscitate orders, determination of death, and nontreatment for impaired newborns.

Patient care consultation focuses more narrowly on these issues as they relate to the care of individual patients. However, the process of facilitating moral reflection is essentially similar in each context. The ethicist facilitates moral reflection by clarifying relevant moral values, conveying significant factual information, identifying alternative solutions, comparing the moral consequences of adopting these alternatives, and making recommendations for resolving the moral problem. Thus, while the particular mode of the ethicist's activity may be more or less connected with immediate patient care decisions, the ethicist's role in each context is to assist the moral reflection of health care administrators and clinical care providers.

Inappropriate Roles for Ethicists

Several tasks might be inappropriately ascribed to or assumed by the ethicist. One is the function of "moral policeman"—identifying instances of immoral behavior by health professionals. The need for ethics specialists is generated by situations in which the morally appropriate course of action is uncertain. The control of immoral behavior represents a distinctively different species of moral problem. Its resolution is more properly assigned to agencies of social control, such as professional peer review groups.

A closely related, but more subtle, mistake is ascribing a "patient advocate" role to the consulting ethicist. A patient advocate represents the patient in efforts to correct a situation in which the latter's interests or rights may be violated. This mistake is more subtle, because there is a sense in which the ethicist should represent the patient's perspective. Part of the process of facilitating moral reflection involves articulation of relevant values, and the ethicist should encourage recognition of those arising from the patient's perspective. But this is part of the process of facilitating cognitive analysis and resolution of a moral problem and is quite different from the task of rectifying certified moral encroachments.

A third mistake confuses the role of the ethicist with a task traditionally assigned to the clergy. One recognized clerical function is to encourage attitudinal changes making persons more disposed toward morally appropriate behavior. The ethicist is sometimes thought to be a "secular clergyperson" having a similar affective function. By contrast, the ethicist's role is predominantly intellectual—facilitating the analytic procedures of moral reflection.

Another inappropriate role conceives the ethicist as a modified psychologist or counselor for health professionals. The general role of the psychological counselor is to assist persons in understanding and resolving their own emotional problems, thereby enhancing their mental well-being. By contrast, the function of the ethicist is to assist health professionals in identifying appropriate norms for patient care. Confusion no doubt arises because moral dilemmas in patient care create emotional stress for health care providers, and the process of reflectively resolving these problems may ameliorate this stress. However, psychological benefits to health professionals are indirect consequences of the consulting ethicist's activities and should not be confused with their primary purpose.

Interestingly, these mistaken views about the role of the ethicist have a common root. Each conceives the ethicist's activities as focusing upon the rectification of particular circumstances that result in failure to treat patients according to commonly recognized norms of conduct. These circumstances are immoral behavior, violation of patients' rights, absence of attitudinal willingness to engage in appropriate behavior, and emotional disability of the health professional, respectively. Thus, proper conceptualization of the role of the ethics specialist requires a clear understanding of the type of moral problem to which his or her professional skills are applied.

QUALIFICATIONS FOR EFFECTIVE ROLE PERFORMANCE

The formulation of qualifications for effective role performance must reflect the elements of the ethicist's role responsibilities and the conditions under which this function is exercised. That is, we should set qualifications assuring that specialists in ethics competently fulfill their responsibilities under typical circumstances of professional practice. Key qualifications involve both intellectual factors and elements of professional style.

Intellectual credentials fall into several categories:

1. The ethicist should have graduate training in ethics or equivalent academic preparation. Knowledge of the purpose and process of moral reflection, familiarity with major moral principles and the historical source of their development, and skill in logical analysis of moral problems are among the qualities the student of ethics should derive from satisfactory graduate level training. These elements of knowledge and skill are obviously essential if the ethicist is to function effectively as a facilitator of moral reflection.

2. Demonstrated current knowledge of the literature of bioethics is also an essential qualification. This knowledge enhances the ethicist's role performance in several ways. It provides information about newly emerging moral issues, such as conflicts of obligations for physicians generated by the DRG reimbursement mechanism. It also provides scholarly analysis and debate about key moral concepts and distinctions useful in analyzing clinical moral problems, such as the properties of competent and incompetent decision making. Finally, the bioethics literature offers information about emerging areas of social agreement (e.g., policies regarding refusal of treatment), and analyzes recent professional guidelines, government regulations, and legal cases.

3. Basic knowledge of medicine and medical terminology is an important requirement. The consulting ethicist cannot identify moral problems, facilitate reflective analysis, or make sound recommendations without an accurate understanding of the medical aspects of particular cases. At a more basic level, the ethicist cannot communicate effectively with health professionals unless he or she is familiar with medical terminology.

4. Ethicists should possess basic knowledge of the psychosocial literature relevant to moral issues in clinical care. Plans for resolving moral problems must interact with existing conditions in producing valued or disvalued consequences. This nexus of conditions includes psychological, sociological, cultural, and economic factors. Consequently, evaluation of alternative solutions may be enhanced by relevant psychosocial data. For example, one recent study analyzed the reasons why patients refuse treatment and the approaches used by physicians in responding to these refusals.[10] This information may be useful in consultation regarding refusal of treatment. Knowledge of relevant psychosocial factors is perhaps the most neglected condition for competence.

Several other elements of professional style enhance effective role performance. The importance of these factors is determined by the special circumstances in which the ethicist must work. First, the ethicist's activities are conducted in a variety of clinical settings—patient care conferences, the physician's office, committee meetings, teaching rounds, and staff seminars. Instruction and consultation in multiple contexts require a flexible and adaptive professional style. Second, specialists in ethics deal with issues that may be emotionally charged for members of the health care team. Facilitating moral reflection in this atmosphere requires the ability to defuse emotional factors and to provide cool, deliberate moral analysis of the issues. Last, clinical ethicists perform a new and unfamiliar role in the hospital setting, dealing with highly sensitive issues. Their presence may provoke mistrust, misunderstanding, and criticism from some health professionals. Hospital ethicists must possess a general professional demeanor that inspires the trust and confidence of health professionals, thereby providing opportunities to demonstrate the usefulness of their special knowledge and skills. In addition, ethicists must be able to respond rationally to criticisms and to explain clearly the activities that do or do not fall within their role.

A REVIEW OF SKEPTICAL RESERVATIONS

At the outset, several common objections were raised to the idea that specialization of health care services and personnel should extend to the creation of a role for clinical ethicists.

The first objection drew its strength from the fact that we lack systematic knowledge of right and wrong to which the great moral systems have aspired. Whereas clinical pharmacologists and nutritionists may utilize organized bodies of scientific information in providing clinical advice, similar resources are not available to the ethicist. This objection involves two mistakes. On one hand, it fails to recognize that ethicists use a variety of conceptual resources in providing clinical assistance. These include knowledge of key moral principles, constituent concepts, and clinically important moral distinctions. The competent ethicist is also familiar with emerging areas of social consensus regarding the resolution of moral issues in medicine. These elements of knowledge can be effectively used in facilitating the moral reflection of health professionals.

More importantly, the objection mistakenly assumes that we cannot resolve moral problems in clinical care without prior systematic knowledge of right and wrong. This assumption misunderstands the very nature of moral reflection itself, which is a process of *constructing* shared norms of conduct. Parenthetically, the objection also seriously overestimates the degree of systemization achieved in our scientific knowledge of medical practice. Not unlike ethics, the growth of medical science involves the continuous development of shared norms for safe and effective patient care.

The second objection expressed doubts about relegating to "moral experts" the task of resolving moral problems of wide social import. The ethicist does not deliver "right answers" to moral questions but rather provides information and analytic skills that members of the health care team can use in developing broadly acceptable and thoroughly considered solutions to moral problems.

The final objection claimed that morally conscientious persons are thoroughly capable of resolving moral problems encountered in professional practice without the assistance of specialists in ethics. It is certainly true that persons who are not morally conscientious are unlikely to reflect carefully upon moral problems. However, the commitments associated with strong moral character are not sufficient to assure satisfactory resolution of moral problems in clinical practice. These problems involve conflicting human values and a lack of social agreement about their relative priority. Their resolution involves a reflective social process in which relevant values are clarified, alternative solutions are identified, and their comparative moral consequences are assessed.

This process is a sophisticated and complex intellectual endeavor. Consequently, professionals who know the relevant principles, concepts, and distinctions and possess skill in their application can facilitate the process of achieving satisfactory solutions to moral issues in medicine.

NOTES

1. See Kai Nielsen, "On Being Skeptical About Applied Ethics," in *Clinical Medical Ethics: Exploration and Assessment,* ed. Terrence Ackerman, Glenn Graber, Charles Reynolds, and David Thomasma (Washington, D.C.: University Press of America, forthcoming).

2. For example, see Cheryl Noble, "Ethics and Experts," *The Hastings Center Report* 12 (June, 1982):7–8.

3. This assumption underlies Mark Lilla's critique of the formal teaching of ethics in professional schools. See "Ethos, 'Ethics,' and Public Service," *The Public Interest* 63 (1981):3–17.

4. The case is drawn, in summarized form, from Terrence Ackerman and Carson Strong, *Clinical Medical Ethics: A Casebook* (New York: Oxford University Press, forthcoming).

5. The solution to a moral problem may be either a "course of action" or a "policy." A "course of action" is a plan for dealing with a moral problem created by a specific situation, such as the case of the elderly stroke patient. A "policy" is a plan for dealing with a set of situations raising the same kind of moral issue, e.g., the use of do-not-resuscitate orders. Since courses of action or policies are assessed in a similar fashion in moral reflection, I use the phrases "solution" or "plan of action" to refer generically to policies and courses of action identified in moral reflection.

6. Often, policies are implemented but do not have the intended effect of securing valued states of affairs. For example, "living will" laws have been enacted to allow persons to prospectively exercise their choice to have life-prolonging treatments limited at a future time when they are no longer competent to make the decision. However, some laws specify that treatment cannot be stopped until 14 days after the patient has been certified by a physician to be in a terminal condition, i.e., a condition in which life cannot be prolonged even with the use of extraordinary medical interventions. Since it is unusual that the presence of a terminal condition (in this sense) can be certified to exist at least two weeks prior to a patient's death, laws with this proviso are singularly ineffectual in broadening the scope of patient autonomy.

7. Among philosophers, the most popular approach to moral reflection involves the deductive application of moral theories to practical moral problems. For a comparison of the latter method with the process of moral reflection outlined in this chapter, see Terrence Ackerman, "What Bioethics Should Be," *The Journal of Medicine and Philosophy* 5 (1980):260–275.

8. Cf. Arthur Caplan, ''Mechanics on Duty: The Limitations of a Technical Definition of Moral Expertise for Work in Applied Ethics,'' *Canadian Journal of Philosophy*, Supplementary Volume VIII (1982):1–18.

9. Similar categories of activities are envisioned for the work of ethics committees. See Ronald Cranford and Edward Doudera, ''The Emergence of Institutional Ethics Committees,'' *Law, Medicine and Health Care* 12 (February 1984):13–20.

10. See Paul Appelbaum and Loren Roth, ''Patients Who Refuse Treatment in Medical Hospitals,'' *Journal of the American Medical Association* 250 (1983):1296–1301.

Chapter 22

Professional Codes and Ethical Decision Making

Susan R. Peterson, MA

Nothing would seem more natural, at least at first glance, than for professionals to require a code of ethics to assist in their deliberations about the proper course of action. This is especially true when moral issues, rather than purely technical or etiquette matters, are involved. However, the fact is that professional codes of ethics are rarely used by professionals in any context. Indeed, it is doubtful that most professionals could lay their hands on a copy of their own code if they wanted to do so, even if most of them could be persuaded that it was worth doing. Given the general neglect of professional codes of ethics, and the fact that professional practice goes on despite their neglect, it might be considered prudent to abandon professional codes. After all, most professionals are morally sensible people desiring the best for their clientele, and those practitioners who are immoral will not be prevented from mischief by the existence of a code anyway. If all such codes do is to enshrine abstract moral ideals having little to do with concrete practice, it would be less hypocritical to discard them than to pay only lip service to them. Naturally, another option would be to revise them in order to make them more useful, functional devices that could enable the modern professional to upgrade his or her services. However, in order to decide which course of action is best, one must first be familiar with the problems besetting them.

Codes of ethics serve other purposes than guiding moral decisions, including promoting a profession's status and prestige, establishing procedures to exclude potential members of the profession, specifying minimum financial fees to guarantee upward mobility of the members of the profession, and guaranteeing peer evaluation. One could almost maintain that guiding decision making is the least significant purpose of an ethical code, given the nature and historical importance of the other factors. In particular, the nonmoral functions of a professional code of ethics appear so self-serving as to actually undermine professional ethics, which is supposed to be based upon a primary concern for the public interest.

There are five main categories of problems facing professional codes of ethics:

1. excess *vagueness* in both prohibitions and prescriptions of conduct;
2. *conflicts of duty* between the various principles within a given code;
3. problems with self-evaluation and peer *enforcement* of provisions in the code;
4. excessive concern with financial and *business interests* in a code of "ethics";
5. *elitism* and exclusionary policies promoting status and prestige rather than moral conduct.

TYPICAL PROBLEMS OF A PROFESSIONAL CODE OF ETHICS

The classical example of a professional code, used for centuries as the very paradigm of professionalism, is the Hippocratic Oath:

> I swear by Appollo Physician and Asclepius and Hygieia and Panaceia and all the gods and goddesses, making them my witnesses, that I will fulfil according to my ability and judgment this oath and this covenant:
>
> To hold him who has taught me this art as equal to my parents and to live my life in partnership with him, and if he is in need of money to give him a share of mine, and to regard his offspring as equal to my brothers in male lineage and to teach them this art—if they desire to learn it—without fee and covenant; to give a share of precepts and oral instruction and all the other learning to my sons and to the sons of him who has instructed me and to pupils who have signed the covenant and have taken an oath according to the medical law, but to no one else.
>
> I will apply dietetic measures for the benefit of the sick according to my ability and judgment; I will keep them from harm and injustice.
>
> I will neither give a deadly drug to anybody if asked for it, nor will I make a suggestion to this effect. Similarly I will not give to a woman an abortive remedy. In purity and holiness I will guard my life and my art.
>
> I will not use the knife, not even on sufferers from stone, but will withdraw in favor of such men as are engaged in this work.
>
> Whatever houses I may visit, I will come for the benefit of the sick, remaining free of all intentional injustice, of all mischief and in particular of sexual relations with both female and male persons, be they free or slaves.

What I may see or hear in the course of the treatment or even outside of the treatment in regard to the life of men, which on no account one must spread abroad, I will keep to myself holding such things shameful to be spoken about.

If I fulfil this oath and do not violate it, may it be granted to me to enjoy life and art, being honored with fame among all men for all time to come; if I transgress it and swear falsely, may the opposite of all this be my lot.[1]

Though a detailed examination of this oath is most interesting, we shall confine ourselves to noting its most obvious flaws, flaws frequently found in other codes of ethics as well.

First, one cannot help but notice the elitism in the oath, which confines its membership to a small "brotherhood." (The sexism is also obvious, but this is not particularly caused by how the code is formulated, rather by social and economic factors.) Second, there is very little moral content in this oath, containing only one general, moral prescription, i.e., to "keep the patient from harm," a principle so vague as to be practically meaningless. For example, physicians argue among themselves as to whether or not to withhold pain-killing drugs from patients in great pain on the grounds that it prevents the harm of future addiction. On the other hand, physicians prescribe painkillers to alleviate suffering and thus avoid harming the patient. This dilemma is not resolved by a reference to a dictum not to harm. The third problem with the oath is its blatant concern for the activities of its practitioners; the promise "not to use the knife" on patients with kidney stones exemplifies the professional concern to maintain rigid divisions of labor among related professions, in this case between surgeons and physicians, protecting the business interests of the profession. The final two concerns in the Hippocratic Oath—confidentiality and avoiding sexual exploitation of patients—are partly moral and partly business oriented; though it is morally wrong to exploit patients and to divulge confidences given within the professional relationship, it is also true that professional practice would be virtually impossible without these assurances. Thus these proscriptions serve a double function, moral *and* business. Finally, there is no mention of what should happen when a physician does violate one of these principles, thus raising the problem of enforcement.

The importance of creating and maintaining professional elitism—usually at the expense of related professions—can be seen in the Florence Nightingale Pledge, until 1950 the code of ethics for nurses:

I solemnly pledge myself before God and in presence of his assembly;
To pass my life in purity and to practice my profession faithfully.
I will abstain from whatever is deleterious and mischievous and will not take or knowingly administer any harmful drug.

I will do all in my power to maintain and elevate the standard of my profession and will hold in confidence all personal matters committed to my keeping and family affairs coming to my knowledge in the practice of my calling.

With loyalty will I endeavor to aid the physician in his work, and devote myself to the welfare of those committed to my care.[2]

This obsequious pledge was memorized by countless nurses for decades before it was updated. It has several interesting features, mostly concerning elitism and matters of professional etiquette, especially with respect to serving physicians loyally. Historically, these features were reinforced by such hospital etiquette as requiring nurses to get off elevators when physicians arrived to board them, curtseying, and having nurses stand together in a group before beginning a hospital shift, all at attention and with hands on their hearts, together reciting the Florence Nightingale Pledge.[3] Though such practices are all but extinct, nurses still feel a loyalty to the physician rather than to the hospital administration, creating problems with conflicts of duty.

The 1976 Code for Nurses[4] remedies the obvious deficiencies in the Florence Nightingale Pledge but still displays problems revealed in the Hippocratic Oath and the AMA Principles of Ethics.[5] Indeed, the American Nurses' Association seemed so aware of these problems, especially vagueness, that they prepared a 14-page interpretative statement on the code to help clarify its principles. For example, Principle 4 of the Code for Nurses, "The nurse assumes responsibility and accountability for individual nursing judgments and actions," is broken down into four components in the interpretative statement: (1) the right of nurses to regulate their own profession (our problems of elitism and enforcement); (2) specification of the nurse's role (a business interest involving division of labor among health care professionals, most particularly the ever-expanding number of technicians required for hospital care); (3) accountability to the law rather than to physicians (creating an obvious conflict of duties); and (4) peer evaluation and its consequent problems of enforcement.

The 1971 AMA Principles of Medical Ethics have problems similar to the Code for Nurses. Consider, for example, Section 3, "A physician should practice a method of healing founded on a scientific basis; and he should not voluntarily associate professionally with anyone who violates this principle."[6] It not only encourages elitism by requiring an extensive university education (and excluding naturalist healers such as herbalists, as well as midwives), but also helps to create a business monopoly designed to increase the financial benefits of physicians. The history of American medicine in particular illustrates the importance of such factors in the creation of a profession.[7] Similarly, Section 6 of the AMA Principles, "A physician should not dispose of his services under terms or conditions which tend to interfere with or impair the free and complete exercise of his medical judgment and skill or tend to cause a deterioration of the quality of medical care," refers not so much to avoiding work with doctors who don't wash their hands as to the increasing desire to locate medical practice in large institutions, particularly the hospital. One could paraphrase Section 6 of the AMA Code as "Physicians should practice as much as possible within hospitals, or at least in private offices having hospital equipment."

Keep in mind that engineering, law, and social work professions face identical problems with their codes; we only refer specifically to the medical codes because they are familiar and they have served as a model for other professional codes. In all professional codes, business interests outnumber moral issues. The AMA Principles have only one truly moral section, Section 1, requiring the physician to render "service to humanity with full respect for the dignity of man."

In a graduate school course in Social Work Ethics,[8] students had great difficulty in *finding* the National Association of Social Workers (NASW) Code of Ethics when assigned to do so. When asked to analyze it, they found that business interests greatly outnumbered moral concerns, and the few moral principles suffered from excessive vagueness; for example, the principle that the client's interests should always be served, when precisely what should be considered in the client's interest is left open to debate. Moreover, the NASW Code of Ethics does nothing to reduce the numbers of conflicts of duty faced by social workers, such as when they are told to use appropriate channels to communicate case information and to preserve the confidentiality of the client. Most professional codes of ethics fail to provide an overall principle to use in resolving conflicts of duty. Violations of the code present problems of enforcement.

THE ACHE CODE OF ETHICS: SOME SOLUTIONS AND SOME NEW PROBLEMS

The American College of Healthcare Executives Code of Ethics[9] exemplifies all five of our problems though it goes some distance toward resolving some of them, most notably conflicts of duty. When the ACHE Code requires "manifest personal integrity" in addition to "capable leadership," it echoes the Florence Nightingale Pledge and the AMA Principles by being vague about the scope of this requirement. Similar to ACHE's "integrity," when the AMA Principles in Section 4 require physicians to "safeguard the public and itself against physicians deficient in moral character," does this mean that doctors committing adultery should be banned from practice? That those neglecting their children should not associate with other professionals? What about those who lie on their income tax returns? In fact, news accounts reveal physicians guilty of felony offenses who continue to practice for years in spite of them. There is some reason to argue that enforcement problems are the root of all difficulties with professional codes of ethics. At any rate, the phrase "deficient in moral character" is so vague as to render it useless for any practical purpose.

The ACHE code reveals some attempt to reduce the usual vagueness found in professional codes, especially by requiring the profession to divest outside interests that could cause conflicts of interest, banning private profit for hospital administrators with privileged information, requiring administrators to coordinate medical professionals to create a proper environment within large institutions, and including a duty to outside professionals in the community.

Unfortunately, these very improvements create new difficulties, especially in the predominance of business interests over moral concerns. The increased specificity of principles does help the professional in decision making, but it does not help with problems of enforcement, and when rules are unenforced, they are frequently ignored. Is it realistic to expect health care administrators to fully disclose their financial dealings just to avoid potential conflicts of interest? Should we expect such administrators to promptly inform a governing authority about potential conflicts by other colleagues? Not only are such expectations unrealistic, they might not be morally justified. This, of course, raises the entire issue of peer evaluation and enforcement, with the related problems of whistle-blowing and the duty to violate even confidentiality under certain circumstances.[10]

We can conclude then, that though the ACHE code reduces vagueness by providing detailed descriptions of roles and conflicts, it fails to provide a principle that can resolve conflicts when they do occur. More seriously still, the level of specificity in the ACHE Code causes it to fail as a moral code at all, because there is so little moral content in it. Moral codes ought to include *at least* such moral terms as justice, fairness, equity, equality, duties, rights, consequences that may justify overruling other rules or duties, and so forth. Admittedly, it is not easy to create an ethical code that will solve all our problems, but some sort of balance between business interests and morality per se ought to be achieved. It should be possible to become more specific about moral requirements without abandoning morality entirely.

CONCLUSIONS AND RECOMMENDATIONS

I hope that this brief analysis can motivate health care professionals in hospital settings to become more active in reforming, discussing, and enforcing codes of ethics. As the ACHE Code reveals, problems of conflicts of duty are the most significant for the hospital professional. Those in middle positions, such as nurses, feel various duties tearing them in different directions—e.g., to the patient, to the hospital, to the physician in charge, and to their own legal accountability for their actions. With the addition of several types of hospital orderlies, the increasing absence of full-time physicians on hand, the presence of residents in training, and so on, hard moral decisions will need to be made to avoid serious organizational discordance and professional violations of ethical codes.

Perhaps many of these problems stem from the tendency of current ethical codes to emulate the Hippocratic Oath and the tradition of the three paradigmatic professions: the law, medicine, and the clergy. Such professions used to be conducted outside an institutional setting and so cannot be productively used as models for today's professional. Most professionals today operate within very complex organizational environments, as the ACHE Code reveals. In addition, professional codes of ethics imply that the professional ought to be motivated solely by altruistic concerns, surely an unreasonable and unrealistic assumption. Perhaps some self-serving requirements in the business interest of the professional are morally justified because they indirectly benefit clients. If so, this ought to be included within a professional code of ethics. For example, professional advertising is frequently prohibited in codes of ethics; it has been argued that advertising can harm clients by enticing them to choose a professional on the basis of financial concerns only. Similarly, an argument for fee schedules can be made; the quality of professional care a client receives should not depend upon the amount of money he or she can provide to the professional. It is important that these issues be discussed by professionals; if codes of ethics ignore them, they will remain problematic.

It would be professionally irresponsible for an ethicist like me to confine the discussion only to problems without making concrete recommendations. For this reason, we will conclude with some specific, though brief, recommendations concerning each of the five problem areas.

1. *Vagueness.* Although excessive vagueness ought to be avoided, professionals should remember that some moral concerns are inherently vague, however important they may be. For example, political liberty is vague enough to have been debated for centuries, but no one would argue that it is therefore meaningless or insignificant. Moreover, if a moral principle is important enough, it is worth including in a code to have an ideal toward which to strive. Much of the excessive vagueness could be eliminated in codes of ethics by merely including more moral language, much of which is very specific.

2. *Conflicts of Duty.* More discussions on this issue should take place within the professional community, in order to reach some form of agreement on how conflicts should be resolved when they occur. It may be helpful to create a code committee made up of representatives of *each* component of the organization (yes, including laboratory technicians and orderlies), so that typical conflicts can be hashed out and resolved in a satisfactory manner. It would help very much if some enforcement power was attached to such a method of resolution.

3. *Enforcement.* Perhaps professional self-monitoring should be abandoned as simply too costly to maintain. Because of the failure of most professionals to take to task members who violate professional rules of conduct,

the public has increasingly resorted to political and legal methods of redress. The current crisis of malpractice insurance is undoubtedly caused, or at least exacerbated, by this problem. A good idea might be creating enforcement committees that represent every important component of a community for enforcement purposes (e.g., professionals, administrators, laypeople, politicians, government officials).

4. *Business Interests.* Professionals and laypeople alike must face up to the fact that professions are businesses. They are not exactly like a normal business, but it is foolish to ignore the business aspect of the professional community. Codes of ethics, therefore, ought to *justify* the business practices of a given profession, not merely disguise them as moral concerns or at best as professional etiquette.

5. *Elitism.* Perhaps social status helps the professional to provide better service to the client. If this is so, this may justify otherwise trivial concerns that appear self-serving and self-aggrandizing, such as ranking various health care professionals on a carefully arranged ladder and making sure that newer professions don't encroach upon "real" (i.e., more established) ones. Professional autonomy is important enough to argue at least for sufficient social status to avoid constant interference in professional conduct.

We may conclude, then, that the professional code of ethics is here to stay and so ought to be reformed to become more relevant and useful to the practicing professional. To do this successfully, however, professionals will have to become more involved in actually discussing moral problems and moral codes—post them around the office, devote committees to them, encourage debate about them, and finally honor them.

NOTES

1. The Hippocratic Oath can be found in *Ancient Medicine: Selected Papers of Ludwig Edelstein*, ed. Owsei Temkin and C. Lilian Temkin (Baltimore: Johns Hopkins Press, 1967), 6.

2. The Florence Nightingale Pledge can be found in Anne J. Davis and Mila A. Aroskar, *Ethical Dilemmas and Nursing Practice* (New York: Appleton-Century-Crofts, 1978), 12–13.

3. These revelations were made by nurses with 15–20 years experience during several courses in medical ethics I taught at C.W. Post Center, Long Island University on Long Island, and at Queensboro Community College in Queens, New York.

4. American Nurses' Association, *Code for Nurses*, 1976.

5. American Medical Association, "Principles of Medical Ethics," *Journal of the American Medical Association* 164, no. 10 (July 6, 1957):1119–1120. Copyright 1957, AMA.

6. American Medical Association, *Judicial Counsel Opinions and Reports* (Chicago: American Medical Association, 1971).

7. An excellent source for the history of medicine in America is Paul Starr's *The Social Transformation of American Medicine* (New York: Basic Books, 1982).

8. Dr. Gary Anderson and I have team taught this course for three years.

9. American College of Healthcare Executives, *Code of Ethics*, February 1986.

10. There are legal requirements for professionals to override duties of confidentiality, as for instance when they know and can prevent a serious crime from occurring by contacting the police about a client.

Chapter 23

Ethical Decision Making and the Health Administrator

Marc D. Hiller, DrPH

INTRODUCTION AND PURPOSE

Health administrators are being forced to confront an increasing number of thorny issues due to a variety of competing external and internal forces.[1] Most of the situations and decisions present several possible options. Moreover, many of these situations pose ethical issues or decisions that hold serious ethical implications for the persons affected by them.

It is important for administrators to recognize consciously that such dilemmas require a process of ethical decision making. Many administrators who perceive their career as decision makers will raise their eyebrows at this statement and ask why ethical decisions are so different from other types. "Does it lie in the methods of decision making? In the conclusions reached? In the assumptions used? In all or none of these?"[2]

What is distinctive about ethical decision making is the centrality of fundamental ethical principles both in the reasoning that leads up to the decision, and because the decision maker accepts the principles in question as part of his or her value orientation. The latter requires a prior clarification of values, often through structured exercises. An administrator "makes an ethical decision, as distinct from some other kind of decision, if and only if he decides what to do by essential reliance upon some ethical rule, principle, standard, or norm."[3] This means that had the administrator not relied on the ethical principle, the same decision may not have been reached; or, had the same decision been made, the reason behind it would have differed and not been based upon an ethical principle. Rather, it would have another basis, such as profitability, business efficiency, or even self-interest.

In making ethical decisions, administrators must also recognize that it is often necessary to prioritize the competing interests to whom they owe accountability. More than a decade ago, Austin noted that health administrators frequently find themselves on the horns of a dilemma, having to juggle a series of competitive obligations.[4] Unlike physicians who usually view their patients as their sole (or at least their principal) responsibility, administrators bear a responsiblity to various additional parties to ensure institutional survival (and, increasingly, a level of profitability demanded by their investors). Toward such ends, they are accountable to the owners, community, staff, third party regulatory and financing bodies (e.g., Health Care Financing Administration, Joint Commission for the Accreditation of Hospitals, private insurance companies, creditors, and sources of capital), in addition to their patients.

Of equal importance is achieving a clear sense of the independent ethical responsibilities of their institution in fulfilling its proclaimed mission.[5] While the ethical responsibility of the institution as an entity has not gained considerable attention, Pellegrino and Thomasma have maintained that the hospital (as an institution) bears collective moral obligations.[6] In claiming that the institution's paramount obligation is to the patient, administrators must exercise the collective moral responsibility of the institution as its representative.

This chapter is not meant to provide the theoretical basis for applying ethics to problems arising in health administration. Nor is it meant to analytically examine or classify the wide range of ethical issues confronting health administrators. Both of these tasks have recently been addressed by the Commission on Ethical Issues in Health Management.[7] Rather, the purpose is to provide administrators with some useful ways, or methodologies, for facilitating ethical decision making. Employing such techniques will strengthen their ability to analyze and justify their decisions, for themselves, their institution and employees, and their communities. Multiple models of ethical decision making have been developed.[8]

FUNDAMENTAL ETHICAL PRINCIPLES

While obvious differences exist in their approaches, essential to all techniques is the recognition of basic normative ethical principles, from which institutional policies and administrative decisions should be derived. Beauchamp and Childress have attempted to illustrate an instructive model of ethical reasoning using four levels of ethical reasoning as exhibited in Table 23-1.[9]

On the basis of general ethical theories, such as utilitarianism or deontology, fundamental principles may be derived to guide administrative decision making (see Table 23-2).

While the precise nature of the distinction between principles and rules is often debated, the former are usually viewed as more general and fundamental. For example, the principle of respect for persons supports many ethical rules such as "it is wrong to lie," "disclosure of confidential information is wrong," and "coercion and deception are wrong." In turn, adherence to such rules facilitates making certain judgments or engaging in particular actions in specific situations. Ethical principles serve as the foundation of most of the more specific

Table 23-1 Hierarchy of Ethical Reasoning in Health Administration

• Theories	Systematically related bodies of principles and rules; used to resolve conflicts between principles
• Principles	Foundation or source for justifying rules that guide administrative decision making
• Rules	Statements that administrative actions of a certain kind ought (or ought not) to be made because they are "right" or "wrong"
• Judgments or Actions	Particular administrative decisions, verdicts, or conclusions

rules that should be employed in making health management decisions in matters involving ethical issues.

Since most situations pose ethical dilemmas to which more than one principle is applicable, in most cases complete analysis requires consideration of several principles in tandem. As this often produces a conflict between, or among, different ethical principles and eventually leads to a prioritization of applicable principles in a given situation, it assures a more adequate and complete examination of all possible alternatives and their respective implications.

No single ethical principle possesses sufficient weight to trump all conflicting ethical claims. It is critically important for administrators to appreciate the plu-

Table 23-2 Fundamental Normative Ethical Principles Relevant to Health Administration

• Beneficence	The obligation to benefit one's institution and those it serves (e.g., community, patients, staff)
• Nonmaleficence	The obligation to bring no harm or injury to one's institution or to those it serves
• Respect for Persons	The obligation to protect and preserve the individual autonomy (self-determination) of those affected by administrative decisions and managerial practices, particularly that of patients and staff
• Justice	The obligation to act in a fair and impartial manner in making administrative decisions that affect one's institution or any party it serves (e.g., in allocating or rationing limited resources and/or services, benefits or burdens, risks and costs)
• Utility	The obligation to balance the above principles to maximize the greatest utility in administrative decision making

ralism of equally weighted principles as a fundamental feature of moral life while concurrently recognizing that the weight, or priority, allocated to specific principles may vary based on the uniqueness of given situations. When applied ethical issues arise in health management (and medicine), the use of ethical principles orchestrates a well-balanced approach toward reaching rational solutions.

Through their application, sound ethical judgments may be distinguished from bad moral claims, or personal attitudes or intuitions, i.e., unreflective and nonobjective principles. Accordingly, Beauchamp and McCullough have claimed that "one must have defensible moral reasons for holding a position, and neither the position nor the reasons that underlie it can be justified if they rest solely on prejudice, emotion, false data, the authority of another individual, or claims of self-evidence."[10]

Nonmaleficence and Beneficence

The principle of *nonmaleficence* dictates: inflict no harm. It reflects the popular medical ethos *primum non nocere* (first of all, do no harm) and instructs that one should engage in no activities known to risk or cause harm or injury to another party. With respect to health administrators, it requires that they avoid any misconduct or wrongdoing. Adherence to this principle by administrators often precipitates conflicts due to their multiple accountabilities. At the institutional level, they are bound to eliminate or minimize any harm coming to the institution, such as financial risk; at the individual level, they are obligated to ensure that harm is not knowingly caused to patients or employees of the institution. Many situations bearing on administrative decision or action force a confrontation between avoiding harm for the institution and for an individual; that is, decisions that are least harmful to the institution may induce harm to an individual staff member or patient (or vice versa).

Beneficence is a more active principle. Whereas nonmaleficence holds that it is the health administrator's responsibility to do no harm, beneficence extends this obligation further toward a more assertive end when situations permit. It obligates the administrator to make decisions that maximize good for (i.e., benefit) the institution and those it serves including the local or regional community, its patients, and its staff.

As with nonmaleficence, adherence to this principle often results in conflicts with respect to what is in the institution's best interest and what is in the best interest of either a patient or a staff member. Among the more obvious examples is the situation in which a particular hospital service (or the operation of a certain department) does not generate sufficient revenues to cover its costs but provides a needed community and patient benefit. Acting in the best interest of the institution might mean eliminating the service (or department) and replacing it with a more cost-effective one. However, an administrative move toward such end would not necessarily be in the best interest of those who might need the eliminated service.

Respect for Persons

The principle of respect for persons, also referred to as autonomy, self-determination, and liberty, serves as the foundation for "individual rights." Using classic medical ethics terminology, such rights are typically referred to as "patient's rights." From a broader managerial perspective, however, administrators are obligated to respect the autonomy of individual staff members as well as patients and ensure that their due respect and independence are not unjustly compromised. Many specific ethical rules and legal doctrines based on this principle have emerged, such as informed consent, confidentiality and privacy, and truth telling.

At bottom, administrators should honor the self-respect and dignity of each individual as an autonomous, free actor. All competent individuals have an intrinsic right to make decisions for themselves on any matter affecting them, at least so far as such decisions do not bring harm to another party. Even when an individual possesses a limited capacity to exercise this right due to a physical or mental condition, this obligation should not be ignored.

Respect for persons offers a clear directive despite its frequent unavoidable clash with beneficence. Common areas of evolving hospital policy exemplify this conflict: policies on foregoing life supporting treatment terminating life (e.g., do-not-resuscitate orders, withdrawal from a respirator) and institutional no-smoking. An institutional policy that will respect a patient's desire to die with dignity protects the right to self-determination. However, some may view such a practice as violating nonmaleficence (if allowing a patient to die "prematurely" is viewed as "harming" the patient). In turn, an institutional ban on smoking may benefit, or at least not harm, those in the institution (e.g., patients, visitors, and staff). Yet, such action might be argued as impinging on the individual right of autonomy for those wishing to smoke.

Justice

What is fair or 'just?' While various concepts of justice are based on a variety of criteria, each demands fairness and impartiality in determining what each individual deserves—be it a burden (or risk) or a benefit.

While many rival theories of justice exist, all major ones share a common element: all cases should be treated similarly, i.e., equals should be treated equally, and unequals unequally.

Each theory of justice subscribes to a different set or combination of material (substantive) or procedural criteria. Beauchamp and Bowie have employed six "material principles of justice" as a basis for many of the theories.[11] While there is no need to accept more than one of these material principles to systematically defend one's interpretation of fairness, usually a combination or prioritization of them is used in defending just decisions.

Interpretations of justice vary with social, economic, and political values. For example, differences of egalitarian, Marxist, libertarian, or utilitarian perspectives influence ethical decision making. Egalitarians emphasize equal access to health care. Administrators holding this material principle would defend programs available to anyone—access would be unlimited for all practical purposes, thus ensuring equity. However, should such an approach ever be economically feasible, services obviously would have to be less than extensive, given that resources are limited. Marxists tend to emphasize need as a basis for allocation. Administrators holding this perspective would advocate that most institutional resources should be allocated for those bearing the greatest need. Advocates of a triage theory would hold that services should first be allocated to those whom they are most likely to benefit; those determined to be beneath an established minimum threshold (i.e., those beyond meaningful recovery) would be denied services. Libertarian theories emphasize that services ought to be rendered on the basis of individual contribution and merit. Criteria vary from the degree of one's community contributions, to the number of one's dependents, to one's ability to pay the price charged for a particular service. Utilitarians support a mixed use of such criteria so that public and private utility is maximized.

Dilemmas frequently arise in terms of what proportion of the health care budget ought to be allocated to particular departments. Of the available resources, how should they be distributed (e.g., for preventive versus curative purposes)? What types of procedural mechanisms could ensure a fair distribution avoiding bias and prejudice; who should decide?

Utility

The principle of utility is unlike the above principles. As a procedural principle, it instructs administrators to "balance" both the good and bad outcomes associated with the various alternatives posed in individual cases. It recognizes that the other principles are not mutually exclusive and often directly conflict with each other. The utility or usefulness of an action is determined by the extent to which it produces the most desired outcome.

For utilitarians, there is one and only one basic principle in ethics, namely utility. It determines the order of activities in a manner that maximizes benefits and minimizes harm. In contrast, for those not holding utility as their sole guide to behavior, it instructs a balancing of the unavoidable conflicts resulting from the application of the other principles.

This principle dictates that administrators carefully weigh the preceding principles with respect to which may hold priority over others amid their inevitable clashes. (For example, to benefit one employee the most will demand sacrificing fairness in treating others; to promote the health of a worker will require denying his or her expressed wishes; to maximize institutional efficiency will force sacrificing that which is in the best interest of an individual employee or patient.)

VALUES CLARIFICATION NEEDED

In addition to ethical principles, which tend to be somewhat rational, objective, and analytic in nature, values often affect decisions that must be made. As values are classically subjective and potentially biased in nature, administrators are obligated to have a clear sense of their own values and how they may influence their decisions. They need to consciously seek to determine why they value some things more than others, and whether they should.

A general consensus holds that certain groups of values exist, such as moral, political, esthetic, religious, and intellectual. While genetic, biological, and cultural influences produce many of these values, there is little agreement with respect to their nature, their relative importance, or any interrelationships.[12]

Among the major factors affecting values is morals. Values may or may not heavily reflect moral or religious leanings. Nonetheless, other factors that strongly contribute to the value formation of administrators include their personal experiences, culture (e.g., race, ethnicity), and peer group (e.g., other health administrators, other members of the American College of Healthcare Executives, others comprising one's socioeconomic class).

For example, administrators who have been hospitalized often bear greater sensitivity to a patient-oriented perspective, or even to "patient rights." If an administrator's culture pays homage to the elderly (e.g., most Asian cultures), then greater attention and sensitivity may be given to the elderly.

At bottom, while values may be common or shared, they remain highly personal. They contribute significantly to administrative behavior and decision making, both consciously and subconsciously. They may or may not contribute to ethical actions or outcomes.

Thus, it is important for all health administrators to clarify their values periodically throughout their careers. Values clarification provides insight regarding values and the valuation process. It provides no set standards, principles, or norms for value formulation but simply offers a descriptive means of identifying and illuminating values. Thus, it permits a critical analysis of how values affect administrative decisions.

LEVELS OF ETHICAL ANALYSIS

Specific ethical problems should be analyzed at multiple levels. At what level does an ethical question lie? As the previous discussion pointed out, part of the administrator's dilemma in resolving ethical issues is due to his or her multiple accountabilities that typically cut across multiple levels.

While ethical problems may exist at only one level, when they hold implications at multiple levels their analysis becomes more complex given the various
perspectives of the different groups that must be considered concurrently. Serious
conflicts often arise when a sound ethical argument to do one thing (reflecting
the application of one principle at one level) is juxtaposed with an equally strong
case to do another (using the same or another principle at another level).

At the macro level, the focus is on the society or community. Issues at this
level typically involve problems or options affecting aggregate bodies and tend
to be of a public policy nature. At the meso level, the orientation is on the
organization or a given profession. Among the priority concerns arising at this
level are those maximizing what is good for the health care institution to facilitate
carrying out its designated mission. In contrast, issues arising at the micro level
focus on individual interrelationships and tend to be most concerned with doing
good for the individual (e.g., the patient or staff member).

In applying these ethical principles, it is important to ensure recognition of
at least three distinctive levels, while recognizing that they are not necessarily
mutually exclusive. This assures that all possible alternatives are identified and
applicable principles employed. While many ethical dilemmas are a function of
the particular problem at hand, additional problems often arise when multiple
ethical implications may be identified as a function of their being viewed from
different levels. Further conflict often becomes more apparent when one level
has priority over another.[13]

Difficult choices must often be made, even after careful ethical analysis, when
one must choose among alternatives that bear incompatible positive consequences. One may produce a social good (i.e., viewed from the macro level)
while another would produce an individual good (i.e., viewed from the micro
level), and a single choice must be made. Similarly, conflicts often arise between
meso and micro levels when one option will maximize an institution's objective
while another may be in an individual's best interest.

For example, implementing an automated management information system
used for both personnel and patient care records may contribute to an institution's
efficiency (meso level). Given increased efficiency, the institution may even
realize additional resources to provide more community services (macro level).
Such a move appears ethical from a utilitarian standpoint. However, such cen-
tralization would require granting access of various authorized (and potentially
unauthorized) personnel to confidential information and increase the risk of
disclosure of sensitive information to undesired parties (micro level). At this
level, the principle of respect for persons would be sacrificed.

Often such clashes cannot be avoided regardless of the application of ethical
principles. In these events, ethical decision making becomes more value-laden
and may simply be resolved based on which level is most valued. Often administrators make decisions perceived to be of a purely managerial nature, failing
to realize the potential ethical implications such decisions may precipitate. That

which makes the most sense for the institution (or one of its departments) may oppose that which might be in the best interests of individual patients or employees.

TYPES OF CONFLICTS CONFRONTING ADMINISTRATORS

Beyond the problem that ethical conflicts are often aggravated by posing different implications at various levels, administrators are increasingly being forced to choose among alternatives that cannot be viewed simply as "good" or "evil." Administrators must not erroneously assume that ethical choices are so clear-cut; few dilemmas pose genuine options that are unquestionably good or bad.

Rather, decisions usually must be made among alternatives that pose a "better versus worse" scenario in which the options are not overly clear. In such cases, decision making becomes progressively more difficult as the determination of which choice is better and which is worse grows more indistinct. This is particularly the situation when units of value are very different, such as when dollars (or an economic benefit) on one hand must be weighed against the degree of fairness or honesty on the other.

Another type of conflict administrators often face is having to choose among "good" alternatives that are mutually exclusive. In this type of situation, no matter which choice is made, the decision will be viewed as bad by some. Conflicts involving multiple good alternatives force administrators to prioritize the ethical principles on which their decisions are based.

A final type of ethical conflict calls upon a more general point, described by Brody as "the principle of 'you can't have your cake and eat it too.' "[14] In situations presenting such dilemmas, administrators must acknowledge that choosing one alternative course of action constitutes a decision not to do others. Most often, such conflicts involve decisions regarding the allocation, either explicitly or implicitly, of scarce finite resources.

Given the wide array of possible ethical issues and related decision-making dilemmas confronting health administrators, several approaches have been developed to assist in assuring a rational process for ethical decision making. While no single method of "doing ethics" can guarantee the resolution of every ethical quandary, each attempts to ensure a systematic examination of alternatives based on the comprehension of fundamental ethical principles and appreciation of personal, institutional, and societal values.

RESOLVING ETHICAL DILEMMAS IN HEALTH MANAGEMENT

The remaining portion of this chapter is designed to provide administrators with two different approaches toward resolving ethical dilemmas. The first reflects a qualitative orientation commonly used in ethical decision making in medicine; the second is strongly grounded in quantitative techniques more often employed in business management. Both approaches reflect the centrality of fundamental ethical principles being employed in resolving ethical problems; the latter, however, emphasizes a mathematical framework.

It is essential, though, that before commencing either approach, administrators must be sensitive to the reality that outcomes (i.e., decisions or actions) often vary as a result of the level prioritized during decision making. While this variation may be considered in employing either of the two approaches, neither truly facilitates the intrinsic consideration of level. Hence, it is important for administrators to acknowledge the potential competition among levels and determine the level at which the analysis is to be conducted (before commencing either approach). Obviously, any effort to justify a final decision where conflict exists between levels could be strengthened if one had conducted similar analyses from the perspective of each level. If the respective ethical outcomes differ, one is able to consciously accept one over the other knowing that both were ethically justifiable but that the final decision was based on a prioritization of levels.

A Qualitative Approach

The first approach, consisting of a six-step process theoretically outlined by Harron, Burnside, and Beauchamp, considers each of the critical elements needed to make an ethically sound decision.[15] It maximizes a rational, systematic examination of alternative courses of action based on the application of fundamental ethical principles. The most successful employment of this process requires that administrators have previously undergone a clarification of their personal values. While personal and professional values will affect ultimate decisions, their influence should be acknowledged and limited (see Step 5).

Step 1. Identifying an Ethical Problem

Identification represents three successive activities: perceive the existence of an ethical problem, identify the problem, and confirm the problem. If an ethical problem truly exists, there must be a real choice between courses of action. In making this assessment, gathering as much relevant information as possible is essential. Should a problem be confirmed, one must be able to attribute significantly different values to the various possible options (i.e., alternatives), or their respective consequences (i.e., implications).

While the above ingredients are essential in confirming the existence of an ethical problem, their mere presence does not ensure such. For example, situations that pose ethical acts on one hand and self-interested (or even illegal) acts on the other do not constitute ethical problems. Furthermore, seeking or obtaining legal resolutions does not necessarily guarantee ethical solutions. Many ethical dilemmas defy legal solutions (e.g., laws or policies governing abortion or foregoing life-sustaining treatments).

Step 2. Determining Alternatives

This step calls for administrators to list all of the identifiable alternative courses of action that could be employed in addressing a problem. Usually, consideration of decision alternatives tends not to produce an exhaustive list; most often, one considers only two.

Human conditioning prefers to limit choice between two alternatives; it is easier to think in terms of "either-or" than in the complexities of multiple alternatives that require juggling or some form of matrixlike analysis. Unfortunately, there are usually more than two, and often it is the third or fourth that provides the optimal solution. Further, limiting decision making to a choice between only two alternatives assumes that one may be weighed against the other. Moreover, in most cases two alternatives exist simply in taking some action or doing nothing. Hence, it is essential that administrators delineate all possible alternatives, even those that may appear somewhat remote.

In considering alternatives, administrators should not immediately discard those that may initially appear in the best interests of others, such as staff members, patients, or the community.

Step 3. Weighing Competing Options

This step involves assessing the respective consequences (i.e., implications) that would most likely result from each alternative, such as the respective strengths and weaknesses of each. It dictates that the implications posed by various alternatives be contrasted and balanced individually and comparatively.

Before initiating the actual weighing process, the more immediate and dramatic consequences of particular alternatives, which usually come quickly to mind, should be examined. Often this is the stage where the varying importance of particular alternatives may be observed as a function of the level from which the analysis is being conducted. When this is the case, administrators need to clarify the level from which they are deciding.

After initially acknowledging the most apparent consequences of each alternative, a further investment of time and effort is required to generate a list of long-range, and not-so-apparent, consequences associated with specific alternatives.

While it is common to think of individual or independent consequences, one must assess the degree to which effects may be interrelated or aggregated as well. At times, resolving conflicting alternatives and consequences requires minimal compromise; in other instances, considerable sacrifice is required at one level or for one party.

Among the most difficult realities that must be reckoned with is that the process commonly generates a degree of uncertainty—given the impossibility of being able to predict every possible consequence for every alternative. Hence, at some point, the weighing process must give way to justification.

Step 4. Justifying by Ethical Principles

It is at this step that the administrator's essential understanding of ethical principles and rules becomes imperative. The justification process involves the application of all relevant ethical principles (and rules) to the identified alternatives and their respective implications.

Justifiable arguments should be constructed to defend particular alternatives using normative ethical principles and rules. Significant effort should be made to critically examine competing alternatives in terms of their respective ability to withstand similar ethical inquiry.

In a genuine ethical dilemma, this justification process permits administrators to prioritize identified alternatives based on their adherence to fundamental ethical principles (e.g., beneficence, nonmaleficence, autonomy, justice, utility). Frequently it also reflects broader ethical theories comprising either a utilitarian view (i.e., being most concerned with the consequences associated with particular alternatives) or a deontological posture (i.e., ranking a certain principle above others independent of the consequences it might precipitate).

To this point, the process has been somewhat devoid of professional or personal values and morals. However, reckoning that most decisions, particularly those involving health care issues, employ a value element, such is considered at this phase. A conscious and sensitive reflection on applicable values, including moral teachings, may at this point have some influence on the pending choices. Having undergone a values clarification process, one must ascertain, control, and defend the extent to which values affect the decision-making process. To the extent that personal values conflict with prior ethical deliberations, further wrestling with the problem at hand may be in order before making an actual choice.

Step 5. Making a Choice

This step in the decision-making process, making a choice, brings a degree of closure. However, many administrative ethical dilemmas require choosing among more than a single good alternative. Legitimate grounds often support multiple alternatives based on different ethical principles. Hence, initial choices frequently reflect how the principles were prioritized in the previous step and therefore may not be agreed upon unanimously.

Inevitably, some if not most choices mirror professional and personal value judgments. Hence, the importance of values clarification cannot be overemphasized.

Step 6. Reassessing Choices

In this step of the ethical decision-making process, the one most often neglected in the haste to reach its conclusion, administrators should identify any unresolved questions, reexamine their choices and their justifications, and compare their choices in this situation to decisions made in similar cases elsewhere at other times.

This final step provides administrators with a valuable opportunity to reexamine their choices and the process by which they were made. It may be characterized as a sort of ''ethical safety net'' that demands administrative reconsideration. It assures that before making what may be an irrevocable decision (or implementing an action) one should be able to firmly support a choice and justify it on sound ethical grounds.

A Quantitative Approach

Given the multitude of possible options frequently encountered in making difficult ethical decisions, some have sought to impose a more structured empirical approach that permits mathematical analysis.[16] While such an approach may possess certain merits, one must be candidly aware that the ingredients used in the process are predicated on many of the same qualitative judgments used in the first approach. Hence, while the methodology reflects many elements similar to those employed in quantitative decision making, such as assigning numerical values to selection criteria and queuing various alternatives (i.e., constructing a decision matrix), it still remains more qualitative than absolute.

Nonetheless, it may be argued that to the extent a quantitative methodological approach is imposed on ethical decision making, its sensitivity to making qualitative value judgments is sacrificed or viewed as artificial. Whether quantitative decision-making theory may be transferred and applied to the resolution of ethical dilemmas, i.e., as the following presentation suggests, is an issue that bears close individual examination. If selected as an approach, however, the decision matrix technique dictates attention to detail and may serve as a rational mechanism for identifying ethically sound administrative alternatives. Hence, the following presentation of this quantitative approach is provided for administrative consideration; its adoption is a matter of personal choice.

In situations requiring choice among a minimum of two alternatives, the use of the decision matrix may facilitate rational problem solving. Further, its efficiency increases as the number of alternatives increases.[17]

Since ethical problems require a minimum of two alternatives, and most usually pose more, application of this approach may provide a meaningful way to resolve complex ethical dilemmas. As a decision aid, it forces administrators to undertake a rather detailed analysis of each alternative in light of imposed ethical criteria and to apply weights to such criteria based on their own personal and professional values.

To illustrate the application of this approach, it is useful to use an example of a common ethical dilemma confronting health care administrators:

Should the hospital in a single-hospital community deny care to indigent individuals (i.e., persons unable to pay for care)?

Step 1. Identifying Alternatives

Not unlike the more qualitative approach, the initial step in employing this mathematically oriented decision matrix technique requires the identification of all possible alternatives that may be justified on ethical grounds. Given serious concern about the outcome, administrators must exercise caution not to exclude any feasible option, since this structured approach does not facilitate later addition or modification. The efficiency of this method is directly related to the number of alternatives included in the matrix. Upon their identification, the methodology calls for listing all of them in a column.

In reference to the sample case, an administrator would initially identify the alternatives that are ethically acceptable. For the purpose of this explanation, the concern rests with illustrating the process rather than conclusions. Hence, only three alternatives are used. If this were an actual case in which the outcome was critical, probably the administrator would identify additional (i.e., all possible) meaningful alternatives, recognizing that the efficiency of employing this method is a function of the number of alternatives analyzed.

Alternative 1: The hospital should establish a policy of denying care to individuals who are unable to demonstrate an ability to pay for it.

Alternative 2: The hospital should establish a policy of providing care for a limited number of individuals who are unable to pay for it by admitting such patients only to the old wing (i.e., a lower class of accommodations) based on the availability of beds located there.

Alternative 3: The hospital should retain its current policy of not denying care to any person based on an inability to pay for it.

Step 2. Determining the Evaluation Criteria

The second phase of this approach requires identifying which criteria (ethical principles, rules, and other selected factors) ought to be employed in evaluating each alternative that was generated in the first step. The objective at hand is to determine the options that are the most ethical based on fundamental ethical principles and rules (as previously discussed).

In doing so, the following seven ethical criteria are commonly employed:

1. *beneficence*, or contributing to the good and welfare of others;
2. *nonmaleficence*, or doing no harm to others;

3. *truth telling*, or being honest and truthful to others;
4. *confidentiality*, or guarding against the dissemination of private (personal) information;
5. *autonomy* (self-determination), or ensuring that individuals are free to make decisions affecting themselves independently and without coercion;
6. *justice*, or ensuring that individuals are treated in an equal (fair) manner;
7. *utility*, or balancing the above in a manner that promises the best outcome in a given situation.

In addition to these ethical criteria, other factors that reflect little if any ethical content (e.g., economic, political, legal, or philosophical) may be added selectively. Rather than ignore such factors and risk criticism as a result, one may consider them with the appreciation that they should be allocated little ethical weight in making actual decisions.

Examining the specific ethical problem at hand, the administrator must determine which of the criteria apply. While any two administrators applying the criteria to a specific problem will most likely reach different conclusions, there should be little question as to the applicability of most criteria.

Step 3. Deriving "Value Statements" from Criteria

From the above criteria, administrators need to determine specific "value statements" (or guidelines) from each that apply to the problem at hand. Using our sample case, the following eight criteria may be deemed relevant: beneficence, nonmaleficence, autonomy, justice, utility, and certain philosophical, political, and legal factors.

Under the principle of beneficence, two value statements (or guidelines) could be identified: (1) The hospital should provide care to patients needing it. (2) We should treat others similar to the way we would like to be treated. Under nonmaleficence, a third might be: (3) The hospital should never deny care to an individual when doing so may result in his or her (further) harm. Under autonomy: (4) Individuals have a moral claim, or right, to health care when they are sick. This value statement may be viewed as having even more validity when an institution benefits from its status (e.g., having charitable tax-exempt status, receiving tax revenues from federal, state, or local governments).

Not surprisingly, in dealing with institutional issues, the principle of justice often precipitates several statements. Such issues commonly reflect conflicts in which the best interest of the institution often does not serve the best interest of either individuals or the community. In this case, we identify only two statements, although there are others that reflect other views of fairness (i.e., what is just). (5) The hospital should promote the equitable distribution of limited resources. (6) Ensuring unlimited care to everyone would result in care being available to no one (i.e., the hospital could not survive financially and would risk closure).

A seventh statement reflects the principle of utility: (7) The hospital should promote maximal community health. In employing such a principle, the hospital commits itself to using its resources to benefit the greatest number (recognizing that in doing so, some may be harmed). This is often actualized by an institution (i.e., through its administrator or governing body) deciding that an unlimited amount of care cannot be provided to a single patient when doing so means that many others will be forced to go without more limited (or less costly) care. While this may not be in the best interest of the single patient in question, such a position is more likely to benefit a greater number of community residents who are also dependent on the hospital.

With respect to other criteria that do not necessarily reflect ethical content, but which may warrant administrative consideration, three have been identified. In the philosophy category, the existing institutional mission may merit some consideration: (8) The hospital will serve all who enter its doors in a state of medical need.

Political sensitivity warrants acknowledging a ninth criterion: (9) The hospital should maintain a positive image in the community to sustain its continued support. This statement reflects the realization that if a policy permits the denial of care, the hospital may face a loss of esteem in the community that may produce undesired consequences.

Finally, at least for purposes of this example, existing law might pertain to the decision at hand. Hence, as a tenth criterion, pertinent law may be included in the matrix analysis: (10) The hospital is legally required to provide emergency room care to stabilize a patient's condition.

Step 4. Ordering of and Calculating Weighting Factors for Value Statements

The next step in formulating the matrix analysis requires determining weights for each value statement (or guideline). This is accomplished first by placing each of the statements in order of importance as judged by the decision maker (i.e., the administrator), and then listing them in reverse order (see Table 23-3).

For example, if there are 10 value statements, the most important is listed first and assigned a ''10''; the least important becomes the tenth statement in the list and is assigned a ''1.'' Should value statements be viewed as having equal importance, they may be clustered together and viewed equally; in such cases, the numbers appearing in the order column will be the same.

Following this ordering of value statements, calculate the weighting factor for each. Derivation of weighting factors is a two-stage process: (1) summation of the numbers found in the ordering column (in the case study, this total is 55); (2) division of the order of each value statement by the total. Should there be any value statements that were assigned the same order, they will also bear equal weighting factors. In other words, regardless of either the order assigned to value

Table 23-3 Ordering and Weighting Value Statements: A Sample Case Study

Value Statement	Order	Weighting Factor
The hospital should promote maximal community health.	10	10/55 = 0.18
Ensuring unlimited care to everyone would result in care being available to no one.	9	9/55 = 0.16
The hospital should never deny care to an individual when doing so may result in his or her harm.	8	8/55 = 0.15
Others should be treated as we would like to be treated.	7	7/55 = 0.13
The hospital should provide care to all patients needing it.	6	6/55 = 0.11
The hospital should promote the equitable distribution of limited resources.	5	5/55 = 0.09
The hospital is legally required to provide emergency room care to stabilize a patient's condition.	4	4/55 = 0.07
Individuals have a right to care when they are sick.	3	3/55 = 0.05
The hospital should maintain a positive image in the community to sustain its continued support.	2	2/55 = 0.04
The hospital will serve all who enter its doors in a state of medical need.	1	1/55 = 0.02
Total	55	55/55 = 1.00

statements or the weighting factor calculated for them, the process remains the same: the order is divided by the total and equals the weighting factor.

Step 5. Rating the Alternatives

In constructing the actual decision matrix as shown in Table 23-4, list the alternatives (or decision options) down the left side of the table. List the value statements across the top of the matrix, starting with the highest value on the left and concluding with the lowest value on the far right. Following this, insert the weighting factor for each value statement into the matrix.

The next step calls for the actual rating of each alternative on a scale of 10 (highest) to 1 (lowest). This rating reveals how much the administrator candidly

Table 23-4 Constructing a Decision Matrix: A Sample Case Study

Value Statements Weighting factors Alternatives	Promote maximal community health	Unlimited care would mean no care	Never deny care if such causes harm	Treat others as we would like	Provide care to all who need it	Promote equitable distribution of resources	Legally required to provide ER care	Right to care when sick	Maintain positive image in community	Serve all who enter doors in medical need	SUM
	0.18	0.16	0.15	0.13	0.11	0.09	0.07	0.05	0.04	0.02	1.0
Deny care to those unable to pay for it											
Provide care for limited number; lower class of care											
Retain current policy of not denying care											

Format from P.H. Hill, et al., *Making Decisions: A Multidisciplinary Introduction*. Reading, MA: Addison-Wesley Publishing Company, Inc., 1978, 1979, pp. 124–126.

perceives that selecting each of the possible alternatives would achieve or promote a particular value. This numerical rating is referred to as a rating factor.

For example, each of the three alternatives, (1) denying care to individuals who are unable to demonstrate an ability to pay for it, (2) providing care for a limited number of individuals who are unable to pay for it by admitting such patients only to the old wing, and (3) not denying care to any person based on inability to pay for it, must be rated on the 10 to 1 scale with respect to achieving or promoting each of the values spread over the top of the matrix. Using each value statement (or criterion), rate each alternative successively.

More specifically, to what extent (10 = most; 1 = least) would the first value of promoting maximal community health be achieved or promoted by choosing the first alternative, denying care to those unable to pay for it? Insert this rating factor in the upper half (i.e., above the diagonal line) of the appropriate square. In a similar manner, determine rating factors, one item at a time, value by value, until each cell has been filled.

Step 6. Completing the Matrix and Making the Decision

In completing the decision matrix, multiply the appropriate weighting factor from the top of each column by each of the respective rating factors that were recorded in the upper half of each square (cell). Then record the product in the lower half of that square below each diagonal line. This simple multiplication process should be completed until each cell is filled with a rating factor in the top of the square and a product of the rating and weighting factors is in the lower half.

Next, add all the products in the lower halves of all of the cells opposite each alternative. Then enter this sum for each alternative in the appropriate box under the "sum" column on the far right side of the matrix (across from each respective alternative). Since all weighting factors must total 1.0 and the highest rating factor is 10, a perfect sum (i.e., maximum score) would be 10 (or 100 percent if reference to a percentage is preferred).

Finally, establish a ranking, or determination of level of confidence, for each possible decision (i.e., alternative) by reviewing the far right ("sum") column. The alternative with the highest ranking should be the most ethical of those considered.

Using the decision matrix to facilitate ethical decision making has the advantage of providing the administrator the ability to both clearly present and document his or her decision to other interested parties. Further, it affords the administrator a personal opportunity to carefully reassess and reaffirm the decision-making process and potentially its outcome.

However, effective employment of this technique demands total honesty and thoroughness from each administrator engaged in resolving difficult ethical dilemmas. Despite the quantitative orientation, many of the variables assigned by the decision maker are predicated on qualitative judgments. Hence, a less than honest administrator may not only fool himself or herself in erroneously justifying a decision but also arrive at a decision that manipulates the technique to justify a predetermined goal.[18]

SUMMARY

Given a meaningful appreciation of fundamental ethical principles and the ability to use them in critical decision-making situations, health administrators should become better prepared to meet their growing institutional and professional challenges. Their skills and expertise in conducting ethical analyses, particularly amid the thorny dilemmas posed by the competing choices inherent in administrative decision making, support an essential professional responsibility. Further, ability to justify decisions on solid ethical grounds contributes to an improved sense of both professional and personal competency. Finally, application of a generic set of normative ethical principles, such as this chapter presents, permits sound decision making without having to depend on a more limited, and often too restrictive and specific, code of ethics, regardless of which of the many approaches to ethical decision making is adopted.

NOTES

1. Marc D. Hiller, "Ethics and Health Care Administration: Issues in Education and Practice," *Journal of Health Administration Education* 2, no. 2 (Spring 1984):147–192.

2. Percy H. Hill et al., *Making Decisions: A Multidisciplinary Introduction* (Reading, MA: Addison-Wesley, 1979), 36.

3. Ibid.

4. Charles J. Austin, "What is Health Administration?" *Hospital Administration* 19 (Summer 1974):14–29.

5. David C. Thomasma, "Hospitals' Ethical Responsibilities as Technology, Regulation Grow," *Hospital Progress* 63 (December 1982):74–79.

6. Edmund D. Pellegrino and David C. Thomasma, *A Philosophical Basis of Medical Practice: Toward a Philosophy and Ethic of the Healing Professions* (New York: Oxford University Press, 1981), 250–253.

7. Marc D. Hiller, *Ethics and Health Administration: Ethical Decision Making in Health Management* (Arlington, VA: Association of University Programs in Health Administration, Commission on Ethical Issues in Health Management, in press).

8. Hill et al., *Making Decisions*, also see Ruth B. Purtilo and Christie K. Cassel, *Ethical Dimensions in the Health Professions* (Philadelphia: W.B. Saunders Co., 1981), pp. 27–29; Howard Brody, *Ethical Decisions in Medicine*, 2nd ed. (Boston: Little, Brown and Co., 1981), pp. 9–15, 353–357; and Frank Harron, John Burnside, and Tom Beauchamp, *Health and Human Values: A Guide to Making Your Own Decisions* (New Haven, CT: Yale University Press, 1983), 4–5.

9. Tom L. Beauchamp and James F. Childress, *Principles of Biomedical Ethics*, 2nd ed. (New York: Oxford University Press, 1983), 3–18.

350   HEALTH CARE ETHICS

10. Tom L. Beauchamp and Laurence B. McCullough, *Medical Ethics: The Moral Responsibilities of Physicians* (Englewood Cliffs, NJ: Prentice-Hall, 1984), 11.

11. Tom L. Beauchamp and Norman E. Bowie, *Ethical Theory and Business*, 2nd ed. (Englewood Cliffs, NJ: Prentice-Hall, 1983), 42.

12. Vincent Barry, *Moral Aspects of Health Care* (Belmont, CA: Wadsworth Publishing Company, 1982), 22.

13. Hiller, "Ethics and Health Care Administration."

14. Brody, *Ethical Decisions in Medicine*, 9.

15. Harron, Burnside and Beauchamp, *Health and Human Values*, 4–5.

16. Hill et al., *Making Decisions*; and Robert T. Francoeur, *Biomedical Ethics: A Guide to Decision Making* (New York: John Wiley & Sons, 1983).

17. Hill et al., *Making Decisions*, 120.

18. *Ibid.*, 127.

Index

About the Editors

GARY R. ANDERSON, MSW, PHD, is a faculty member of Hunter College School of Social Work, City University of New York. He has an MSW from the University of Michigan and a PhD from the University of Chicago School of Social Service Administration. Dr. Anderson is a children's services consultant and lecturer, and is involved in training and program evaluation in child welfare. In addition to teaching graduate courses on ethics and ethical practice, Dr. Anderson has published articles on ethical issues, including an article on ethical decision making for health care supervisors. He is a member of the peer review board of *Child Welfare* and has published numerous articles on children's issues.

Dr. Anderson has also taught at the University of Chicago School of Social Service Administration and George Williams College. Prior to his career in education Dr. Anderson worked with abused and neglected children and their families.

VALERIE A. GLESNES-ANDERSON, MHSA, is acting president of West Essex General Hospital in Livingston, New Jersey.

Mrs. Glesnes-Anderson has been a senior health care executive with the Health Corporation of the Archdiocese of Newark since 1982. In her career as a hospital/health care professional, Mrs. Glesnes-Anderson has held positions in state government, served on the executive staffs of five hospitals, worked in international health care, and directed the American Hospital Association's publication *Health Law Vigil* as editor-in-chief.

In 1985 her book *Hospital Management: Winning Strategies for the 80's* was published by Aspen Publishers, Inc., adding to the articles she has published on health care topics. Mrs. Glesnes-Anderson has a master's degree in health service administration from the University of Michigan and speaks regularly on hospital and health care issues.

About the Contributors

FREDRICK R. ABRAMS, director of the Center for Applied Biomedical Ethics at Rose Medical Center, is also assistant clinical professor of obstetrics and gynecology at the University of Colorado Health Sciences Center, and privately practices gynecology. He received his MD from Cornell University Medical College in New York City in 1954. He serves on the ethics committees of Rose Medical Center, the Denver Medical Society, The American College of Obstetricians and Gynecologists, and the Council for Professional Education of the Colorado Medical Society. He is also on the Advisory Board on Institutional Ethics Committees of the American Society of Law and Medicine.

Dr. Abrams has conducted workshops, lectures, and conferences on ethical issues and has written book chapters on ethical issues in high risk pregnancy and on ethical issues in the control of reproduction. Articles have appeared in the *AMA News, Journal of Medicine and Philosophy, Saturday Review, People and Policy,* and *Colorado Medicine.* He has appeared on national television and is executive producer of an award-winning video cassette on the functions and formation of Institutional and Infant Bioethics Committees. He has written *Guidelines in Ethical Decision-making,* a teaching device for applying ethical principles in an orderly pattern, and *A Physician's Affirmation,* his version of a contemporary personal code for the medical practitioner.

TERRENCE F. ACKERMAN is associate professor and chairman of the Department of Human Values and Ethics, College of Medicine, University of Tennessee, Memphis. He is also chairman of the Hospital Ethics Committee, Regional Medical Center at Memphis. Dr. Ackerman has contributed numerous articles on moral issues to the literature of both medicine and medical ethics, including several papers on bioethical inquiry and ethics consultation. He is coauthor of the forthcoming volume entitled *Clinical Medical Ethics: A Casebook.*

MICHAEL D. BROMBERG has been the executive director of the Federation of American Health Systems since 1969. The federation is a national trade association representing 1,300 investor-owned hospitals, hospital management companies, and health systems.

Prior to joining the federation, Mr. Bromberg was campaign manager and subsequently legislative and administrative assistant to former U.S. Representative Herbert Tenzer (D-NY). He also served as the Washington representative for Nassau County, NY.

An attorney, Mr. Bromberg practiced as New York and Washington counsel for the New York law firm of Tenzer, Greenblatt, Fallon, and Kaplan. He graduated from Columbia College in 1959 and received his LLB from New York University Law School in 1962. He is a member of the bars of the state of New York, the District of Columbia, and the U.S. Supreme Court.

He serves as a member of the Executive Committee of the National Health Lawyers Association. He is the author of numerous published articles about national health care policy and the hospital industry.

E. RICHARD BROWN is associate professor of public health in the UCLA School of Public Health. He received his PhD from the University of California, Berkeley. He has studied and written extensively about a broad range of health policies, programs, and institutions, with particular emphasis on issues that affect the access of low-income people to health care. These have included articles, book chapters, and monographs on Medicare and Medicaid, cost containment reforms and cutbacks in Medicare and Medicaid, problems and policy options facing public hospitals, the rationing of health care, and state policies and community strategies to influence local government health policies. He has also authored *Rockefeller Medicine Men: Medicine and Capitalism in America* (University of California Press), about the role of foundations and the medical profession in shaping medical education and medical research. Dr. Brown is currently expanding his analyses of rationing in health care and the organization of health care as a market system and is studying the recent development of health care for profit and its consequences for access, quality, and costs of care.

MICHAEL R. CALLAHAN is a partner in the health care department of Katten, Muchin, Zavis, Pearl, Greenberger & Galler. He specializes in patient care issues, risk management, medical staff credentialing, and antitrust and is former chairman of the Health and Hospital Law Committee of the Chicago Bar Association. He has given numerous lectures and speeches on these topics and is currently working on an article on staff credentialing.

SUSAN N. CHERNOFF is an associate of the law firm of Gardner, Carton & Douglas, specializing in health and hospital law. Ms. Chernoff received her AB degree, with honors, in 1978 from Duke University. She received a JD and an MBA in 1983, both from Washington University in St. Louis.

Ms. Chernoff is a member of the American and Chicago Bar Associations, chairman of the Health and Hospital Law Committee of the Young Lawyers

Section of the Chicago Bar Association, and a member of the American Academy of Medicine. She is a coauthor of *Medical Records and the Law* and has been a contributing author to *Topics in Health Record Management*.

LEAH L. CURTIN is the editor of the journal *Nursing Management*. She received her MS in health planning and health administration from the University of Cincinnati, and MA in philosophy from Anthenaeum of Ohio. She is a Fellow of the American Academy of Nursing and the American Academy of Political and Social Sciences. In addition to over three hundred articles and editorials, Leah Curtin has authored or coauthored several books on ethics, including *Nursing Ethics: Theories and Pragmatics* and *The Mask of Euthanasia*.

CAROL ESTWING FERRANS is a research associate at the University of Illinois at Chicago, College of Nursing. A recipient of national awards for research, Dr. Ferrans has focused her investigations on the quality of life of various illness groups, with a specialization in end-stage renal disease patients. Her findings have been presented nationally in numerous publications and presentations. She also has served as a consultant on quality of life issues for the Veterans Administration and the End-Stage Renal Disease Network Coordinating Council funded by the U.S. Health Care Financing Administration.

RUTH L. GARVEY is director of social work services at Saint Michael's Medical Center, Newark, NJ. She has served on numerous advisory boards at local and state levels.

She has participated on ethics panels discussing termination of life supports, AIDS, and discharge planning. She served as moderator and presentor on a Health Information Network cable television show titled "AIDS: Perspectives."

THOMAS G. GOODWIN is director of public affairs for the Federation of American Health Systems (FAHS), which represents 1,300 investor-owned hospitals and health systems. Mr. Goodwin is the official spokesman for the federation. In addition, he is responsible for the organization's communication and educational activities—public affairs, media relations, promotions, and advertising.

Prior to joining FAHS, Goodwin served as director of government affairs for the National Association of Pharmaceutical Manufacturers. Mr. Goodwin served as an editor with F-D-C Reports, independent publishers of weekly newspapers in the health care field. During his tenure, Goodwin covered such federal agencies as the U.S. Food and Drug Administration, the Health Care Financing Administration, and Office of Management and Budget. Upon receiving his communications degree from The American University in Washington, D.C., in May 1974, Goodwin served as press secretary to (former) U.S. Representative Paul W. Cronin of Massachusetts.

LUKE GREGORY is vice president for professional services at Northeast Georgia Medical Center in Gainesville, GA. Mr. Gregory earned an MBA and MHA from Georgia State University. He has previously published on issues of management ethics in the *Journal for the American College of Healthcare Executives*.

MARC D. HILLER is associate professor in the Department of Health Administration and Planning, School of Health Studies, University of New Hampshire in Durham. He received his DrPH from the University of Pittsburgh Graduate School of Public Health. In addition to teaching and research, he has provided professional consultation and technical assistance to organizations concerning ethical issues and dilemmas. He was a visiting scholar at the Institute of Society, Ethics, and the Life Sciences—The Hastings Center. The author of several books and monographs and numerous articles, he is a member of the American Public Health Association's Forum on Bioethics.

GEORGE A. KANOTI is director of the Department of Bioethics at the Cleveland Clinic Foundation, adjunct professor in the Religious Studies Department at John Carroll University, and research professor at the Northeastern Ohio Universities College of Medicine. He is a consultant on ethical issues in medicine locally, nationally, and internationally. He has served as an ethical consultant on institutional review boards, ethics committees, and animal research committees.

Dr. Kanoti is also a trustee of the Society for Animal Welfare, a member of the Cleveland AIDS Task Force, and a founding member of the Society for Bioethics Consultation. He has published numerous articles, books, and audiovisual materials on the subject of medical ethics. Most recently he coedited a book entitled *Ethical Moments in Critical Care Medicine*.

ANDREW M. KAUNITZ is director of family planning/ambulatory care in the Department of Obstetrics and Gynecology, University Hospital of Jacksonville, FL; assistant professor, Department of Obstetrics and Gynecology, University of Florida; and consultant, Western Hemisphere Region, International Planned Parenthood Federation.

Dr. Kaunitz received his undergraduate education at Brown University and his MD from the College of Physicians and Surgeons, Columbia University. He completed a residency in obstetrics and gynecology at Northwestern University and served two years in the United States Public Health Service as an epidemic intelligence officer at the Centers for Disease Control, Atlanta, GA, before assuming his current position in Jacksonville.

He has contributed to the literature in subjects including fertility regulation, maternal mortality, and a variety of medicolegal issues.

KAREN ROSE KOPPEL KAUNITZ is assistant vice president for legal affairs at Methodist Hospital, Inc., Jacksonville, Florida. Ms. Kaunitz has a JD from the Albany Law School of Union University, Albany, NY, and an AB from

Goucher College, Towson, MD, where she graduated with general and departmental honors and was elected to Phi Beta Kappa. She spent four years as a senior staff attorney at the American Hospital Association and two years as attorney/advisor at the office of the general counsel, Centers for Disease Control.

Ms. Kaunitz is a member of the bars of New York, Illinois, Georgia, District of Columbia, and Florida. She has published and lectured throughout the country on health law issues and serves on numerous national and local health law committees.

BARBARA SUE KOPPEL is an attending neurologist at Metropolitan Hospital of New York City. She is on the faculty of New York Medical College. Dr. Koppel received her BA with distinction from the University of Rochester, NY, and her MD from Columbia University College of Physicians and Surgeons, where she received the Kaufman Prize for "the graduate who exemplifies the humanitarian spirit in the art and practice of medicine." She received her training in neurology at the Neurological Institute of New York, Columbia University, and is a member of the American Board of Psychiatry and Neurology.

Dr. Koppel was responsible for establishing the criteria for establishing brain death at her hospital and is involved with educational efforts to implement them. She serves on numerous committees, including the bioethics committee at Metropolitan Hospital. She has published and lectured on a variety of subjects including brain death.

REV. JOSEPH W. KUKURA is a member of the corporate staff (V.P. Ministry and Ethics) of the Health Corporation, a sponsored corporation of the Archdiocese of Newark. From 1973 to 1985 he was an associate professor of Christian ethics at Immaculate Conception Seminary of the Archdiocese located at Seton Hall University. He has been the moderator of the Newark Archdiocese Medical Moral Committee and ethical consultant to many local hospitals and the Franciscan Sisters of the Poor Health Care System.

WALTER J. MCNERNEY is the Herman Smith Professor of hospital and health services management at the J.L. Kellogg Graduate School of Management, Northwestern University, and the managing partner of Walter J. McNerney and Associates, a management consulting firm in the health field. He served as president of the Blue Cross Association from 1961 to 1978 and as president of the Blue Cross and Blue Shield Associations from 1978 through 1981.

Prior to 1961, Mr. McNerney was in hospital and medical center administration and held faculty appointments at the Graduate School of Public Health and the Graduate School of Management, University of Michigan. He is past president of the International Federation of Voluntary Health Service Funds and of the National Health Council. He has published three books, *Hospital and Medical Economics, Regionalization and Rural Healthcare*, and *Working for a Healthier America*; two monographs; and more than 50 journal articles.

He is the recipient of numerous awards, including the Award of Honor and Justice Ford Kimball Award, American Hospital Association; Yale Medal; Outstanding Achievement Award, University of Minnesota; Special Award for Meritorious Service, AMA; Silver Medal Award, American College of Hospital Administration; Secretary's Unit Citation, HEW; and Doctor of Humane Letters, Rush University.

MARK D. NELSON has been associated with Wood, Lucksinger & Epstein since 1982. He received his BA from the University of Illinois and JD from the Wake Forest University School of Law and the University of Illinois Law School. A substantial portion of Mr. Nelson's practice is in the areas of labor and employment discrimination law. He has lectured before the American Hospital Association and other organizations on numerous employment matters.

Mr. Nelson is the coauthor of "Implementing Layoffs and Reductions in Force: A Practical Guide," *EEO Today*, Spring 1983, and has coauthored "Substance Abuse and Health Care Institutions: Issues and Strategies," *HealthSpan*, October 1986. He is a member of the American, Chicago, and Illinois State Bar Associations and the Labor Law Section Council of the Illinois State Bar Association. He is a member of the Illinois Hospital Association task force on AIDS.

J. PHILLIP O'BRIEN is a partner with the law firm of Katten, Muchin, Zavis, Pearl, Greenberger & Galler, Chicago, where he specializes in health care law. Prior to joining the Katten firm, he was corporate counsel with the American Hospital Association. He has written numerous articles on legal issues affecting hospitals and other health care organizations.

KEVIN D. O'ROURKE, a member of the Dominican Order, is director of the Center for Health Care Ethics, St. Louis University Medical Center, and professor of medical ethics, St. Louis University Medical School. Before establishing the Center for Health Care Ethics in 1979, he served as vice president for medical-moral affairs for the Catholic Hospital Association. Working with several health care corporations and health care facilities, he has helped design ethical programs and institutes for the wider integration of ethical values into the profession of health care.

DAVID A. OGDEN is director of nephrology at the University of Arizona Health Sciences Center, Tucson, and is a professor of medicine at the University of Arizona College of Medicine. He has been involved in clinical care in dialysis and renal transplantation for over 25 years and is a frequent contributor to the literature concerning artificial kidney technology and transplant function.

Dr. Ogden has served as a national consultant to the Regional Medical Program Service, the U.S. Veterans Administration National Renal Transplant Consultant Group, and has served as a member and chairman of National Kidney Foundation's Council on Dialysis and Transplantation, Committee on Health and Scientific Affairs, and Executive Committee. He has been a trustee of the National Kidney Foundation since 1978 and served as vice president of that organization in 1981 and 1982 and president in 1983 and 1984.

SUSAN R. PETERSON has taught ethics at a variety of metropolitan New York schools including Adelphi University, Nassau Community College, and Hunter College. She received a masters degree in philosophy at San Francisco State University, has done doctoral work at the University of Toronto, and is completing her doctorate in philosophy at the City University of New York Graduate Center.

In addition to higher education teaching, Ms. Peterson has specialized in communicating ethical content to nonphilosophic audiences, including nurses, social workers, and engineers. She has authored numerous articles in ethics, including works on women's issues and on professional codes of ethics. She is a member of the American Philosophical Association.

WILLIAM H. ROACH, JR., is a partner and chairman of the health law department of the law firm of Gardner, Carton & Douglas. Mr. Roach's health law practice specialties include mergers and acquisitions, corporate restructuring, tax-exempt organizations, health finance, certificate of need, medical staff by-laws and contracts, medical records, patient rights and responsibilities, health industry joint ventures, and legal audits.

Before entering private practice, Mr. Roach was vice president for legal affairs at Rush-Presbyterian-St. Luke's Medical Center and senior staff counsel at Michael Reese Hospital and Medical Center. He received an AB from Columbia College of Columbia University, a JD from Vanderbilt University, and an MS from the Health Law Training Program of the University of Pittsburgh. Mr. Roach is a former president and founding director of the Illinois Association of Hospital Attorneys and is a member of the American, Illinois, and Chicago Bar Associations, the American Academy of Hospital Attorneys, the National Health Lawyers Association, and the American Society of Law and Medicine.

JAMIE A. SAVAIANO is an associate at the law firm of Katten, Muchin, Zavis, Pearl, Greenberger & Galler. She is a member of the health care department, which represents numerous hospitals, hospital networks, and physician and hospital joint ventures throughout the United States. Ms. Savaiano has a JD from the University of Wisconsin and a BSW from Valparaiso University.

ROBERT L. SCHWARTZ is an attorney and health care consultant. As vice president/general counsel of Hotel Dieu Medical Center, El Paso, TX, his responsibilities ranged from risk management to strategic planning. He was editor of *Hospital Law*, the newsletter of the American Academy of Hospital Attorneys from 1978 to 1982, and now divides his time among health care consulting, a private law practice, and academic activities.

K. BRUCE STICKLER received his BA and JD degrees from Southern Methodist University. He is a partner in the law firm of Wood, Lucksinger & Epstein, engaged exclusively in representing management in equal employment and labor relations matters. Mr. Stickler has practiced employment and labor law before federal and state courts and agencies, including the EEOC and NLRB. He lectures throughout the country on employment law and has published extensively on the subject. He is the author of "Labor Relations Reports" published biweekly in the American Hospital Association's *Health Law Vigil*.

Mr. Stickler serves as special labor counsel to the American Hospital Association, Illinois Hospital Association, the Greater Houston Hospital Council, and several religious orders, hospitals, and health care institutions. He is also a clinical faculty member of St. Louis University Department of Hospital and Health Care Administration.

In addition to memberships in the American, Illinois, Texas, and Chicago Bar Associations, Mr. Stickler's professional affiliations include the American Society of Hospital Attorneys, the National Health Lawyers Association, and the Federal Mediation and Conciliation Service Health Care Industry Labor-Management Committee.

JENNIFER A. STILLER is an attorney in private practice with the health law department of Wolf, Block, Schorr, and Solis-Cohen, Philadelphia. The author of numerous articles on health law topics, Ms. Stiller was previously general counsel of the Illinois hospital rate-setting authority, manager of the American Hospital Association's Department of Federal Law, and a deputy attorney general in the Pennsylvania Department of Health. She is a graduate of the University of Michigan and the New York University School of Law.

JANICEMARIE K. VINICKY is program coordinator for the Department of Bioethics at the Cleveland Clinic Foundation and a law student at the Cleveland Marshall College of Law. Ms. Vinicky is also a certified physician assistant and has served as the director of the Physician Assistant program at the Cleveland Clinic Foundation. She has a master's degree in human services with a concentration in bioethics. She is an instructor in allied health ethics at Cuyahoga Community College.

Ms. Vinicky is also a consultant to several local institutions in the area of medical ethics and continues to teach adult education courses in ethical decision making.

SYLVIA RIDLEN WENSTON is assistant professor in social work at Hunter College School of Social Work, City University of New York. Previously she taught social work at the University of Wyoming and the University of Wisconsin Eau Claire. She has worked in social work in both hospital and outpatient psychiatric settings. She served as social work consultant to hospitals in Wyoming and a health-related consumer group in Wisconsin. She has written, lectured, and conducted research on ethics in social work practice and education. She has a particular interest in ethics in interdisciplinary settings.